Multifamily Groups in the Treatment of Severe Psychiatric Disorders

WILLIAM R. McFARLANE

Foreword by
Harriet P. Lefley

Afterword by
C. Christian Beels

THE GUILFORD PRESS
New York   London

© 2002 The Guilford Press
A Division of Guilford Publications, Inc.
72 Spring Street, New York, NY 10012
www.guilford.com

Paperback edition 2004

Printed in the United States of America

This book is printed on acid-free paper.

Last digit is print number: 9 8 7 6 5 4 3 2

Library of Congress Cataloging-in-Publication Data

McFarlane, William R.
  Multifamily groups in the treatment of severe psychiatric disorders /
by William R. McFarlane.
     p. cm.
   ISBN 1-57230-743-9 (hc.)   ISBN 1-59385-095-6 (pbk.)
   1. Family psychotherapy. 2. Group psychotherapy. 3. Mental
illness—Treatment. I. Title.
RC488.5 .M3945 2002
616.89′156—dc21   2002003730

In memory of
H. Peter Laqueur,
who first saw the power of small healing communities
to transcend the artificial categories
of patients, clinicians, and families.

About the Author

William R. McFarlane, MD, is Professor of Psychiatry at the University of Vermont and Director of Research and former Chairman, Department of Psychiatry, Maine Medical Center. Previously, he was Director of the Biosocial Treatment Research Division of the New York State Psychiatric Institute and an Associate Professor in the Department of Psychiatry, College of Physicians and Surgeons, Columbia University. His main interests are in developing and testing family and psychosocial treatments for major mental illnesses and determining their application in the public sector. Dr. McFarlane edited *Family Therapy in Schizophrenia* (Guilford Press, 1983) and has published more than 40 articles and book chapters. He is an Associate Editor of *Family Process* and *Families, Systems and Health,* and has served on the Board of Directors of the American Orthopsychiatric Association, on the Council of the Association for Clinical Psychosocial Research, and as President of the Maine Psychiatric Association.

Contributing Authors

Cynthia B. Berkowitz, MD, Walker Home and School, Needham, Massachusetts

Susan M. Deakins, MD, New York State Psychiatric Institute, New York, New York

Lisa Dixon, MD, MPH, Department of Psychiatry, University of Maryland, Baltimore, Maryland

Laura M. Drury, MSW, Butler Hospital, Providence, Rhode Island

Edward Dunne, PhD, Ackerman Institute for the Family and Pride Institute, New York, New York

Susan Gingerich, MSW, Delaware Psychiatric Center, Newcastle, Delaware

Sandra Gonzalez, PhD, Department of Family Medicine, Harbor–UCLA Medical Center, Torrance, California

John G. Gunderson, MD, Department of Psychiatry, McLean Hospital, Belmont, Massachusetts

Bonnie T. Horen, MA, Department of Psychiatry, Columbia University College of Physicians and Surgeons, New York, New York

Gabor I. Keitner, MD, Department of Psychiatry, Rhode Island Hospital, Providence, Rhode Island

Ellen P. Lukens, MSW, PhD, Columbia University School of Social Work, New York, New York

Ivan W. Miller, PhD, Department of Psychiatry, Rhode Island Hospital, Providence, Rhode Island

David A. Moltz, MD, Sweetser/Shoreline, Brunswick, Maine

Margaret Newmark, MSW, private practice, New York, New York

William H. Norman, PhD, Meadows Edge Recovery Center, North Kingstown, Rhode Island

Jules M. Ranz, MD, Department of Psychiatry, Columbia University College of Physicians and Surgeons, New York, New York

Christine E. Ryan, PhD, Department of Psychiatry, Rhode Island Hospital, Providence, Rhode Island

David A. Solomon, MD, Department of Psychiatry, Rhode Island Hospital, Providence, Rhode Island

Peter Steinglass, MD, Ackerman Institute for the Family and Cornell Medical College, New York, New York

Gail Steketee, PhD, Boston University School of Social Work, Boston, Massachusetts

Barbara Van Noppen, MSW, Angell St. Wellness Collaborative, Providence, Rhode Island

Foreword

For more than 10 years I have been conducting a weekly educational and support group for families of persons with severe mental illness at a large medical center in south Florida. Numerous people have come and gone according to their needs, but a core group of families has participated for many years. Edie (a pseudonym), whose son, Harry (also a pseudonym), has severe schizophrenia, had attended almost from the beginning. A difficult woman, garrulous, oppositional, and given to tangential thinking, Edie often behaved inappropriately and sometimes alienated newcomers with words such as "Just wait, you're in for a lifetime of hell!" Other members had to squelch her and quite a few members wanted her extruded from the group. But Edie had estranged many people, and except for her only child, Harry, she had no one—no friends, no relatives, no social network other than the members of the group.

Several years ago, Edie developed a lump in her breast but refused to seek medical attention. Dragged to a specialist by two women in the group, she adamantly rejected a biopsy. The lump grew visibly, but Edie persisted in her opposition and stated that she preferred death to chemotherapy or surgery. She lost weight and weakened, with no apparent change in her resolve. The group then insisted that she go to an attorney to make a will and set up a special needs trust for Harry. She agreed that this was a good idea but resisted going. Accompanied by two insistent couples, Edie finally did this, barely 2 weeks before she died. The group tended Edie in her final days, arranged her funeral and the funeral repast, helped Harry with his anxieties and grief, and assisted him in managing his affairs. Following Edie's death, group members visited Harry at his boarding home and during several rehospitalizations. Now, a year later, Harry has access to funds he surely would have lost, a case manager, and ongoing support persons concerned with his welfare.

The full import of this type of anecdote cannot be captured in quantitative outcome data. But this book comes closest to suggesting both the human dimensions and empirical validation of the multifamily group experience. William McFarlane, of course, has been one of the pioneers of family psychoeducation as a major psychosocial intervention for schizophrenia. Superseding the older, sometimes damaging models of family therapy, with their presumption of systemic dysfunction, family psychoeducation addresses lack of knowledge with no presumption of family pathology. As noted in the first two chapters, schizophrenia is presented as "a biologically based vulnerability to stress," including the stressors of ordinary family interactions. Families are taught how to reduce complexity and overstimulation in the social environment, as well as how to learn management techniques and problem-solving strategies.

The materials on the concepts, psychobiology, and social ramifications of the schizophrenic condition that are taught to families are also ideal for professional training, and for training of other caregivers involved with patients. McFarlane's goals, like those of other psychoeducators, are to minimize the type of sensory input that might generate hyperarousal in persons with the core deficits of schizophrenia, with attendant rises in fear and suspiciousness and defective attentional capacity, and to provide the environmental resources for optimal functioning. It is state-of-the-art information, mostly presented with the caveat that all knowledge is fluid and subject to change. The research suggests an empirical linkage between the conveyance of psychobiological information, together with an array of family coping skills, and reduction of early relapse as well as functional improvement of patients. However, as McFarlane points out, knowledge alone is insufficient. His findings suggest that the context of knowledge transmission may be even more important than content. Even with minimal psychoeducation or behavior management techniques, there is a powerful long-term effect of the multifamily group format on symptom stabilization.

Research-based psychoeducational interventions have measured outcome in terms of patients' progress. In recent years, there have been attempts to distinguish between psychoeducation, which focuses on patient outcomes, and family education, which targets the well-being of the family as a whole.[1] The National Alliance for the Mentally Ill (NAMI) has for years offered its members mutual support groups that help families cope with the multiple problems of the illness. Because most families have contended with years of unremitting or cyclical symptomatology and functioning, positive effects on the patient are a hoped-for but secondary consideration. The finding by McFarlane and colleagues that the multifamily group is superior to single-family interventions empirically weds the two desiderata. The group gives an added benefit to families: mutual support, a profoundly empathic understanding of shared experiences, information exchange on resources and coping strategies, and a social network. These features are extremely important to families who tend to be isolated by the demands, burdens, and stigma of mental illness. McFarlane endows the group experience with an enhanced problem-solving capacity, an antidote to overinvolvement, and a more positive environment than the single-family format. He also adds stigma reduction, cross-parenting, communication normalization, and crisis intervention. Many of these attributes may be seen in the true story with which I began this foreword.

The chapters in Part II, written by leading psychoeducators, provide a comprehensive how-to manual for clinicians, fleshing out the techniques of multifamily group treatment. There is a superb, time-phased discussion of the interfaces and integration of family psychoeducation with clinical treatment, community reentry and adaptation, and long-term rehabilitation. Problems and solutions are offered from actual practice. Because most research on psychoeducational interventions has been restricted to families and has focused on schizophrenia, and to a lesser extent affective disorders, Part III is of exceptional interest to an expanding field. The development of a staff training model in other contexts, such as assertive community treatment or supported housing programs, is an important innovation. In outlining specific applications to other conditions, the book brings an innovative technology to the treatment of borderline personality disorder and obsessive–compulsive disorder, as well as a range of chronic medical disorders.

There have been difficulties in implementing family psychoeducation in real-world settings, well described by Lisa Dixon and Edward Dunne (Chapter 17). Managed care and Federal reimbursement procedures discourage education as opposed to therapy, and for agencies dependent on third-party payors, there are few monetary incentives for multifamily groups. Additionally, support from organized family groups has been sporadic and inconsistent. Some NAMI members still view psychoeducational interventions as inextricably linked to the expressed emotion (EE) research. Although many family members resonate to the EE concept and have used the research findings to temper their own behaviors, others view the continuing emphasis on the toxic effects of high EE as perpetuating the destructive tradition of blaming families.[2] Indeed, some clinicians have reinforced old prejudices by equating high EE with schizophrenogenesis. Most seem ignorant of research findings that the distributions are highly culture-bound and that low EE is modal in the majority of families of persons with schizophrenia throughout the world.[3] An additional complaint is that psychoeducational interventions have focused on families as presumably permanent caregivers, ignoring the more widespread educational needs of alternative caregivers in clinical and residential settings. This book implicitly answers some of these criticisms. It neutralizes the EE concept and is exceptionally valuable in its application of psychoeducation to staff training in multiple contexts.

Unfortunately, most mental health facilities still lack family education of any type. NAMI has developed its own Family-to-Family educational program that attempts to offer education allied to support groups and, I hope, involve families in advocacy to improve mental health systems.[4] However, lay organizations can serve only a small portion of the thousands of families who need education and support in dealing with an array of difficult behaviors and an essentially incomprehensible life stressor. We need widespread acceptance of multifamily psychoeducation throughout mental health systems, with intensive staff training and adequate reimbursement procedures, for a demonstrably effective psychosocial intervention. This book provides both empirical data and a comprehensive manual of techniques to support this much-needed effort.

HARRIET P. LEFLEY, PhD

Preface

This volume is being published 20 years after the death of the person generally acknowledged as the pioneer of multifamily groups, H. Peter Laqueur. Remarkably, it is the first book devoted to this approach, and it is long overdue. It could be faulted for being a little late on the scene. For one thing, an entire generation of therapists has been trained and entered practice with little exposure to these groups, with their remarkable capacity to heal and lift the spirits of families, patients, and, very often, the groups' leaders. Conversely, recent refinements in the practical technology of these groups have revolutionized the outcomes that have been reported and can now be routinely expected. In other words, it was probably a good idea to wait until a theoretically sound model and the empirical evidence for its efficacy were available.

The early approaches to multifamily groups were rooted in notions that the family needs to be treated—that is, fixed in some nebulous way—and that groups of families might be more efficient in doing so. Laqueur viewed his groups from that perspective. However, simple mathematics added up to a different process and a better outcome. Relatives outnumbered the therapists. Therefore, they usually succeeded in shifting the focus to their own travails and their need, if not their right, to have more information, guidance, respect, and, in the end, empathy. Furthermore, they tended to insist, usually with the concurrence of their peers, that they were trying to help their ill family members, in the only ways they knew, to return to being the people whom they knew and loved. For reasons that seemed to have little to do with the actual techniques used to conduct them, these early groups tended to promote unprecedented improvements in the social functioning of the patients who participated in them, to say nothing of the clear improvement in the families' morale. Many patients had been on medication for many years without improvement in social or cognitive functioning before entering these groups. I had the pleasure of watching these results evolve firsthand, working with Laqueur at the Vermont State Hospital between 1973 and 1975. It was clear to me and to several other observers that something different was happening to these patients, especially in comparison with family and patient group therapy.

The later arrival of neuroscience and psychoeducational and behavioral approaches to the family radically redefined the role of the family, from source of pathology to a key resource in treating pathology, now understood to be brain disorders rather than the catastrophic results of poor parenting. The first ongoing psychoeducational multifamily groups for schizophrenia of the type described here started in 1979, in the South Bronx, and we have been refining and testing them since then. This volume is the product of those 20 years of development, which happily is still proceeding. Even more important, this remarkably cost-effective treatment has proven to be adaptable to many disorders and even to nonfamily social environments and rehabilitative functions. Though all the results are not yet in, it looks as if they will bring about as much of an improvement in these other maladies as they have in schizophrenia.

Horen and Ranz, Moltz and Newmark, Keitner and colleagues, Berkowitz and Gunderson, Van Noppen and Steketee, Dixon and Dunne, and Gonzalez and Steinglass have applied a great deal of wisdom and practical, empirically driven design effort to building new treatments that focus on the key particulars of various disorders. They have done so in a way that is new and rooted more in science than in theory; that is, their treatment models arise from empirical observations about the relationship of family factors to outcome and the special problems faced by families in each disorder. These models are all being applied in the field, with careful examination of outcome before claims of effectiveness are made.

This book is organized into three parts. Part I reviews the science that undergirds, and the results that have been demonstrated for, multifamily group treatment for the schizophrenic disorders. Part II describes in detail that approach to treatment and rehabilitation. It includes strategies that have been developed by these groups for addressing the most common predicaments and issues faced by those with schizophrenia and their closest relatives. Part III describes adaptations of multifamily groups to other disorders, some of which are described here in detail for the first time.

We hope that this book serves a need that has been unfulfilled since 1960: a practical guide to the successful application of these methods. The contributors have provided details that more experienced clinicians can use to begin to offer treatment to their patients and clients. All of the material provided to the research clinicians who have achieved the results summarized in Chapter 4 is presented in Part II. In addition, it attempts to explain the rationale for conducting the groups in these particular ways. Each approach is supported by a review of the literature and a theoretical justification for the techniques and perspectives that are applied. The book will also be of use to students who anticipate working in settings in which severe psychiatric disorders are treated. Those disorders have generally not responded to the psychotherapies so often taught to psychiatry, social work, psychiatric nursing, and psychology trainees. The multifamily group approach offers an interesting, gratifying, and sustaining and sustainable means for alleviating the many symptoms and disabilities that these disorders create.

The size, density, sophistication, and adaptability of the members of the social network of those with chronic illness are powerful predictors of outcome. Indeed, these same phenomena are predictive of onset of disorder in those who are predisposed. C. Christian Beels, writing in response to these findings in relation to schizophrenia, developed the concept of the "invisible village": Clinicians should organize a therapeutic social network to counteract the fragmenting and isolating tendencies of both schizophrenia and postmodern industrial society. The multifamily group offers the opportunity to create visible villages—prosthetic social networks—in contrast to invisible villages; that is, these groups become healing communities constructed by the healers initially to benefit the patients, then to support the families, and, in the end, to sustain the healers themselves. One of the things that makes it difficult to categorize multifamily groups as a group, individual, or family therapy is that it is not clear who among the participants benefits most. Experienced practitioners often describe the phenomenon that, in spite of its greater initial complexity, the burden imposed by each patient's illness seems to be divided by the number of participants, and *not* multiplied by the number of patients in the group. Some of the more effective groups are very large, especially once clinical stability has been achieved. In short, camaraderie may be much more powerful as a healing and rehabilitative force for treating severe mental illness than has been previously appreciated.

There is probably no other way to explain not only the multifamily groups' efficacy and cost-effectiveness but also the nearly universal tendency for therapists, families, and patients to want so strongly for them to continue, often for years. In the end, misery loves company. Multifamily groups supply that company to the point that real relationships, neighbor-like assistance, and group identity emerge, suggesting that these social networks cease being prosthetic or artificial and indeed become real, indistinguishable from their natural counterparts. Using this potent format to deliver psychoeducation and coping skill training is additive to its therapeutic impact. Some of the data suggest that, over time, the interaction of psychoeducation and multifamily groups becomes synergistic, as a culture of treatment adherence, hope, and belief in rehabilitation begins to amplify coping skills and even the effects of medication. Dennis Dyck, at the Washington State Institute for Mental Health Research and Training, has documented that psychoeducational multifamily groups reduce *negative* symptoms in schizophrenia, while patients in the control group—receiving standard outpatient therapy and medication—experience increasing negative symptoms over the same period of time. In other words, a highly social treatment may be capable of reversing the very symptoms that lead to the deterioration in social functioning so dreaded in that disorder, proving what many were seeing over 20 years ago in Vermont—inexplicable improvement in social functioning. Our hope is that this volume will assist readers in seeing the same or better outcomes in their own practices.

Acknowledgments

I would like to thank the New York State Alliance for the Mentally Ill for its support and encouragement, as well as its vision in supporting a clinical research effort involving families, when that effort seemed risky. This trust has led to benefits for thousands of families, now extending well outside the boundaries of New York State. In addition, a full measure of gratitude goes to the senior staff of the Biosocial Treatment Research Division at the New York State Psychiatric Institute, including Susan M. Deakins, MD, Edward Dunne, PhD, Bonnie T. Horen, MA, Margaret Newmark, MSW, Ellen P. Lukens, MSW, DPhil, Robert Dushay, PhD, Peter Stastny, MD, Joanne Toran, and Susan Gingerich, MSW. For their indispensable assistance in further developing the vocational approach, Richard Balser, MS, CRC, Brenda Harvey, MS, CRC, and Renee Leavitt, OTR, of the Maine Medical Center deserve abundant recognition. I am indebted to all the site directors and clinicians who have been involved in the outcome studies represented in Part I. There is no way to acknowledge them here individually, but their efforts have advanced the field in ways that they began to experience for themselves but whose significance often seemed, in the midst of the work, to be remote at best. Finally, my appreciation goes to the Center for Mental Health Services and its predecessor, the Community Support Program of the National Institute of Mental Health, for support of the research demonstrating the efficacy of multifamily groups in vocational rehabilitation.

Contents

PART I. Theoretical and Empirical Foundations
The Scientific Basis of Multifamily Group Treatment

1   The Psychobiology of Schizophrenia   3

2   Families, Social Networks, and Schizophrenia   18
Ellen P. Lukens and William R. McFarlane

3   The Therapeutic Social Network: A Healing Community   36

4   Empirical Studies of Outcome in Multifamily Groups   49

PART II. The Practice of Multifamily Group Treatment in Schizophrenia
A Psychoeducational Approach to Developing a Healing Social Network

5   An Overview of Psychoeducational Multifamily Group Treatment   71

6   Joining with Families and Patients   104
William R. McFarlane, Susan Gingerich, Susan M. Deakins, Edward Dunne, Bonnie T. Horen, and Margaret Newmark

7   Educating Families: A Multifamily Workshop on Schizophrenia   113
William R. McFarlane, Susan Gingerich, Susan M. Deakins, Edward Dunne, Bonnie T. Horen, and Margaret Newmark

8   The Initial Sessions of a Psychoeducational   127
    Multifamily Group: Forming a Healing Network
    William R. McFarlane, Susan Gingerich, Susan M. Deakins,
    Edward Dunne, Bonnie T. Horen, and Margaret Newmark

9   Problem-Solving in Multifamily Groups: 142
    A Psychoeducational Approach to Treatment
    and Rehabilitation
    William R. McFarlane, Susan Gingerich, Susan M. Deakins,
    Edward Dunne, Bonnie T. Horen, and Margaret Newmark

PART III. Applications in Other Disorders and Contexts
Expanding the Range and Relevance of Multifamily Group Treatment

10 Family-Aided Assertive Community Treatment   175
    William R. McFarlane and Susan M. Deakins

11 Training Staff of Supportive Housing Programs   198
    in Principles and Practices of Psychoeducation:
    Creating a Family-Like Social Environment
    Bonnie T. Horen and Jules M. Ranz

12 Multifamily Groups for Bipolar Illness   220
    David A. Moltz and Margaret Newmark

13 Multifamily Group Treatment for Major Depressive Disorder   244
    Gabor I. Keitner, Laura M. Drury, Christine E. Ryan,
    Ivan W. Miller, William H. Norman, and David A. Solomon

14 Multifamily Psychoeducational Treatment   268
    of Borderline Personality Disorder
    Cynthia B. Berkowitz and John G. Gunderson

15 Multifamily Behavioral Treatment of   291
    Obsessive–Compulsive Disorder
    Barbara Van Noppen and Gail Steketee

16 Application of Multifamily Groups in Chronic   315
    Medical Disorders
    Sandra Gonzalez and Peter Steinglass

17 Implementing Multifamily Groups in the Real World: 341
The New York State and Ohio Training
and Dissemination Programs
Lisa Dixon and Edward Dunne

Afterword 359
C. Christian Beels

References 363

Index 395

MULTIFAMILY GROUPS IN THE
TREATMENT OF SEVERE PSYCHIATRIC DISORDERS

Part I

Theoretical and Empirical Foundations

The Scientific Basis of Multifamily Group Treatment

Chapter 1

The Psychobiology
of Schizophrenia

Biological and scientific information about schizophrenia is included in a book on a psychosocial treatment for two reasons. First, the psychoeducational and family behavioral approaches are based on the core concept that schizophrenia is a biologically based vulnerability to stress, manifest as positive symptoms and cognitive deficits. All clinicians who work with people who have schizophrenia should have a working knowledge of that biology, in order to understand symptomatic behavior and to focus treatment efforts on specific deficits. A basic grasp of what the brain does and how brain abnormalities affect functioning makes the work not only more effective but also more satisfying. Second, this treatment approach requires that all clinicians understand psychiatric disorders well enough to educate those individuals' families. Much of this material is shared with families, so that they, too, can base their interactions and plans on a solid, empirically based, and relatively consistent body of knowledge.

The information presented here is relatively new, and it is constantly in flux and under development. Some of it is still controversial. Most critically, few findings apply to every person with the disorder. In fact, research now suggests that it is likely that there are several diseases that cause the disorder. Thus, schizophrenia is looking more like diabetes or mental retardation: a serious illness mediated by psychosocial stresses and caused in large part by a host of biological disorders of several types. With that caveat, however, an increasingly consistent picture is evolving across studies and is increasingly confirmed by rigorous empirical studies.

A BRIEF HISTORY OF THE
CONCEPT OF SCHIZOPHRENIA

Concepts of schizophrenia and psychosis have changed over time in ways
that mirror the philosophical and social predilections of the respective eras
that spawned them. That is a problem for persons suffering this disorder
and their families. For at least two generations in the United States, most
clinicians have assumed that mental difficulties stem from the experiences
that one has in one's family in the first few years of life and/or from the intrapsychic conflict that ensues. This view, of course, began with Freud and
some of his earlier writings on paranoid psychosis, and was amplified repeatedly by American clinicians and psychological theorists. These assumptions were challenged by empirical and clinical evidence that conventional individual and family therapies are not effective in alleviating
symptoms or improving the course of the disorder. Those theories and therapies are being replaced as the study of schizophrenia shifts from phenomenological and theory-driven methods to scientific methods, with dramatic
and often surprising results. The psychoeducational approach is part of this
larger enterprise. The dominant paradigm, supported by tens of thousands
of research reports, is that schizophrenia is a disorder of brain function and,
in many cases, the result of major alterations in normal brain anatomy.

With that biological understanding as a given, this family supportive
approach arose largely from experimental evidence that clarified the role
that family interaction plays in relapse and recovery, and the devastating
impact that the disorder has on families. Because the illness itself leaves its
victims exquisitely sensitive to sensory stimulation and cognitive overload
from any source, families may unintentionally stimulate the very symptoms
that they are usually trying to alleviate. The psychoeducational multifamily
group model is an approach that, among several other goals, intends to alter ongoing brain function by altering the psychosocial environment to fit
more closely the specific needs and biological vulnerabilities of people with
schizophrenia. In fact, it is assumed that clinical improvement and rehabilitation can only occur if abnormal brain functioning is compensated by
psychosocial and pharmacological means.

THE CLINICAL SYMPTOMS OF SCHIZOPHRENIA

Most readers of this volume will be familiar with the diagnostic symptoms
of the disorder: hallucinations, delusions, and thought disorder, accompanied by functional deterioration lasting at least 2 weeks in the acute form

and 6 months in a residual form.[5] These have been termed positive symptoms, because they are added to usual mental functions. While they are dramatic and lead to relapse, hospitalization, and occasionally violence, they generally respond to antipsychotic medications and in many patients tend to diminish naturally over time.[6-10]

Less commonly recognized and understood are negative, or deficit, symptoms: normal functions that are lost, usually after an acute episode, and lost more profoundly as the illness worsens over months and years. In fact, evidence suggests that these symptoms accumulate with each succeeding acute episode.[11, 12] They include anhedonia, alogia, apathy, amotivation, and attentional deficit. What is lost encompasses a broad range of human experience, including most of what is enjoyable, or at least interesting, about being conscious. In the most severe form, the deficit syndrome involves a flatness of feeling, thought, sensation, and desire that is hard for most of us to comprehend.[13] It contributes to difficulties in taking initiative or carrying out responsibilities. Since it includes loss of pleasure and sensation, actions that are actually carried out are not accompanied by internal reward. The schizophrenic attentional deficit includes a general inability to direct and maintain mental focus on external and internal objects and processes. Bleuler emphasized these negative symptoms as the fundamental disorders in schizophrenia, because they were more consistent over time and led more directly to disability, personal misery, and family and clinician distress.[14] They are what patients themselves most often complain about, especially the absence of pleasure in events, interactions, and achievements. Family exasperation can be linked to negative symptoms; family members attribute them to character flaws such as laziness or manipulativeness.[15, 16] Understanding negative symptoms accurately and gradually alleviating them are two of the central goals of psychoeducational multifamily groups. They are also important because they are now well known to reflect the more fundamental functional and structural aberrations of the schizophrenic brain. In fact, their presence is more predictive of later positive symptoms than positive symptoms themselves.[17] Thus, a scientific perspective on schizophrenia regards negative symptoms as markers of the primary disorder.

SCHIZOPHRENIA OVER TIME

The Course of Recovery from an Acute Episode

For many younger patients, alleviation of psychotic symptoms is a rapid process, usually occurring 5 to 15 days after medication is started. However, closer analysis of risk for relapse over time[18] and of return of cognitive function[19] suggests that negative symptoms increase during the acute episode and then, if relapse does not occur, slowly decline over the ensuing 12 to 36 months. This course may be reflected in loss of nerve cells in prefrontal cortex during unstable periods and in cortical cellular breakdown early in the illness before drug therapy.[20] The implication is that tolerance for stress and readiness for rehabilitation are low after an acute episode and increase very gradually thereafter.

A Review of the Various Courses

Strauss emphasized that schizophrenia takes one of several course types over the lifetime of those afflicted. Some people have one episode, recover, and never have another, though little is known of the middle and later years of these more fortunate lives. A few begin deteriorating functionally early in childhood and remain profoundly disabled and psychotic for most of their lives. The range in between is occupied by myriad variations. The most common, statistically, is the person who has repeated episodes in early adulthood, losing functional capacities and gaining negative symptoms with each episode, often becoming chronically though mildly psychotic on a permanent basis. (Repeated relapses have become common with deinstitutionalization and the inability to guarantee that medications are used adequately and consistently enough to prevent relapse and deterioration.) However, several studies have found that about 50% of all those with schizophrenia recover to the degree that they can function independently and have few or no positive symptoms by the time they reach their fifties.[9, 10, 21] Another 25% are able to function, but with persistent symptoms. Only about 25% across these studies manifest a poorer course indefinitely.

A similarly encouraging view is now emerging with regard to the fate of persons having their first episode. It appears that the earlier the impending or emerging psychosis is recognized and the earlier it is treated, even if with low doses of medication, the better the long-term outcome.[12, 22, 23] A plausible interpretation is that the fewer days a given person spends in a psychotic state, the less chance there is for development of long-term deterioration and treatment resistance.

THE BRAIN AND ITS ALTERATION IN SCHIZOPHRENIA

Alterations in brain function have consistently been shown to be associated with schizophrenia. By the end of this chapter, the reader will have a working knowledge of a multilevel, empirically derived model of brain function and dysfunction that can be highly useful in guiding family and patient education, adaptation to community life, and rehabilitation. This is termed the biosocial model, because it assumes reciprocal influences of both the social environment on the brain and the dysfunction of the brain on the social environment. Leaders of multifamily groups should be expert in the interaction of these seemingly distant spheres.

The Brain Stem, the Midbrain, and Their Activation Centers

We start with the brain stem and its upper portion, the midbrain. Over the course of evolution, more complex functions have generally been added by laying new structures on top of older structures. So, it is not an oversimplification to say that the most basic, though primitive, functions are mediated by the brain stem, which lies at the base of the skull, just above the spinal cord, and that the most elegant and complex functions are mediated by the prefrontal cortex, which, as the name implies, lies just behind the forehead. Likewise, during fetal development, the lower centers are organized first, while higher order centers, especially the prefrontal cortex, arise last and involve the migration forward and upward of cell groups that start life directly adjacent to the brain stem. Migrating cells maintain important physical connections, mediated by electrical and chemical activity, with cells in the structures that gave rise to them. So prefrontal cells have important connections to cells in the brain stem and in the diencephalon, especially the principal sensory integration center, the thalamus. Their functions are interrelated as well. Schizophrenia affects parts of all these structures.

The brain stem regulates the level of activation of the nervous system, primarily through the action of three neurotransmitters—dopamine, serotonin, and noradrenaline. Four small structures, composed of groups of neurons and lying near each other in the midbrain (the upper portion of the brain stem), regulate the activity of other parts of the brain using these neurotransmitters. Those neuronal groups are the ventral tegmentum, the substantia nigra (both use dopamine), the raphe nuclei (serotonin), and the locus coeruleus (noradrenaline)(see Figure 1.1). They determine the level of consciousness as well as the varying levels of activity in almost all other higher brain structures.

The dopamine system controls the level of activity in both the prefrontal cortex and in the limbic cortex and other limbic structures, including the hippocampus and the amygdala, all of which are affected in schizophrenia (discussion follows). Dopamine was the first neurotransmitter to be linked directly to schizophrenia, because antipsychotic drugs de-

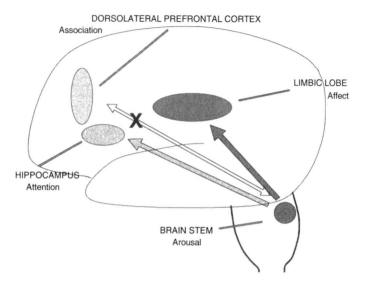

FIGURE 1.1. A simplified view of the interaction of the principal anatomical components of the dopamine system in the schizophrenic brain.

crease dopamine activity. These medications mimic the molecular shape of dopamine sufficiently to occupy the receptors, thus preventing the usual activation of this system.

Thus, it should be no surprise that schizophrenia is characterized by excess levels of dopamine activity during the acute episodes and periods of clinical instability, and by abnormally low levels when negative symptoms and extreme apathy predominate.[24, 25] One effect is that the limbic system tends to be overstimulated during acute episodes. Dopamine activity normally also increases the activity of the prefrontal cortex, but this does *not* occur in schizophrenia. Usually, when the dopamine system is activated, so is the noradrenaline system, with the result that heart and respiratory rates, blood pressure, anxiety, and agitation are also increased.

It is too early in the progress of brain research to provide a clear understanding of the serotonin system and its role in schizophrenia. However, serotonin is widely distributed in the entire cortex and to many subcortical structures. It appears to inhibit the dopamine system, modulating its influence.[26] Also, in the schizophrenic dorsolateral prefrontal cortex, there are increased neurotransmitter receptors for some forms of serotonin and decreased receptors for others.[27] It is clear that drugs that block serotonin at the receptor, such as clozapine, have better negative symptom outcomes and fewer Parkinson's disease-like side effects, reflecting complex effects on a variety of receptor subgroups and brain areas. The rest of the serotonin story is very complex and as yet far from clear.

It is now considered likely that other neurotransmitters are involved in the disorder, including gamma-aminobutyric acid (GABA), glutamate, and N-methyl-D-aspartate (NMDA), a subtype of glutamate. The last appears to be reduced in activity in the cortex in general, in some subcortical areas,[28] and in connections between the thalamus and the cingulate cortex, both of which are involved in processing more complex sensory information.[29, 30] Drugs that reduce activity in the glutamate system have been found in normal volunteers to induce thought disorder and negative symptoms that cannot be distinguished from those of patients on structured interviews of thinking.[31] Alterations of glutamate and/or NMDA have been found in the prefrontal and superior temporal cortex, and in the hippocampus, the areas most directly implicated in schizophrenia.[32-34] Remarkably, amino acids that regulate this neurotransmitter system, glycine and D-serine, have been found to improve positive and negative symptoms substantially for patients already taking antipsychotic medication.[35, 36] GABA precursors (messenger RNA [mRNA]) and levels of GABA itself have been found to be markedly reduced in the prefrontal cortex, reflecting reduced neuronal activity in this important region.[37] Recently integrated models for the interaction of some of these neurotransmitter systems have been proposed, explaining both biochemical findings and the differences in effects and efficacy among various antipsychotic drugs.[29, 32, 38-40]

The key concept is that the midbrain is impaired in its ability to adjust the activation of the brain and nervous system in ways that are normal or appropriate to the situation at hand. Although the means by which this adjustment occurs are unclear, the brain under normal circumstances can very precisely change its activation to match the environmental, social, or internal demands imposed by exercise, infection, metabolic imbalance, and cognitive and emotional input. In schizophrenia, the dopamine and norepinephrine systems are both unstable, tending toward overactivity when stress is present. This abnormal activation then radiates its effects through at least three other neurotransmitter systems to the rest of the brain in ways that are complex but that nearly always undermine mental and emotional well-being. At the other extreme, negative symptoms tend to be associated with underactivity of dopamine-driven systems,[24] as well as reduced activity on the part of activating neurotransmitters, especially GABA and the glutamate/NMDA system. Studies of the excitatory neurotransmitters—glutamate, NMDA, and GABA—have great promise for development of new drug and perhaps nutritional treatments for this disorder.

The Limbic System and Thalamus

The next higher strata, above the brain stem, include the limbic cortex and the thalamus, as well as several other nearby structures. The limbic system is a way station among the prefrontal cortex, the thalamus, and the temporal lobe. Two of its components, the amygdala and the cingulate cortex, generate more primitive and life-sustaining affects and emotions, especially anger and fear, the classic fight-or-flight pattern of response. It is the limbic system that is most directly affected therapeutically by antipsychotic medications; that effect is mediated by dopamine blockade. The drugs alleviate labile emotions and delusional thinking, which are more extreme forms of fear and suspiciousness. The limbic system has consistently been found to be hyperactive during psychosis and underactive in conjunction with negative symptoms.

Another limbic structure of great importance is the hippocampus. This tiny, seashell-like structure mediates all short-term memory registration and many crucial components of attention, especially establishing and maintaining focus. In schizophrenic patients it has been found to be atrophied and its very cell structure disorganized.[41, 42] The effect is a partial, but consistently confirmed, disability in directing attention appropriately, focusing attention, and ignoring distracting stimuli when necessary. Furthermore, this defect creates marked difficulties with storing information long enough to be transferred for longer-term retention, resulting in subtle and erratic memory deficits.

The thalamus, which serves as the central control system for integrating sensory input, has been found to be underactive in schizophrenia, resulting in an inability to screen out sensory stimuli and a tendency for all sensory information to be experienced as excessive, inappropriately generalized, and overwhelming.[43, 44] One recent study has found that portions of the thalamus are reduced in size in schizophrenia, suggesting an anatomical basis for this impairment.[45] In schizophrenia, defects in the limbic and thalamic systems create a state of sensory hypersensitivity, combined with a tendency toward excessive levels of fear, suspiciousness, and anger.[46–48]

Disorders of the limbic, thalamic, and midbrain systems are functionally linked in schizophrenia; that is, as arousal increases in response to outside or internal sources of stimulation, attention deteriorates. As attention deteriorates, arousal increases reactively, leading to a downward spiral that ends in hyperarousal in the entire limbic system, with resulting extreme states of primitive emotion, increasingly heightened sensory sensitivity, and severely limited attentional capacity. This cycle is termed the distraction–arousal hypothesis and is central to the psychoeducational approach.[49]

Higher Cortical Areas Affected: Prefrontal, Superior Temporal Gyri, and Postcentral Areas

Modern imaging methods (CT [computed tomography], PET [positron emission tomography], SPECT [single photon emission tomography], and MRI [magnetic resonance imaging] scans) have demonstrated in schizophrenia an increase in the size of the ventricles, the usually small channels through which flows cerebrospinal fluid from brain to spinal cord to bloodstream.[50] Increased ventricular size usually indicates loss of cerebral tissue, though it says little about the site of loss; that is, in many people with schizophrenia, living brain tissue has been replaced by spaces filled with fluid. These studies show that in many persons with schizophrenia, the cerebral cortex is reduced in size and has less total volume.[51-55] Indeed, some studies, though not all, show that the entire brain tends to be smaller on average.[56] The changes are similar in type to dementias, though far less dramatic and less progressive over time. The most pronounced changes are concentrated in prefrontal, medial and superior temporal, and cingulate cortices. The differences noted do not seem to be acute, because there is only the weakest correlation with age or number of episodes. These changes are present even at the first episode in young adults.[57] Studies of children with schizophrenia, followed into adolescence, show some enlargement of ventricles over a 2-year time span, suggesting that some degradation of brain structure may occur in the early years of adolescence in cases with a very early onset.[58] Many studies have shown correlations of ventricular enlargement with negative symptomatology and cognitive impairment.[47, 59] *This indicates, perhaps more clearly than any other single set of findings, that functional disability in some persons with schizophrenia is secondary to structural defects in the brain itself.*

PET and functional MRI scans provide an increasingly coherent picture in several studies. Most important, the prefrontal cortex has been found to be less active than normal, especially when the subject is challenged to do complex and frustrating mental tasks, such as the Wisconsin Card Sort, a test of abstracting and problem-solving capacity under social duress. The dorsolateral prefrontal cortex appears to be the brain area that activates to accomplish the test. However, in schizophrenia, there is dramatically lower activation to the test and poor performance as well.[60] Recent work has shown that the prefrontal area is less active in proportion to the degree of negative symptoms, verbal task demands, and cognitive impairments, and in the presence of delusions, hallucinations, and stereotyped ideas.[46, 48, 61–63]

The left superior temporal area tends to be overactive in association with thought disorder, negative symptoms, and verbal tasks, even while having reduced physical volume. However, it is less active in the presence of delusions and hallucinations.[64–68] This last insight is particularly useful, suggesting that this area may be deficient in processing, inhibiting, and modulating auditory stimuli, predisposing patients to alterations and misperceptions in the auditory sphere. It is not clear how verbal hallucinations are formed, but given what is known, it may be that reduction in temporal brain tissue removes some key monitoring functions and leaves open the way to spontaneous verbal perceptions.

Another key finding is that activity is increased in the posterior portions of the cerebral cortex, in the parietal and occipital areas. These have long been known to be the processors of visual and other nonverbal sensory input, elaborating, correlating, and interpreting sensory data. A possible model is emerging: The thalamus is impaired and releases the parietal and occipital cortical areas to overprocess, underinhibit, and overreact to sensory information, creating a tendency toward relative overactivity, in turn leading to the well-demonstrated heightened sensitivity to sensory stimuli so characteristic of this disorder.

To summarize, a picture is emerging from hundreds of studies, using scanning techniques, metabolic studies and the direct examination of brain tissue and cells. Physical and biochemical abnormalities correlate with symptoms and functional difficulties. Specifically, the functional axis comprising the midbrain, the thalamus, and the limbic, superior temporal, and prefrontal cortexes is disordered and in many patients is clearly but not severely damaged, with secondary effects on the parietal–occipital/sensory cortical areas. The neurotransmitters involved in this axis—dopamine, serotonin, noradrenaline, glutamate, GABA, and some neuropeptides—tend to be deranged complexly. Dopamine in excess appears to mediate psychosis and, when decreased, mediates the deficit state, while excess serotonin that may be serving as an antipsychotic in reaction to excess dopamine activity may be deficient in some patients and in some receptor subsystems. The antipsychotic drugs act by down-regulating dopamine in the limbic cortex and perhaps serotonin in the prefrontal cortex. However, this is a partial and, in some areas of research, confusing picture. It is sure to be revised and expanded in the near future.

THE SCHIZOPHRENIC BRAIN MANIFESTED
IN PSYCHOLOGICAL FUNCTIONING

These biological abnormalities exert a major influence on the psychic state and psychological capacities of the person with schizophrenia. During periods of heightened activation and/or psychosis, arousal dyscontrol leads to pervasive anxiety and tension, often described as a sense of impending doom. Heart rate and respirations are more rapid than usual. In more extreme states, this can become fearfulness, then terror, then suspiciousness, and can end in delusional thinking and fixed delusional beliefs. Sufferers complain of difficulties focusing their attention. They say that minor distractions seem larger, and more intense and pressing than when they were well. Everyday experience becomes subject to hundreds of extraneous stimuli, which cannot be ignored, but which also cannot be processed and integrated. Psychophysiological research has explained this phenomenon by showing that the brain in schizophrenia cannot damp multiple, repeating stimuli, as can the unaffected brain, so that adaptation cannot occur as readily.[43, 69, 70] Reaction time is slowed and there are often minor degrees of difficulty with motor coordination and other "soft" neurological abnormalities.[71, 72] Perception is altered, leading to distorted and often very intense visual sensations and louder, hard-to-ignore auditory experiences. These can lead to frank hallucinations. Thinking becomes more fragmented and less under conscious control. Harrow and Quinlan demonstrated that loose associations are rather like computer output that has been cut into pieces then randomly put into a new and chaotic sequence.[73] As arousal increases, attention deteriorates, and anxiety and arousal rise further, often with psychosis as the end result.[49] This process can only be interrupted by medication or by unusually positive social support and isolation from stimuli, or preferably a combination of both.

In the aftermath of a psychotic episode, as negative symptoms predominate, there is less conscious thought altogether. It remains at a more rudimentary, concrete level, without affective meaning or expression. Motivation diminishes and *la belle indifférence* becomes the substitute for desire and concern. Capacities for problem solving, sequencing of behavior and action, planning, and even self-care are increasingly impaired. Emotional interaction becomes bland or anxiety-provoking and engenders fearfulness or suspiciousness. The ability to recognize emotional states in others is lost, reducing the appropriateness of emotional responses.[74] All these cognitive deficits result in a significant loss of social skills and difficulties in working.[75] The end result is social withdrawal and cognitive disability that can become as enduring as it is pervasive. As stresses impose themselves, the process can begin again, traversing prodromal symptoms, mild then severe psychotic experiences, agitation and loss of behavioral control, and then on again, into the deficit state. Recent evidence strongly points to increasing negative symptoms, disability, and reduced responsiveness to antipsychotic treatment with each episode, and probably with each day spent in a psychotic state.[22, 76-78]

What cannot be forgotten in our increased understanding of the linkages between biology and psychology is that the psychotic experience also happens to an individual human being, whose unique personality and prior experience will influence how much control he or she gains over the illness. In particular, outcome will be influenced by the person's desire to regain sanity and stability, and his or her resilience in the attempt to retain and rebuild social relationships and a career. The less that psychotic symptoms and experiences totally replace the personality and erode intellectual abilities, the greater the chance that the process of recovery will not be undone.[79] Even more important influences in recovery, however, are the ability and willingness to participate in drug and other therapies, and the influence of the immediate environment, both social and physical. One of the most basic insights gained in the last two decades of research is that schizophrenia is a disorder of the capacity to tolerate, defend against, and manage sensory stimulation, negative social interaction, and the stresses of life, with its complex chain of events and demands. We turn in Chapter 2 to those influences and the research supporting that perspective.

PRESENT UNDERSTANDING OF THE CAUSES OF THE DISORDER

The causes of schizophrenia remain unknown at the present time. However, increasingly strong evidence for a variety of types of causes, from genetics to fetal viral infection, to autoimmune disorders, provide support for the view that schizophrenia can now be viewed as a neurological and/or developmental disorder, with the same kinds of causes as many other such disorders. For instance, evidence for genetic factors includes the fact that identical twins have a high concordance for schizophrenia, at least 40% in most studies.[80-83] Recent studies using large population data sets and newer analytical methods put the variance explained by heritability at 83% and that of the environment at 17%.[84] Beyond genetics, an increasingly likely explanation for several of the documented brain abnormalities is that development of the prefrontal cortex is delayed or deranged just enough to lead to the disorder we know as schizophrenia, but not so much as to leave the person disabled intellectually or physically. In this model, events during the late first trimester through the second trimester leave the prefrontal cortex without key connections that become important in early adulthood, especially those related to higher cognitive functioning and complex information processing.[60, 85] Another proposed mechanism for these findings is that the normal pruning of cells, which occurs throughout the cortex as an integral part of brain development, is excessive and leads to the brain overreducing its cell census.[86, 87]

Several studies have correlated complications at birth with later onset of schizophrenia.[88–94] Spinal anesthesia, low Apgar scores, hypoxia, and other seemingly less serious complications have also predicted schizophrenia.[95] This was especially true for women patients[96] and for those *without* genetic risk.[97] Furthermore, there appeared to be more people born with schizophrenia during the winter.[98] Further research found that this effect was largely restricted to those without a family history of schizophrenia.[99] The implication is that an environmental factor, especially an infection prior to or just following birth, was the likely culprit. Prominent among these possible causes is infection with influenza, especially during well-identified epidemics.[89, 96, 100–102] Another among the increasingly likely causes of schizophrenia is autoimmune disease.[103, 104] Most telling is the presence of antibodies to brain cells associated with other abnormalities, suggesting an autoimmune process directly involving brain structures known to be abnormal in schizophrenia.[105] Other recently documented causes include Rh incompatibility[106] and severe malnutrition.[107]

The parallels with understanding about the causes of mental retardation are most telling. That, too, was once viewed as a single disease, but there are now over 100 known causes. If schizophrenia is similar, it will be something of an embarrassment for a field that saw psychosis as rooted in early childhood experience or family interactional aberrations. However, the reward would be that many of those causes may be treatable, and a few may be preventable.

IMPLICATIONS FOR AN OPTIMAL ENVIRONMENT

The psychoeducational approach of Carol Anderson and her colleagues at the University of Pittsburgh advanced treatment outcomes, linking a biological understanding of schizophrenia with a design for the social and physical environment that specifically compensates for many of the known vulnerabilities and deficits.[108] This approach has proven to be especially acceptable for families and patients, while proving itself to be a powerful means of fostering adaptation to community life and guiding rehabilitation. The newer psychosocial methods, including the psychoeducational multifamily group approach, assertive community treatment (see Chapter 10), and atypical antipsychotic medications are achieving a different kind of illness course in younger adults.[109] Here, episodes become more and more rare, negative symptoms decrease slowly but steadily, and functional capacities and some degree of mental liveliness and ability to work and study return over time. We explore this in more detail in Chapter 4 but summarize it here.

- To compensate for difficulty in regulating arousal, the people closest to the susceptible person can create a relatively quiet, calm, and emotionally warm environment.
- They can attempt to protect against sudden intrusions, confrontational conversations, arousing entertainment, and simultaneous and multiple kinds of sensory input.
- To help with information-processing difficulties, conversations can be shorter, less complex, and focused on everyday topics.
- Complexity in the environment and stressful life events will overwhelm cognitive capacities: These need to be protected against and buffered as much as possible.
- The optimal emotional tone is in the middle range, not intense and especially not negative, but also not overly distant, cold, or rigid.
- To compensate for delusions, family and friends can be encouraged to change the subject and not dwell on delusional ideas, but rather focus on less stressful topics.
- Sensory overload can be avoided by these same means, and also, for example, by reducing background noise, keeping light levels moderate, and having only one conversation going at a time.
- Negative symptoms can moderate with time but not under conditions of high stress: Rehabilitation should be carried out in small, careful steps, using reductions in negative and positive symptoms as indicators of safety and success.
- There is a biological and psychological relapse recovery process that cannot be accelerated without risking another relapse or at least stalling progress toward functional recovery; slow, careful, and

steady rehabilitation can achieve remarkable degrees of functional improvement without relapse.

- Time, rather than an enemy that leads inevitably toward deterioration, is on the side of recovery.
- Stresses and demands are taken seriously and steps toward recovery are paced to keep stress below the threshold for symptom exacerbation.

Multifamily groups address the many complexities and difficulties in applying these principles through ongoing problem-solving techniques that help families to use and individualize these ideas.

Our experience has shown that different families can use and understand various aspects of this information. Although the knowledge requirements for each family seem to be unique, the overriding message is universal, essential, and powerful in its therapeutic impact: This is a complex, serious, and ultimately biologically based disorder that can be ameliorated by those who know and care about the person affected when their effort is combined with optimal drug therapy and psychosocial rehabilitation.

Chapter 2

Families, Social Networks, and Schizophrenia

ELLEN P. LUKENS AND WILLIAM R. MCFARLANE

Over the course of the 20th century, many factors influenced, and to some extent limited, our understanding of the external or environmental processes that ameliorate and contribute to the course and outcome of persons with schizophrenia. In providing this overview of the psychosocial influences on schizophrenia, our goal is to facilitate a paradigmatic shift from an illness-based, "we–they," adversarial perspective to a strengths-based collaborative approach in which families, patients, and professionals are key players in promoting rehabilitation. All of the treatments described in this volume are based on this core strategy.

Schizophrenia manifests itself in different ways. Onset may be insidious, evolving over a number of years with prodromal signs suggesting varying degrees of difficulty. Or it may be acute, appearing rather suddenly, and sometimes dramatically, in a person who had previously functioned well. Regardless of presentation and course, it has a major impact on both the family and the individual with illness, and on relationships among family members. In those cases in which it manifests as a chronic illness, it must be confronted again and again, in many guises by both the individual with the illness and his or her social support system.

Schizophrenia is a disorder of the brain and as such it attacks the self of the person. To varying degrees, it affects the person's sense of reality and

18

ability to form and sustain relationships, develop insight, and engage emotionally. As Zubin and colleagues[110] state,

> The biological challenge posed by the current *Zeitgeist* views schizophrenia as something one *has*, not what one *is*, and that what one *has* is a biological disease. However, unlike some physical disorders, which are confined to specific organs, schizophrenia permeates the entire personality. From a basic conceptual standpoint, targeting only the biological focus and ignoring the psychosocial penumbra will not be an adequate solution. (p. 17)

The impact of environment on course and outcome is critical to understanding the complex nature of the illness itself. In this chapter, we address some of these profound environmental challenges as a means of guiding the reader through the complexity of the literature, and as a platform for the subsequent chapters on psychoeducational approaches to intervention with the entire family. We propose, based on a review of the literature, that the family needs an extremely strong system of support if its members are to maintain a sense of perspective and emotional balance in the face of such a complex and emotionally devastating illness. Expecting family members to respond in the most helpful manner to the often confusing and provocative symptoms of schizophrenia without some knowledge base and understanding is, at best, unrealistic.[111, 112] Without this perspective, both family members and patient are easily trapped in an interactive pattern that hinders rather than promotes maximum levels of functioning. Until recently, such negative patterns were reinforced by hostile attitudes and behavior on the part of mental health providers. Throughout this volume, the reader will find descriptions of treatments that can prevent or reverse these patterns, if present, and facilitate and enhance rehabilitative processes.

SCHIZOPHRENIA AND STRESS

It is well established that the course, outcome, and symptoms of both medical and psychiatric illnesses are worsened by stress. So understanding the nature of the relationships among biological factors and the environment is central to the development of effective treatment models throughout medicine.[110, 113–115] For someone with schizophrenia, which so profoundly affects the self, the combined impact of external or environmental stressors and internal or illness-based stressors is particularly complex and debilitating.

The stress–diathesis or stress–vulnerability model provides a useful frame for the relationships among provoking agents (stressors), vulnerability and symptom formation (diathesis), and outcome.[110, 115] Thus, a vulnerable person whose tolerance for stress is incompatible with exposure to either internally or externally generated stimulation may be thrown into a first or a recurring episode of illness.

Moving from this assumption, successful treatment depends on a careful assessment of a specific person's mix of symptoms, the course of illness, and a planful use of medication. To a significant extent, the level of stimuli in the environment can also be identified and adjusted. However, this is not a simple endeavor. It is critically dependent on the person's self-awareness and the availability, responsiveness, sophistication, and sensitivity of those who provide social and practical support.

The positive effects of stress include growth, reprioritization of goals, increased self-esteem, and expanded or strengthened networks; the negative effects include, initially, heightened arousal, anxiety and psychosis, then withdrawal, apathy, depression, and diminished sense of self-worth and self-efficacy.[116] The absence of meaningful stimulation can be stressful as well; too little stress can lead to boredom and anergia.[117] Because schizophrenia is often characterized by apathy and social withdrawal, there is a continuous struggle between maintaining a safe existence and the dangers imposed by attempting even minimal change or challenge.[118–120] Monitoring this balance requires careful attention to individual assets and limitations (e.g., level of cognitive functioning, available coping skills, strength of social network, availability and nature of family and professional supports) to determine therapeutic strategies best suited to the patient.

DOMAINS OF OUTCOME

As early as 1974, Carpenter and Buchanan noted that assessing outcome for persons with schizophrenia should not be based on relapse of psychotic symptoms alone. They identified three other measures, including social functioning, vocational functioning, and quality of life. Nonetheless, until recently, outcome has been measured by the relapse of psychotic symptoms of the illness, particularly delusions, hallucinations, or bizarre behavior. But with the addition of the negative symptoms as first-rank symptoms in DSM-IV,[5] increasing attention has been given to how these other symptoms affect the person's day-to-day functioning and course of illness. Attending to all of these outcomes creates new possibilities for support and may indirectly or directly influence rates of relapse.

Recent work adds credence to the argument that symptomatology and social functioning should be considered separately and that they have differing impacts on the individual.[121] Through examining the relationship between sense of self and psychosocial function, Brekke identified a two-tiered model of functioning, measured by self-esteem, subjective distress, and life satisfaction. The first tier included symptoms; the second, functional status variables, particularly those related to employment, social skills, and living situation. Although intrapsychic deficits contributed to both, the symptoms had a more powerful impact on self-concept, distress, and perception of overall life satisfaction than did the functional variables. However, positive experiences at work, in social interactions, and in living situations were more strongly related to self-esteem.[118, 122] These findings support the conclusion that attending directly to improvement in functioning is ultimately essential to achieving positive outcome and well-being.

SOCIAL NETWORKS, SOCIAL SUPPORT, AND THE COURSE OF ILLNESS

Depending on severity of symptoms, a person with schizophrenia needs varying degrees of vigilance and constancy of care if he or she is to function adequately in the community.[123, 124] This requires cooperation and knowledge on the part of the key players involved, including the patient, the available family (primary) support, community (secondary) support, and professional support. Involving the patient in this process is critical but may be hindered by stage of illness or by a decline in social functioning or awareness.[125]

Four dimensions are traditionally considered central to the concept of social support, including emotional (caring, trust, empathy), instrumental (performing concrete tasks), informational (imparting knowledge and skills), and appraisal or feedback support.[126] Breier and Strauss[127] include reciprocity of communication and caring (i.e., give-and-take between individuals), material support, constancy, opportunity for ventilation, social approval, and integration. Various aspects of support are provided by family members, friends, community members, or professionals, but their level, nature, and quality may vary tremendously.

For the healthy population, supports external to the family contribute to stability, well-being, and a sense of community. In contrast, the long-term mentally ill have small social networks, and these networks largely consist of family.[128] Professionals also play a key role[129, 130] and may be perceived as informal providers of care by people with schizophrenia,[131] filling in for roles typically reserved for family and friends among the healthy population. The end result is that for most people with this disorder, the actual, and therefore key, social network is a small, dense one, consisting of family, paraprofessionals, and professional clinicians.

Supports are also affected by the emotional availability of the person with the illness and complicated by the configuration of symptoms and cognitive deficits. Both symptoms and deficits interfere with reciprocity and provide an added stressor to what can easily become strained relationships.[132, 133] Although withdrawal may serve as a protection against stress, it also reduces the potential for social engagement and hence for support.[129, 134] Assessing the adequacy of support is further complicated by the observation that patients tend to (inaccurately) perceive their own support systems as sufficient, which may be a reflection of a diminished ability to establish and maintain relationships,[131] or an unwillingness or inability to admit the extent of deficits associated with the illness.[135]

The literature on social support and networks addresses the question of how the social environment affects the capacity to cope. Supportive relationships are crucial to sustain one through life crises and chronic internal and external stressors; the absence of support leads to increased psychiatric and physical distress among both the general population and those suffering from mental illness.[126, 136–138] The availability of a social network and support is essential in restoring equilibrium within the family.[139, 140]

The social networks and social supports of individuals with schizophrenia have been well studied, as have those of their families. The findings are consistent across studies: Patients, and very often their families, are more socially isolated than their peers. Pattison and colleagues,[141] Hammer,[132] and Garrison[142] found that patients were living in smaller social networks than their unaffected peers. Garrison also noted that the family members of the most severely ill patients seemed to be isolated, and preoccupied with, and burdened by, the patient. Brown and colleagues,[143] noted that 90% of the families with high expressed emotion were small in size and socially isolated. In a study (unpublished) of patients with a schizophrenic disorder evaluated during an acute psychotic episode, we found that isolation of mothers correlated with emotional overinvolvement and with their own experience and sense of having been stigmatized by friends, neighbors, and relatives. Anderson and colleagues[144] did not find the same association but did demonstrate that family network size diminished with length of illness, a finding consistent with a study by Lipton and colleagues,[146] in which network size for patients appeared to decrease in the period immediately following a first episode. Tolsdorf[146] found smaller network size at the time of first admission, suggesting that individuals with schizophrenia and their families have already lost social supports before the onset of manifest symptomatology. A typical survey of families[147] demonstrated that family members report having withdrawn from their own social circles, and vice versa.

Beyond size, other characteristics of networks have been found to affect, and to be affected by, schizophrenia. For instance, when density is low—when the various clusters in a network are not known to each other, independent of the patient—network shrinkage is more likely. Lower density and fewer social contacts are associated with relapse and rehospitalization.[148, 149] Dozier and colleagues[150] concluded that, compared with high and low density, *moderate* density correlated with the lowest rates of rehospitalization. In other words, high density in a small network may lead to excessive burden and reduced endurance among its caretaking members.

The evidence across several severe and chronic illnesses indicates that ongoing access to social contact and support prevents the deterioration of such conditions and improves their course.[138] Social network size, emotional support, perceived support, and functional support, especially the availability of information, have been shown to predict cardiac disease and mortality, incidence of certain cancers, cancer mortality, death from stroke, complications of pregnancy and childbirth, and responses to, and disability from, rheumatoid arthritis. This relationship was recently confirmed prospectively in a sample of 32,624 professionals followed for 4 years: Social network size predicted cardiac mortality, accidents, suicides, and incidence of stroke.[151] Brown and Harris demonstrated a strong association between size and availability of a friendship and family network, and the onset and duration of depression.[152] Social support buffers the impact of adverse life events.[153] It is one of the key factors influencing medication compliance,[154] as is the stance of the immediate family regarding compliance.[155] Heller and colleagues[156] found that information was actually provided through the families' natural, preexisting social networks, even though they were in educational support groups.

Wanting, but lacking, social attachments predicted schizophrenic relapse over 4 years, while available social support at the time of life events yielded fewer relapses than when it was lacking.[157] As might be expected, the quality of life of mentally ill adults living in the community was strongly associated with social network size, especially if it was in the midrange.[158–160] The subjective burden experienced by relatives was explained by severity of stressors, social support, and coping capabilities.[161] Coping capabilities, in themselves, were shown to be a function of affirming social support, the density of the social network, and participation in a support group.[162] Availability of social support to the family was one of the factors associated with successful community tenure of individuals with chronic schizophrenia.[163] Negative symptoms have often been associated with social network size, which includes relatives, but this has been assumed to be determined by negative symptoms.[17, 164, 165]

Most studies have also found that among persons with more severe and chronic illnesses, patient networks contain fewer family members, although the *proportion* of the network that is comprised of family is higher over time.[130, 142, 166] The landmark World Health Organization Study found that after baseline measures of severity, social support was the strongest predictor of symptom status 2 to 5 years later.[167] Outcome was significantly better in areas where there was a traditional village social structure in India, Nigeria, and Colombia. In traditional cultures, one finds that ill individuals are routinely in contact with and cared for by families, which in turn are themselves embedded in a more dense and extended social network.

LONG-TERM OUTCOME, SOCIAL SUPPORT, AND CONTINUITY OF CARE

A study by Hogarty and Ulrich[18] found that relapse risk declines with time, especially during the second year after an episode. That result is consistent with findings from the Harding and colleagues study[10] and several other long-term studies[8, 9] that after two or three decades, symptomatology and functioning substantially improve in nearly three-fourths of chronic cases. Long-term social support accounted for some of the positive outcome, because outreach staff maintained contact for up to 5 years after discharge. It is noteworthy that earlier psychosocial intervention studies by Pasamanick and colleagues[168] and Stein and Test[169] found that deterioration began after the test treatments were discontinued. As for long-term outcome in family psychoeducation trials, in a follow-up study of patients who had participated in a controlled trial of family crisis intervention[170] the authors found that relapse was remarkably rare 3 to 6 years after termination of therapy. In another study by McFarlane and colleagues, half the patients treated in psychoeducational multifamily groups had not relapsed during the 6 years after discharge.[171]

Continuity of social context may be as important to outcome as continuity of care, especially when that context includes treatment interventions. Conversely, disruption of social networks leads to destabilization and relapse. Steinberg and Durrell found that the vast majority of first episodes in an Australian sample occurred after separation from home and family—on entering college or the military.[172] It is widely recognized that therapist departure, even for vacation, often precipitates relapse. The data on life events and their relation to relapse suggest a strong association. Indeed, most adverse life events involve disruption of social support and the membership and organization of a social network.

COGNITIVE DEFICITS AND SCHIZOPHRENIA

Recent work on the cognitive deficits associated with schizophrenia helps to explain the fundamental barriers a patient confronts in attempting to form social alliances or build relationships (see Chapter 1). Even for persons without mental illness, the environment serves as an important frame of reference in which family, friends and co-workers, external structures, schedules, and events help to ground, remind, cue, and orient. For someone with schizophrenia, the milieu is particularly critical, because it can compensate for the cognitive deficits and associated symptoms and behaviors of the illness.[60, 173] Depending on the person and the nature of the surroundings, these structures and guideposts could occur in the family home, in a well-structured and sensitively run community residence, or in a day hospital or inpatient unit. When these supports—essentially, a prosthetic ego—are not in place, the patient is most likely to flounder.

The ability to use external social structure as a reference point is initially learned in the family. A family provides its children with a way to learn to recognize external cues and signals, internalize these cues and modulate appropriate social responses, achieve increased mastery and comfort with associated skills, and adapt them for a range of situations. Persons who function within the healthy range can transfer the skills learned in this safe, or "holding," environment to other settings. But when a person develops schizophrenia, associated cognitive deficits interfere with the ability to recognize and modulate both internal and external cues, and to make this transfer, that is, to generalize a cognitive set.[174] This interrupted process is itself a stressor: symptomatic behaviors or incongruent or inappropriate social responses can be triggered or exacerbated. Moreover, these cognitive functions usually remain deficient or worsen even after the symptoms have remitted.[175] This is frustrating, both for the individual and for those with whom he or she interacts, particularly if this process is misinterpreted or poorly understood. It sets the stage for functional disability.

During the last decade, research has begun to explain how schizophrenia interferes with the very simple internal or external (i.e., social) cues that serve to ground and orient. Silverstein uses a reciprocal model of cognitive processing to explain these complex social response sets.[176] He postulates that feedback loops across a series of processing stages appear to explain the interaction between ongoing behaviors and cognition. These stages include (1) encoding both internal and external cues; (2) realistic appraisal of the cues; (3) decision making regarding both immediate and long-term goals; (4) remembering acceptable responses; (5) evaluating these or new responses; and (6) carrying responses out appropriately. Other cognitive factors complicate the process. For instance, neuropsychological deficits can interfere with the ability to recall past responses and place them in context. Formulating goals requires the ability to draw on abstract thinking, while affect (e.g., anger, hostility) can interfere with how a situation is interpreted, the cues attended to, and the appropriateness of responses generated.

Environmental factors clearly help or hinder this process. For example, Penn and his associates found that when patients were given a focused task situation (such as a role play) with clearly structured parameters, they were able to stay on task and respond more appropriately than when faced with the more undefined task of functioning socially on a hospital ward with less structure and uncontrolled levels of (often) extreme stimulation. Data from this and other studies suggest that patients who can improve their ability to respond appropriately to differing environmental cues are more competent socially and are less likely to relapse.[123, 176, 177] Therefore, attending to deficits at this cognitive level is an important consideration in designing rehabilitation programs, but is clearly complicated by the very presence of such deficits.[174]

Various environmental interventions have been introduced to help the patient overcome the social impact of the cognitive deficits at the stages outlined by Silverstein.[176] These include teaching coping mechanisms, such as how to use simple daily schedules, compartmentalized pill boxes, or other organizational aids as check points, to help recognize external cues and structure appropriate responses. Training in problem solving[178, 179] or communication and other social skills[119, 180, 181] are other effective but more complex interventions. Over the past 15 years, Hogarty and his colleagues have developed a targeted therapy for schizophrenia referred to as Personal

Therapy.[182–184] They used individualized, staged but traditional behavioral techniques, as well as joining, gradual reentry, and graduated assumption of responsibility and reintegration—the cornerstones of his and Anderson's psychoeducational interventions,[108, 185] to improve both mood and behavior. The family appeared to serve a protective function regarding relapse; their informal care freed up clinicians to focus on treatment of symptoms per se.[183, 184]

FAMILY STRESS

The most prominent stressor for the family and the patient alike is the illness itself. Given the evidence we have reviewed, it would be difficult to ignore or minimize such stress. One can easily imagine how it can dominate family life. Additional family stressors include current and remote life events and chronic stress conditions, including lack of access to resources, and personal and professional supports.[186, 187] For the patient, the stress manifests itself through an increase in symptoms, an inability to work or to maintain relationships, or to participate fully in the activities of everyday life.

The impact on the family is enormous, exacerbated by the very nature of the illness. Lefley writes movingly about the hurdles that families must face and the stressors with which they must contend on a daily basis.[188] At the societal level, she cites negative cultural attitudes and labeling of families and patients based on ignorance and stigma, which results in service deficiencies, indifference, or outright neglect. At the service level, she describes legal constraints for both hospitalization and discharge, premature discharge, inadequate community support and housing, and, increasingly, diversion to the criminal justice system. This is worsened when mental health care professionals fail to provide adequate or even minimal support or information, breach confidentiality, reject and label the family and patient, or display lack of knowledge. Lefley also describes the intensity of the situational burden and the existential impact of living with mental illness in the family. This burden includes loss and sorrow, a kind of "mourning without end,"[189, 190] negative impact on children and siblings,[191] economic burden, social isolation, fear for the patient's future, the patient's rejection of treatment, and erratic or dangerous behavior. Not surprisingly, the cumulative impact can include grief, confusion, anger or self-blame, isolation, disruption, frustration, guilt, or weakened defenses, both emotional and physical.[188, 189, 192]

Available coping strategies, especially comprehension and knowledge

of schizophrenia and correct attribution and appraisal of the situation, contribute to the family's ability to handle the stress.[186, 187] For the families, as
well as the patients, stressors may be perceived as negative, reflecting loss
or threat of loss, or conversely, as opportunities for growth or change.[193, 194]

STIGMA

Stigma is a concept derived from labeling theory. Although labeling can
have both positive—through accurate diagnoses and effective treatment—
and negative outcomes—through associated stigma,[195] stigma usually refers
to a set of negative beliefs regarding any one group and reinforced by society and especially the media. Such beliefs or attitudes contribute to stereo-
typing, prejudice, and spoiled identity. For a person labeled with mental
disability, stigma can be associated with a withdrawal of social support, demoralization, and loss of self-esteem, and can have far-reaching effects on
daily functioning, particularly in the workplace. With the availability of
new medications and concomitant emphases on improved functioning and
rehabilitation, stigma becomes a more important focal point for intervention.[118] As Link and his colleagues[196] observed, stigma has a strong continuing impact on well-being, even though proper diagnoses and treatment improve symptoms and levels of functioning over time.

Stigma affects the family in a negative fashion as well.[197–199] In many
ways, family responses parallel those of the person with illness. They include withdrawal and isolation on the part of family members, which in
turn are associated with a decrease in social network size and emotional
support, increased burden, and decreased quality of life. Self-imposed
stigma and labeling change family identity and contribute to lowered self-
efficacy and increased burden. In some studies, relatives tried to conceal
their family member's illness from friends,[200, 201] whereas in another survey,
very little concealment or shame was reported.[197] The difference appears to
relate to chronicity. This fits with clinical experience in which relatives of
younger patients may feel more shame and personal stigma than those of
older patients. On the other hand, stigma on the part of friends and more
distant relatives may play a role in the shrinking network phenomenon. In
the pilot study by the authors mentioned earlier,[168] stigma experienced by
mothers of patients was associated with overinvolvement with the patient,
but only in the presence of a smaller social network. From these and other
studies, it appears that stigma is not experienced universally among family

members, but it may be important as a factor in shaping the social network on the one hand, and relationships within the family on the other.

For professionals working with families and those challenged by mental illness, understanding the impact of stigma is essential to the psychoeducational approach. Once someone is labeled with mental illness, a whole set of characteristics is quickly assigned to him or her, which may have little to do with that person's experience of illness or presentation of symptoms. Sorting out the reality from the label by attending to strengths requires that the clinician learn who the individual is, distinct from the illness, a person *with*, or *suffering from* schizophrenia, as opposed to a "schizophrenic." Helping all members of the family focus on these strengths is key to rehabilitative effectiveness.

QUALITY OF LIFE AND EXPERIENCED BURDEN

As we have emphasized, the mere existence of mental illness within the family results in changes in structure and challenges normal functioning and patterns of interaction in many ways.[202] Burdens cited by families, both objective and subjective, include interference with social and leisure activities and daily routine, deterioration of one's own health and mental health—including symptoms such as insomnia, headaches, irritability, and depression—confusion, learned helplessness, and difficulty in communicating with the person with illness. As illustrated in Figure 2.1, these variables interact. Tensions inevitably arise from unpredictable behavior and the associated need for supervision[188, 203, 204] and secondarily increase the tendency toward patient relapse, and social and vocational dysfunction.[161, 205–209] As symptoms in the ill person become more pronounced and persistent, family burden increases.[210] Families seem to have the greatest difficulty with negative symptoms, particularly if the person had functioned relatively well prior to onset of illness.[211, 212]

Such responses are complicated by loss, mourning the person who existed before the illness struck and what he or she might have become.[213–215] Burden seems to be at least in part a function of the number and density of social supports available.[216, 217] An inverse relationship has been observed between (1) satisfaction with the total social network and the degree of burden experienced, and (2) network density and burden.[161, 162, 207] Burden is further complicated if family members, including the individual with schizophrenia, deny, or fail to acknowledge or accept, the illness among family members.[16, 218] Without resources and support, both professional and

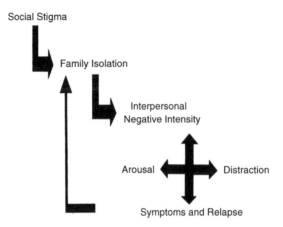

FIGURE 2.1. Interaction of principal biological, psychological, and social factors in schizophrenia.

personal, the intensity of this interaction can contribute to the experience that families describe of being drawn into an bottomless "sinkhole."[189]

HISTORICAL PERSPECTIVES

A full understanding of the range of familial responses to mental illness, the differential impact on family life, and the complexity of family attitudes toward professional support requires an understanding of how attitudes toward families have changed over time. Until the late 1950s, the predominant approach to treatment for the severely mentally ill was custodial management, characterized by poor prognosis, institutionalized and dependent behavior, and limited functioning. Since it was assumed that psychiatric illness emerged from unhealthy relationships among family members and could best be treated though a private relationship between therapist and client, clinicians tended to avoid and discourage contact between patients and their relatives.[219] Families were separated from the hospitalized person and were directly or indirectly excluded from treatment. During this same period, a series of case studies on family dynamics and schizophrenia suggested that behaviors within the family, and particularly by the mother as primary caregiver, contributed to the onset and course of psychiatric illness among children.[220–224] Another series of case studies examined the relationship between family dynamics and illness, and strongly influenced the growing family therapy movement. In 1956 Bateson and his colleagues[225] described what they referred to as the "double bind," while Lidz and colleagues coined the term "marital schism and skew."[226] Both were said to be associated with poor generational and role boundaries, and were causally linked with development of schizophrenia by the child. These ideas permeated the literature, reinforcing negative stereotypes regarding the relationship between schizophrenia and the family at many different levels.

Given the rapid shift that occurred from hospital to community in the 1960s and 1970s, inadequate organization and knowledge, and insufficient funding across system levels quickly created serious gaps in service, particularly in the outpatient clinics.[227] As a result, families were forced to step in, and they became increasingly immersed in providing care and lodging for the adult patient. Since there was little professional or institutional support for caregiving families, they were unprepared for the profound challenges involved in living with and caring for patients, many of whom many had been chronically institutionalized. Not surprisingly, researchers and clinicians began to revisit the question of how family attitudes and behavior might be related to the cause or course of illness. The ironic, if not tragic, result was that families were held responsible for daily monitoring and care, while they were excluded from participation in the treatment or decision-making process, and from information regarding illness or intervention.[228] They were held responsible for both care and cause.

EXPRESSED EMOTION

In parallel, an interest in what came to be referred to as "expressed emotion" (EE) appeared in the literature in the 1960s. Preliminary research on EE, conducted in Britain during the 1950s, focused on the clinical observation that the family atmosphere of some people suffering from schizophrenia was characterized by overstimulation, dominance, overprotection, rejection, criticism, and contradictory messages,[229, 230] language familiar from the earlier case studies on mother–child relationships, parenting, and schizophrenia. Data were collected through a lengthy series of semi-structured interviews, sometimes as long as 3 or 4 hours, conducted in the home, audiotaped, and coded by trained raters. Initially, the family environment was characterized by parameters that included criticism, hostility, dissatisfaction, warmth, positive comments, and overinvolvement, as expressed by both family and patient, but most of these scales were eventually dropped because of lack of findings. As a result, EE has typically been measured by a dichotomous summary variable reflecting either high or low EE (i.e., presence or absence of criticism and/or overinvolvement), as expressed by relatives in regard to the ill family member.

The initial findings in Great Britain and subsequent replication in the United States suggested that high levels of emotion were strongly associated with the exacerbation or relapse of symptoms.[143, 231, 232] This work has been replicated many times over, and in many cultures. In an extensive meta-analysis, Bebbington and Kuipers[233] cited the overwhelming evidence among 25 studies, representing 1,346 patients in 12 different countries, for a predictive relationship between high levels of EE and relapse of schizophrenia.

In some families, it appears that emotional overinvolvement (EOI) by relatives may impede functional progress, especially when greater interpersonal and physical distance between patient and relative are required. While dependence-inducing interaction was considered ubiquitous in families of schizophrenic patients in psychodynamic and family systems theories of etiology, the experience of the clinicians who have worked within a psychoeducational framework is that this kind of interaction is markedly rare, *after families are reassured and supported in dealing with the illness.* Miklowitz and colleagues[234, 235] found that only one-third of families rated high on EOI, and that EOI was associated with single mothers, with sons as patients, poor premorbid adjustment in the patient, high levels of residual symptomatology, and higher levels of communication; that is, what has been called overinvolvement is often a reaction to very serious symptomatology and functional disability in the patient or is secondary to isolation and relationship difficulties that are nearly inherent in certain family constellations (e.g., single mothers living with, and caring for, male adult, mentally ill children). Furthermore, much "over"involvement can be more reasonably seen as compensation for major deficits in the social domain. In any case, the degree of involvement that is appropriate and rehabilitative is very much a controversial issue in the rehabilitation field, so that it is unlikely that most relatives will have spontaneously achieved the optimal balance between compensation and challenge toward autonomy. A positive feedback interaction in which poor premorbid functioning elicits overinvolvement, which in turn may exacerbate poor adult functioning, seems likely and is, at the least, the most parsimonious and least blaming explanation.

To address these apparently powerful findings, concerned clinicians and researchers designed various educational interventions to teach families, particularly those described as high in EE, how to provide a low-key and less stressful environment in the home. The results have been striking: Multiple studies suggest that when the families are educated, trained, and supported, relapse rates among patients are remarkably low (see Chapter 4).

FAMILY RESPONSES TO EXPRESSED EMOTION

Beginning in the 1970s the increasingly active and outspoken grassroots family advocacy movement, led by the Alliance for the Mentally Ill (AMI; now the National Alliance for the Mentally Ill), began to gain prominence. Family advocates interpreted the emphasis on high EE as yet another form of arrogance, blame, dominance, and paternalism among the professional elite. They interpreted the studies as a means of holding families responsible for maintaining patient stability, and as a mechanism for diverting attention and dollars from biological research and critically needed community supports (such as housing and rehabilitation) for the patients.[188, 203, 212, 236–240] EE has been criticized for other reasons as well, including the stigmatization and labeling inherent in defining it as a dichotomized variable, the inconsistent definition of relapse in the intervention studies, the emphasis on relapse as the primary outcome variable to the exclusion of other measures of functioning, and vague descriptions of the educational interventions.[241–243]

In response to the challenges regarding a direct causal relationship between EE and relapse, more inclusive reciprocal models have been proposed to increase the accuracy of the construct.[243–245] These cover both internal and external stressors, including the cognitive challenges described earlier, coping mechanisms and other personality variables, and the family's external supports and resources.[246, 247] For example, Strachan and colleagues[248] and Goldstein and colleagues[249] examined EE among key relatives as a reflection of transactional processes between the patient and family. They observed that patients who interacted with relatives having low EE made significantly fewer critical and more autonomous statements than those who interacted with relatives described as high in EE. The authors observed that the quality of behavior for both the families *and* the person with illness was associated with subsequent functioning for the subject. Wuerker has demonstrated that high EE is associated with tighter linkage between patient and relative interactional responses, and with more competition for control, much of it initiated by the patient.[250, 251]

The attribution or understanding of illness has also been associated with EE. In these studies, relatives described as critical or hostile perceived the patient as somehow responsible for unpleasant behavior, whereas more accepting relatives saw identical behaviors as characteristic of the illness it-self.[252, 253] As we have stated before, an individual who is cognitively im-paired, denying illness, paranoid, angry, hostile, socially withdrawn, or showing signs of anhedonia will be much less available to receive the sup-port needed to function at an optimal level.[112] If the family member con-fronted by such symptoms has little formal knowledge of the illness, he or she might respond with increased involvement, intensity, and criticism. Life-cycle variables play into this situation as well. Under normal circum-stances, adult children do not require ongoing attention, supervision, or in-tervention from immediate family members (i.e., the nature of the relation-ships changes as well).[188, 254]

Unfortunately, the anger engendered by the literature on EE has lim-ited opportunities to explore fully the crucial function that families and other intimates can serve for the patient. As a result, little emphasis has been placed on low EE and either how it might affect outcomes or positive aspects of family involvement, or how it might serve both the family and the person with illness.[188, 238, 255] Low EE may be protective, as some research-ers have contended, or it may be dysfunctional, signifying withdrawal, helplessness, or even despair.[188] The involvement and attentiveness associ-ated with high EE may provide a self-protective function for families, par-ticularly given hostile and exclusionary professional attitudes toward the family.[255] The "over" involvement component of expressed emotion may also help to keep the patient grounded and on track, and even foster reha-bilitation, given the nature of the cognitive deficits discussed earlier. In re-cently reported work, King and Dixon found that EOI among family mem-bers was actually associated with improved measures of social functioning at 9-month follow-up.[256] This replicates our finding that overinvolvement among fathers was correlated with the vocational achievement of their sons with schizophrenia (McFarlane et al., 1984). Analysis that examines EE in relation to outcomes other than relapse is sorely needed. Finally, only spo-radic attention has been paid to the relationship among availability and continuity of services, perceived support, and the emotional environment of the family.

SUMMARY: THE NEED FOR FAMILY
AND PROFESSIONAL ALLIANCES

Given the serious nature of schizophrenia and the responsibility for care that families continue to shoulder, creating caregiving alliances of professionals and families is no longer optional. In her studies of comparative approaches to case management, Pescosolido and colleagues reflect on the roles of the treatment system, the social service system, and the lay community in providing a safety net or "community of care" for the client.[257] Achieving a balance between necessary needed support and unwelcome intrusion, oversolicitation, or coercion is as much a dilemma for the professional caregiver as for the family provider. For professionals, this means reflecting on where and how to place supports, while still promoting self-determination and growth for the person with illness.

To achieve improved outcomes and quality of life, social isolation, stigma, burden, EE, and misattribution must be addressed. As described in Part II, the role of the mental health professional is to work to reestablish some semblance of balance in the face of the major life disruption created by the presence of mental illness.[254] The psychoeducational models offer a rich forum in which families and professionals may share and use knowledge to reduce the impact of severe mental illness. Connecting with people who have faced common challenges helps to normalize the experience and provides an opportunity to anticipate situations and cope with them more effectively.[112, 258-260]

Chapter 3

The Therapeutic Social Network

A Healing Community

Multifamily therapy originated nearly four decades ago in attempts by Laqueur[261] and Detre[262] to develop an improved psychosocial treatment approach for hospitalized schizophrenic patients. Unlike family therapy during its early period, the emphasis in multifamily groups was more pragmatic than theoretical. The earliest reported experiences with the modality arose, in fact, from a need to solve ward management problems. Laqueur noted improved ward social functioning in patients who insisted on attending a group organized for visiting relatives (personal communication, October, 1973). Detre and his colleagues started a multifamily group in order to encourage cooperation between resident psychiatrists and social workers on an acute inpatient service but quickly found a high level of interest in the group among patients and family members alike, as well as improvements in family communication and morale. Though use of this modality has grown steadily, most of the focus has continued to be on the major psychiatric disorders.[263] The clinical efficacy of psychoeducational multifamily groups, even when compared with single-family psychoeducation, requires an explanation. This chapter explores the theoretical underpinnings of these groups. The most basic question is this: Why are outcomes better when there are more people in the room during treatment sessions, compared to outcomes, when a clinician meets with one family and their ill member? A derivative question is whether adding other families, and thus more people, to single-family psychoeducation or family behavioral management introduces a new treatment intervention or simply enhances those already operating. A set of more technical questions involves an explanation for findings outlined in Chapter 4: Multifamily groups, compared to single-family psychoeducational treatment, have greater efficacy with high expressed emotion (EE) families, in poor responders to antipsychotic medication, in first episodes, and in Caucasian, compared with African American, families.

The multifamily group, with its unique social structure, enjoys an especially effective congruence with specific social and clinical problems in schizophrenia and several other psychiatric disorders. The psychoeducational variant of multifamily groups described in this volume attempts to capitalize further on that congruence by emphasizing the natural therapeutic and rehabilitative processes characteristic of, and perhaps inherent in, that format. This new form of multifamily group incorporates the advantages of each of its source treatments—psychoeducation,[108] family–behavioral,[178] and multifamily therapy. That is accomplished by expanding the number and variety of individuals, families, and patients that bring their collective resources to bear on a given clinical or human dilemma. This approach also diminishes the negative features of the single-family approaches, yielding synergistic effects that enhance efficacy. Like the psychoeducational family approach of Anderson and her colleagues,[108] the model presented here has attempted to reflect contemporary understanding of schizophrenia from biological, psychological, and social perspectives, on the assumption that an effective treatment should address as many known aspects of the illness as possible, from as many perspectives as possible. Because pharmacological therapy and family psychoeducational and behavioral management have multiple effects at the biological, psychological, and family levels, the discussion here focuses on the family and social aspects of schizophrenia, and the ways in which the specific social structure and group process in multifamily groups affect the course of illness, the patient, and the family.

THE MULTIFAMILY GROUP AS A THERAPEUTIC SOCIAL NETWORK

The social networks and social supports of individuals with schizophrenia have been well studied, as have those of their families, as was shown in Chapter 2. The findings are consistent across studies: Patients and their families are more socially isolated than their peers. Furthermore, their networks are often overly dense, although their smaller size correlates with higher EE and vulnerability to stress, more frequent crises, and even effects on physical health. Smaller networks also lead to lack of social support and diminished sense of well-being, as well as poorer access to information and help with coping skills. Conversely, ongoing access to social contact and support prevents the deterioration of such conditions and improves their course.[138] Social support buffers the impact of adverse life events[153] and also influences medication compliance.[154] Larger networks of moderate density enhance long-term capacity to provide ongoing secondary support to primary caretakers. From a clinical perspective, the most effective psychosocial treatments for schizophrenia are those that expand the patient's and the family's social support and, because they are long-term approaches, ultimately expand their social network.[264, 265]

Therefore, enlarging the social network, as in a psychoeducational multifamily group, addresses one of the principal determinants of outcome, one that in other group modalities is accomplished by assembling only patients. The key difference in multifamily groups is that the majority of those participating—families and clinicians—do not have brain abnormalities that interfere with social interaction and joint therapeutic effort. Psychoeducational and family behavioral methods in these groups enhance the therapeutic effects of expanding the network; that is, coping skills training occurs within a social support network in which members often make significant contributions to the quality and quantity of available ideas. That creates a therapeutic social network, involving several entire families, which is both a goal in itself and the means to conducting other aspects of the treatment. Continuity of social context may be as important to outcome as is continuity of care, especially when that context includes treatment interventions. A major weakness of single-family models of treatment is that they are vulnerable to the vicissitudes of the therapist's professional career, which often lead to disruption. For that and other reasons, the design of a psychosocial treatment requires some means for ensuring as much continuity of social support and clinical care as possible.

In psychoeducational multifamily groups, families are provided an artificial social support system in addition to encouragement in maintaining or expanding their natural network. A multifamily group satisfies the technical requirements for a natural social network: The other family members are not kin and are heterogeneous as to age sex, personality, ethnicity, and class, yet they share a vital common experience and concern: mental illness in one member of the family. The family's network increases in the multifamily group, because the other families provide many different, more varied relationships, real and potential. These new relationships are, on the whole, much less intense than family relationships and usually remain less intense than most close friendships. Because only a few relationships in a multifamily group evolve into close friendships, the network expansion that occurs tends to be in the realm of what have been termed "weak ties," which have a greater than expected degree of importance to human functioning.[266] It is these very relationships that can provide burden relief but are often attenuated by chronic mental illnesses.[144]

Network density approximates the normal, midrange level, because all the families in the group become interconnected. With time and therapists' encouragement, the multifamily group can become a natural network, with formal characteristics similar to those that arise spontaneously. Given the evidence that many families are socially isolated, and that isolation may be associated with high EE and relapse frequency, it seems possible that resocialization of the family may be a key element in achieving the goals of psychoeducational approaches. The fact that family members have begun to band together in self-help organizations[113] is a testament to the need for, and value of, illness-induced network expansion. The other therapeutic effects described here depend on therapeutic network expansion for their effectiveness.

Because multifamily groups easily persist for years, they provide the kind of long-term continuity that in other treatment approaches is too often disrupted by therapist turnover and departures by members of the family. The multifamily group is resilient and less vulnerable to changes in the participation of any one member. Not only do multifamily groups consist of the same social groupings as traditional villages—multiple generations from several families, led by clinicians with significant expertise and socially constituted authority and responsibility, they often continue long enough to allow the social structure and interactions to approximate more natural, traditional networks. Thus, the multifamily group provides a specific correction for an empirically known deficit—isolation—that is frequently cited by family members themselves as one of the more demoralizing and burdensome, long-term consequences of the disorder.

FROM STIGMA TO A MASTERY-BASED GROUP IDENTITY

As was evident in the studies reviewed in Chapter 2, experienced stigma is an important factor in shaping the social network on the one hand, and relationships within the family on the other. Anderson, Falloon, Leff, and others have noted that education appears to reduce the family's sense of shame and guilt. It has long been recognized that relief and higher morale result from group members sharing their difficulties openly and discussing with others who are in similar straits the experience of living with a relative who has a mental illness. In this process, there is often such a profound sense of relief and acknowledgment that stigma is reversed, replaced by a kind of pride in being able, as a group, to understand and master the illness that until then has been a great burden. If members have experienced social rejection or discrimination as a consequence of the illness, the group becomes a source of social acceptance. To the extent that the psychoeducational multifamily group induces improved social functioning among the patients, it becomes a source of pride, promoting a sense of achievement, improved morale, and cognitive mastery in family and patients alike.

RELIEF AND COPING IN CAREGIVING

Nearly all families experience severe burdens, whose extent seems to be at least partly a function of the number and density of social supports available.[216, 217] Multifamily groups have equally positive effects on family burdens. The subjective aspects are somewhat relieved by the shared realization that schizophrenia has predictable and common effects on family members. The perception that other patients do improve in treatment produces a sense of impending relief. By ventilating specific anxieties and receiving support and encouragement, family members experience an increase in morale that allows them to carry on. As for objective burdens, group members trade experiences and advice, develop new coping strategies, arrange to relieve one another, and bring pressure on the therapists and their institutions to provide sorely needed services. Finally, to the extent that the group succeeds in alleviating positive and negative schizophrenic symptoms, and in developing new family coping strategies, both the sense *and the reality* of burden are reduced. These phenomena of reversal of stigma and reduction of burden go a long way toward explaining the enthusiasm and loyalty that families come to feel about a psychoeducational multifamily group and the high retention rates that have been noted.

FAMILY COPING WITH NEGATIVE SYMPTOMS AND FUNCTIONAL DEFICITS

Negative symptoms, and social and vocational disability seem to be largely untouched by neuroleptic medication. Indeed, negative symptoms are associated with reduced dopamine metabolism, making dopamine blockade unlikely to be an effective long-term treatment for a crucial aspect of the disorder.[24] The psychoeducational multifamily group model is based on several findings and one theoretical principle that suggest a more promising outcome.

A central consideration is that schizophrenia makes it remarkably difficult to make discrete transitions from one context to another, especially from home to work, school, or peer relationships. These transitions can be seen as requiring more control of arousal and greater information-processing capacity than many patients may possess. Thus, it could be argued that family members need to be present initially to provide a kind of social bridge to nonfamily contexts, much as occurs in traditional village societies. Reiss and Costell documented this family-to-society acculturation process in multifamily groups for hospitalized adolescents.[267] Using direct, interactional measurement techniques, they found that even when the adolescents sat in a group separate from their parents, cues from family members and the social structure of the senior subgroup determined speech dominance patterns and other structural aspects of the adolescent subgroup. The implication is that adolescents and, by extension, younger patients with schizophrenia have much of their behavior organized by the behavior of other family members, particularly parents, but in ways that are more indirect than usually assumed. To the extent that interaction between families in psychoeducation multifamily groups is socially appropriate (i.e., normative), it appears to promote more normative behavior by patients within, and later across, family boundaries.

Falloon[268] and his colleagues found that behavioral family intervention was most successful when families developed more effective coping strategies, an outcome that contributed more to outcome than changes in EE. Because that approach relies on a problem-solving strategy, the larger the pool of available solutions from which to choose, the greater the likelihood of a workable solution. Furthermore, a multifamily group contains a great variety of personal experiences, including those of the participating relatives and of the clinicians. That variety promotes the nonfamily ties and increases the efficacy of problem solving.

Another way in which multifamily groups assist families in coping is a process that involves "indirect learning." It is much more acceptable and validating to some families than overt suggestions or interpretations, and it is also more useful to those who are less verbal and more action- or visually oriented. Family members are remarkably attuned to the structural and interactional problems in other families, while empathetic to the stresses of coping with a mentally ill member. When the problem-solving method is used, families appear to apply the concrete solutions arrived at for another family, as well as their underlying lessons, to their own family, without having to acknowledge the similarity explicitly. Of course, the same process can occur overtly, but that may be too threatening for some families. It seems that insight and direct instruction may not always be necessary to change coping skills, but exposure to other families in a process of mutual change may be.

ESTABLISHING A THERAPEUTIC SOCIAL ENVIRONMENT

The EE studies strongly suggest that, for persons with schizophrenia, it is now possible to describe optimal, though atypical, social environments. These environments are characterized by interactions that are calm, benign, relatively simple, and flexible, with known social structure and behavioral limits, carefully controlled performance expectations, continuity of membership, and a high degree of predictability. That is also the conclusion from studies on arousal, attention, and dysfunctions of the dopaminergic system. It is also increasingly clear that much of the EE observed in families is contextual in origin (see Chapter 2). It derives from high levels of symptoms and disability; hostility and loss of interpersonal competence on the part of the individual with the illness; the family's existing coping capacities and social, educational, and professional supports available to the family; and, ultimately, the beliefs held by members of the family, community, and culture.

While a great deal of attention has been paid to helping families to establish a home environment based on these empirically based principles, the psychoeducational multifamily group model attempts to go one step further and build these optimal characteristics into the treatment context and new social network. The concern driving this effort is to avoid presenting the patient with an overwhelming stimulus load in the treatment situation. Patients often seem to prefer the mixture of family and nonfamily membership, possibly because of previously observed tendencies for members of different families to develop remarkably tolerant and supportive relationships toward the patients in the group. The ambient tone is often close to the optimal "emotional expression" described by Spiegel and Wissler,[269] who found that family members' positive feeling of acceptance toward patients was predictive of a longer remission interval. In addition, the education, continued training, and updating alleviate the confusion that attend this illness, which helps families to attribute difficulties to the illness itself rather than to personalities, misbehavior, and/or poor parenting. These processes and interfamily interactions all contribute to reducing exasperation and EE.

BALANCING INTRA- AND INTERFAMILY BOUNDARIES

To the extent that emotional overinvolvement (EOI) hinders functional improvement, a successful intervention would have to address this process, if it were present. However, unlike critical comments, EOI may reflect a long-standing interactional pattern in the family and may therefore be slower to change as a result of direct intervention.[15] Because one study suggests that EOI is also associated with social isolation and stigmatic rejection of the caretaking family by more distant relatives and friends,[270] a more benign and effective approach would expand social networks and reduce feelings of stigma among relatives, while offering substitute extrafamilial relationships. Since direct confrontation by the therapists is often perceived as blaming, suggestions or criticisms should come from other families who have been struggling with the same issues.

The psychoeducational multifamily group approach offers ample opportunities for each of these more indirect and, ultimately, more effective strategies. The social structure of a multifamily group provides a non-intrusive alternative to the problem of family overinvolvement, an important element of high EE. Family members can develop new, less intense, and more functional and satisfying relationships in the group, *while preserving and validating intrafamily bonds*. With time, these new relationships gradually attenuate enmeshed interaction, particularly between parents and their offspring with schizophrenia. The either–or choice presented by more straightforward psychoeducation approaches (i.e., overinvolvement vs. disengagement) is avoided in psychoeducational multifamily groups by providing readily available substitutes for intrafamily relationships, while in no way attempting to disqualify or interrupt them. The rate of disenmeshment can be controlled by the family, so that change can proceed at a non-threatening pace. Note that this process imitates nature: Most young adults gradually increase their interpersonal distance with their parents, at a rate that is more or less tolerable for all family members. In both generations, parent–child interaction is replaced by extrafamilial social interaction and relationships. Here, therapy imitates nature; that is, external relationships replace their overcharged and countertherapeutic internal counterparts.

Almost all the literature and our consistent clinical observations concur that overinvolved families become more functional as they develop relationships with members of the other families in multifamily groups.

Rigidity in family relationships is difficult to preserve indefinitely in a multifamily group, because group interaction tends to be increasingly complex and unpredictable, usually in positive ways. Cross-family relationships wax and wane, depending on circumstances, and gradually open family boundaries. This process is almost universally welcomed, with the partial exception of a very few highly secretive families, with tendencies toward paranoia or histories of intrafamily abuse. Family members are often surprised and relieved by the different ways their intimates behave in the multifamily group, especially the patients, who are usually more responsible and responsive in the group than at home.

Beyond these indirect effects, specific processes tend to occur that reduce overinvolvement. In a well-established group, relatives are often blunt in their criticism of overprotective, disengaged, or rejecting behavior in other families. Such comments are usually received with acceptance and sometimes appreciation, but only because the source is a fellow sufferer. These confrontational interactions are tolerated because someone almost always steps forward to provide emotional support for the individual receiving criticism.

Another subtype of this process is termed "cross-parenting." Relatives who have become involved in tense, overstimulating relationships with their patient–offspring will often show remarkably sensitive and supportive attention to the patient members of other families. That attention may be quite therapeutic for the recipient, but it seems as well to become the basis for new and more adaptive interaction with that parent's own ill relative. At the same time, the recipient's relatives see that other kinds of behavior are not only possible, but that they also evoke a very different response in their supposedly intractable and disabled offspring. Thus, a multifamily group allows family members to try new, more adaptive, and empathetic relational styles with members of other families before attempting to use them within their own family. The group-based problem solving used in the psychoeducational multifamily group approach is a structured variation of this mechanism, in which clinicians actively involve other families' members in dealing with the sensitive and complex issues encountered as families begin to implement the family management guidelines. It is a natural extension of processes that occur spontaneously in multifamily groups: cross-family, problem-solving methodology seems to enhance cross-parenting, and vice versa.

PROMOTING EFFECTIVE FAMILY COMMUNICATION

Improvements in family communication were the first and most consistently reported therapeutic effects of multifamily therapy. The psychoeducational multifamily group model, with its overt emphasis on certain prescribed modes of communication, is a synergistic combination of seemingly intrinsic multifamily group therapeutic processes and a structured communication skills methodology. Harrow and colleagues[271] demonstrated the effects of multifamily groups empirically: More family members spoke spontaneously, more problem solutions were offered, more family issues were openly discussed, and more comments were made about others' interactions than in conventional patients' groups. Patients, themselves, spoke more. The apparent efficacy of a psychoeducational multifamily group in improving patients' social performance seems to relate to this aspect: The group is an ideal setting for patients with schizophrenia to practice being in a complex social environment, without being expected to perform normally until they are able, while having available the bridging support of family members.

Singer and Wynne[272] described a family characteristic that they termed "communication deviance." It usually means that relatives of patients with schizophrenia especially in conversations with each other in test situations, manifest higher degrees of either vague and amorphous or anxious and fragmented communication patterns than relatives in other psychiatric conditions. Because it appears to have a linguistic structure similar to formal thought disorder, it most likely represents a subclinical manifestation of a heritable cognitive disorder, and there is increasing evidence that relatives, especially first-degree relatives, share some of the more subtle cognitive and psychophysiological characteristics of clinically ill patients.[273]

The implication of these findings is that the treatment, through technique and social structure, should compensate for difficulties that patients and some of their family members may have in sustaining a conversational focus during a social or therapeutic meeting. Furthermore, to the degree that communication problems are a function of social isolation, it is important to offer social contact that reinforces communicational effectiveness. The psychoeducational multifamily group approach attempts to address these issues specifically, both in the structure of the treatment—by exposing participants to a large group in which many individuals will communicate normally—and in technique—by providing an extra measure of structure and predictability, with an emphasis on clear communication and task completion without distraction. By virtue of its social structure, it reinforces the communicational norms of the dominant culture, while substituting communication across family boundaries for the potentially redundant and less adaptive patterns within some of the more socially isolated families.

Difficulties in communicating diminish in a multifamily group if the family remains in the group for several months. The group process evokes societal norms for speech and discussion that then influence members to conform to them. In addition, the majority of family members do not manifest the full syndrome of communication deviance and tend to set norms that are more linguistically adaptive. Thus, most groups are composed of a majority of people who do not have difficulties in thinking or communication. The fact that this is the only type of treatment in which patients interact extensively with large numbers of others who are not impaired may well account for the consistent observation that patient and family communication in multifamily groups increases and improves over time. This process is an example of the well-studied and powerful influence of groups in enforcing conformity to group and societal norms for styles of communication, behavior, and even the structure of thought.[274–277] As to whether family psychoeducation affects communication deviance, there is only one study in the literature that addresses the question.[278] Family behavioral management was not demonstrated to reduce family communication deviance in single-family treatment, but that approach lacks entirely the interfamily processes that are a distinct feature of multifamily groups.

EDUCATIONAL, DIRECTIVE, BEHAVIORAL, AND EMOTIONAL PROCESSES

The educational and directive processes arise directly from the psychoeducational aspects of the approach. The process of establishing a collaborative alliance with family members, providing information about schizophrenia, and giving instruction in family management reduces guilt, anxiety, and confusion in family members and thereby reduces family tension. Furthermore, the content of the family management advice is specific to certain aspects of schizophrenic psychophysiology, particularly vulnerability to sensory stimulation, stress, and cognitive disability. Thus, teaching family members to give the patient psychological space, to reduce expectations, to set limits on extreme behavior, and to use a straightforward and more positive communication style with the patient are all methods designed to reduce pressure and create a more emotionally neutral, supportive, environment that reduces the risk of relapse. By encouraging family members to maintain or develop their own social support network, we hope that they will be better able to sustain an optimal environment over a prolonged period. In essence, the family is recruited as a therapeutic ally. In the psychoeducational version of multifamily groups, other families and patients are engaged as collaborators in the treatment effort by being involved consistently in a group-centered, problem-solving process. For most families, the group itself becomes a key element of their social network, because it meets so many needs. The net result is that families' coping capacity increases, as does their morale.

There are other mechanisms that explain the therapeutic effects of multifamily groups, including (1) expanded problem-solving capacity, (2) positive emotional tone, and (3) capacity to absorb anxiety. The first is the result of social network expansion: The problem-solving process is quite different in single- and multifamily group formats. For instance, with their large and diverse membership of people from different backgrounds, perspectives, and life experiences, multifamily groups generate a greater variety of alternatives during problem solving. Second, multifamily groups are usually characterized by more humor and warmth than single-family sessions, easing the gradual engagement of some of these families in the group and in more open relationships. The tone of multifamily groups is usually more positive and lighthearted than single-family sessions. That tone appears to support improvements in participating patients' social skills and to decrease tendencies toward criticism within families, by both the ill members and their well relatives. Finally, multifamily groups absorb anxiety and stress generated by psychotic symptoms and disability in a given family's midst, especially among patients who respond poorly to medication and family members who respond to mental illness with exasperation, anxiety, or resentment. In the next chapter, it is demonstrated that multifamily groups interact specifically with high residual symptoms and EE in families to yield remarkably good outcome in these higher-risk cases. Conversely, the same level of symptomatology in a single-family session tends to generate more family tension than the clinician and an already stressed family can dissipate with available techniques.

In the end, it could well be the similarity of multifamily groups to traditional, and perhaps prehistoric, social forms that explains and underlies these specific mechanisms. A therapeutic social network ultimately relies for its efficacy on the relationships between those who are initially strangers and from diverse social groups, as opposed to family or patient groups. Of all therapies only multifamily groups provide this wide diversity of relationships across categories of age, class, and, especially, life experience. Clinical experience as well as the processes described here suggest that there is indeed therapeutic power in exactly that kind of diversity, if the clinicians have the techniques and skills that allow it to gradually emerge. In Part II, we review the techniques that capitalize on the natural capacities and tendencies of these groups, and share the skills that have been found to realize their potential.

Chapter 4

Empirical Studies of Outcome in Multifamily Groups

There have been claims of impressive results in multifamily groups (MFGs) from the earliest anecdotal and clinical reports. In 1961, Laqueur and Detre pioneered the modality, independently starting groups at a state hospital in Queens, New York, and at New Haven's Grace–New Haven Hospital in Connecticut, and reporting their outcomes.[262, 279] Beels and his colleagues, in the Bronx, New York, developed an entire community treatment program for patients with schizophrenia, with MFGs as a major component.[280] Various clinically rich and promising reports have described therapeutic processes and positive outcomes that appeared specific to the modality.[281–285] Most, but not all, have described closed, long-term family groups, with patient participation, led by two clinicians.

There is a striking consistency of therapeutic effects across this early literature. Articles describe group loyalty and cohesion; rapidly developed feelings of support and reassurance, openness of families and patients to suggestions and criticism from others, increased and improved communication within families, improvement in patients' symptomatology, and particularly, social functioning. Several authors noted that the groups diffuse intrafamily intensity and validate the family's identity and strengths.

However, as important as these findings were, they were not accompanied by thoroughgoing quantitative analysis or scientific validation. Nonetheless, 1-year relapse rates in five of the early articles fell in the 0–21% range, well below rates reported for antipsychotic medication alone.[281–285] While none of these studies were controlled trials, the consistency among them and the contrast to relapse rates of 30–40% for maintenance medication are suggestive of a substantial clinical effect. Because these effects oc-

49

curred regardless of the therapeutic content or strategy used within the MFGs, a leading explanation for such results could be the expanded, varied social network created by the groups.

Nevertheless, there had been no empirical trials of the typical version—an ongoing, closed, long-term group led by clinicians, involving both patients and their families. Furthermore, all reviews of the modality[263, 286, 287] lamented the absence of truly scientific outcome studies. Given the consistent claims for efficacy, the absence of more rigorous testing was a deficiency from two perspectives—as a guide to techniques for clinical application, and as an opportunity to test the therapeutic efficacy of artificial expansion of the patient's and the family's social network.

The advent of new, family-based educational and behavioral management treatment models presented opportunities for additional variants on MFG techniques. The psychoeducational approach of Anderson, Reiss, and Hogarty; family behavioral management, developed by Falloon, Liberman, and others; and the family crisis therapy model, developed by Goldstein and his colleagues, showed clear-cut efficacy and appeared to be adaptable to the MFG format,[108, 268, 288] although their impressive effects were achieved in a single-family format. Because those studies had included contact between families in ways that were uncontrolled, it was unclear what portion, if any, of their reported outcomes might have been caused by interfamily interaction and support. An experimental comparative study, with the content of the sessions held constant, was needed to delineate specific effects of the MFG format.

It was reasonable to expect that the MFG approach in combination with psychoeducation would yield superior results. Many patients with schizophrenia and their families have diminished social networks[132, 134, 145] and there was some evidence that the smaller the network, the greater the expressed emotion.[144, 270, 289] Clinical experience had strongly suggested that families find the peer support available in a MFG important and beneficial. A number of specific social processes in longer-term, closed MFGs appeared to foster high morale and improved coping skills in families and to enhance interpersonal functioning in patients.[179, 262, 271, 290] In theory, these effects could be additive, combined with those of the newer, primarily single-family approaches of Goldstein, Anderson, and Falloon. Furthermore, because the psychoeducational approach focuses on developing individualized, disorder-specific management strategies, it seemed likely that the MFG would offer a larger pool of experience from which to draw new, adaptive suggestions. The cost-effectiveness of the group format for psychoeducation would make it more attractive to hard-pressed mental health agencies.

THE BERGEN COUNTY TRIAL:
4-YEAR RELAPSE OUTCOME

For all the reasons outlined previously, a clinical trial of psychoeducational MFGs was undertaken in 1981, in Bergen County, New Jersey, a suburb of New York City.[171] This was a small-sample experiment that compared symptomatic relapse outcome in single- and multifamily versions of the same family psychoeducational intervention over 4 years, an unusually long period of observation. This study tested (1) the direct effects of lowering family anxiety and emotional overinvolvement and enhancing problem solving, and (2) the indirect effects of providing a larger social support system. These effects would, in theory, lead to better outcomes. But would the specific processes in the group format counterbalance the dilution of the more individualized single-family intervention method?

Design and Methods

Forty-one patients were selected during symptomatic relapses that had required hospital admission. The patients met Research Diagnostic Criteria[291] for schizophrenia or schizoaffective disorder and had at least 10 hours of contact per week with a family member. They were randomly assigned to one of three treatments: a psychoeducational multifamily group (PMFG), a psychoeducational single-family treatment (PSFT) or a family-dynamic multifamily group (FDMFG). To isolate the interfamily contact, the PSFT clinicians fostered no contact between families. The study allocated psychoeducational intervention and social network expansion in the following manner:

- Social network expansion: Family-dynamic multifamily groups
- Psychoeducation alone: Psychoeducational single-family treatment
- Both components combined: Psychoeducational multifamily groups

The sample represented the type of psychiatric patients usually seen in public, acute general hospitals: young (average age, 29.0 years), mostly male (71%), averaging 13.6 months between admissions and 3.9 previous admissions over 6.4 years of illness. They came from middle- and working-class backgrounds.

The treatments used in this study were based on the psychoeducational family-based model developed by Anderson, Hogarty, and Reiss at the University of Pittsburgh.[108] The MFG treatment model is described later, in Part II, and the single-family version, elsewhere.[108] The protocol for PSFT included, in sequence, (1) a minimum of three sessions for the family engagement process, (2) two or three educational sessions devoted to informing family members about schizophrenia and illness management, and (3) regular sessions with one clinician, focused on implementing these guidelines using problem-solving techniques. The multifamily version of the psychoeducational approach was designed to follow as closely as possible the PSFT treatment, conducted in a group. The FDMFG treatment condition was included to examine the effects of "pure" social network expansion, without psychoeducational treatment. In this modality, the supervisor and therapists provided no education about schizophrenia, avoided discussion of mental illness or medication compliance, and used no structured problem solving. Instead, they emphasized opening intrafamily communication, sharing emotional responses, and attempting to resolve family conflicts. The treating psychiatrists in each modality were instructed to use the most effective antipsychotic medication, continued at the lowest effective dose. The first and second symptomatic relapses occurring after the index hospital discharge were the principal outcomes.*

Results

Of the three treatment approaches, the PMFG cohort yielded the lowest relapse rate after 4 years, exactly 50% versus 78% of the patients in the PSFT cohort and 57% in the FDMFG cohort. The risk for relapse in the PMFG cell was 33% of the rate in the PSFT cell ($p < .05$). These outcomes contrast sharply with the 16-month interepisode remission interval observed in the 2 years prior to the study. Clinicians reported that after the first year of treatment, patients who did relapse tended to readmit voluntarily and to recompensate quickly. Finally, the long period of remission enjoyed by 50% of the PMFG patients allowed them to make significant functional progress:

---

*Relapse was defined as the reemergence of major psychotic symptoms persisting for 7 days or more. Eight cases did not complete the 4 years of treatment but were tracked for outcome.

Half became employed by the end of the second year, and most of those remained employed for the remainder of the trial. Among patients who continued in treatment after the 4-year trial, *nonrelapsers averaged over 7 years in remission*, most having been in family treatment for the duration. The average period of remission was 59 out of a possible 90 months (65.8%) in PMFGs, 35 out of a possible 73 months (48.5%) in PSFTs, and 50 out of a possible 96 months (52.5%) in FDMFGs.

This study suggested that better long-term outcome may result from the multifamily factor than from psychoeducational aspect. Furthermore, outcomes in both multifamily modalities converged over time and increasingly diverged from the PSFT modality. Thus, the larger social network treatment format yielded superior outcomes over the long period of time required for recovery.

THE NEW YORK STATE FAMILY PSYCHOEDUCATION STUDY: A 2-YEAR FIELD TRIAL AT SIX SITES

The New York State Family Psychoeducation Study compared single- and multifamily psychoeducational treatment over 2 years at five state psychiatric hospitals and one city hospital, using a large representative sample of patients with schizophrenia.[186] The study was designed to replicate the Bergen County trial and, additionally, to evaluate the efficacy of the multifamily approach with different types of families.

Design and Methods

The key factors in MFG treatment—social network expansion and problem solving in a group format—were tested, while psychoeducation was held constant. The treatment also assessed interactions between treatment type, and family and patient variables relative to outcome. Patients had to have a diagnosis of schizophrenia, schizoaffective, or schizophreniform disorder according to DSM-III-R criteria.[292] At four of the five state hospitals, the patients had been transferred from brief-stay acute inpatient units in general hospitals. The mean age in the patient sample was 27 years; 74% were men; 37% had a documented history of substance abuse. One-third were high school graduates, while 27% had attended college. Forty-one percent were African American. Eighty-three percent lived with relatives, and 87% had never married. Forty-six percent of the families were rated as high in EE. The families and patients represented a wide variety of working-class to lower-middle-class people.

Patients and their families were randomly assigned to PMFG or PSFT for 2 years of treatment. In contrast to the Bergen County study, all participants received psychoeducation; both multi- and single-family treatment included formal and systematic problem solving as described by Falloon and his colleagues,[178] focusing on coping skills for managing schizophrenic illness. The "family clinicians" were regularly employed members of the social work, psychology, or nursing staff at the site hospital, supervised via videotape by the study supervisors.

Results

Symptomatic relapse rates for one and two years are shown in Figure 4.1. The PMFG relapse rate was exactly one-third less than the PSFT rate: 27.7% compared to 41.6%. In treatment, controlling for medication compliance (a significant predictor of relapse), PSFT cases had a 60% higher risk of relapse than PMFG cases. Positive symptoms at baseline markedly influenced relapse outcome in PMFGs and PSFTs ($p < .05$). Remarkably, for each 1-point increase in the score on the discharge Brief Psychiatric Rating Scale (BPRS), the

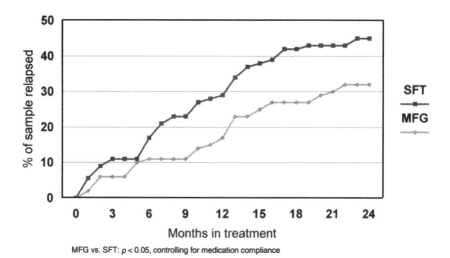

MFG vs. SFT: $p < 0.05$, controlling for medication compliance

FIGURE 4.1. Symptomatic relapse rates in multi- and single-family psychoeducational treatment over 2 years.

risk of relapse increased by 39% in PSFTs, but, in stark contrast, *decreased* by 42% in multifamily groups. For those 76 cases who were only partially remitted (BPRS > 2), the difference was marked: 19% of PMFGs relapsed versus 51% of PSFTs. In PMFGs, the *best* outcome occurred in patients with the *greatest* degree of initial residual positive schizophrenic symptoms: PMFG relapse risk was only 28% that of PSFT ($p < .01$). Similarly, in families scored as having high expressed emotion (rated using a modified form of the Camberwell Family Interview[293]) at baseline, relapse rates were *lower* in PMFGs than in the low expressed emotion PMFG subgroup, whereas in PSFTs, relapse rates were greater in high expressed emotion families, as expected. That is, in PMFGs, the higher the risk of relapse from baseline symptoms or expressed emotion, the lower the actual rate of relapse; the opposite relationship occurred in PSFTs. Minority patients, almost all African American, fared better on average in PSFT, regardless of expressed emotion.

Combining treatment effects and their interactions with three factors (baseline symptoms, expressed emotion, and ethnicity) yields a model for prediction of relapse. In Figure 4.2, relapse rates in the two treatments are shown for cases with zero, one, two, or three factors. For instance, an African American patient with a good response to antipsychotic medication during an acute episode and a low-expressed emotion family would be expected to have very low risk for relapse in PSFT (22% vs. 42% in PMFG, over 2 years). By contrast, a Caucasian patient who did not fully remit on

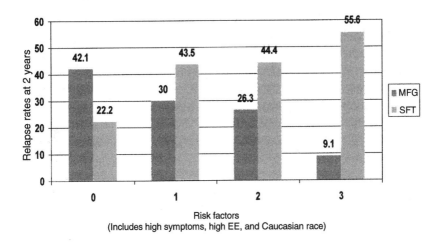

FIGURE 4.2. Interaction of risk factors and treatment format on relapse rates.

medication, and who had a family member with high expressed emotion, would be expected to have unusually good outcome in a PMFG. *For this subgroup with three factors, the difference at 2 years is stark: 9% versus 56%, favoring PMFG.* Contrary to expectations based on symptoms and expressed emotion, this seemingly high-risk subgroup was all but completely protected against relapse in PMFGs: Their expected rate of *clinical* (remaining psychotic for 1 week or more) relapse was 3% per year. The most powerful predictor was baseline patient symptoms, followed by family expressed emotion, whereas ethnicity, the weakest predictor, was largely a function of the better medication response and lower expressed emotion levels in the African American cases.

There are other, completely opposite relationships between single- and multifamily formats for risks and outcome. Even among cases in which a family member entered the program with low expressed emotion and ended with high ratings (12% of the sample), relapse rates were lower in PMFGs—20% versus 44% among the single-family cohort. For cases with high expressed emotion ratings at *any* time during the study, the difference is even greater (17% vs. 49%). Furthermore, 36% of those with high ratings on both expressed emotion components—critical comments and over-involvement—relapsed in PSFT, while *none* relapsed in PMFGs.

Other findings included the following:

1. Relapse rates were significantly lower in PMFGs than in PSFT when families and/or patients participated in the test treatment for a full 2 years: 31% in PMFGs versus 48% in PSFT ($p < .05$). (Twenty-nine percent were lost from the PMFG cohort and 25% from PSFT. Only 11% of those dropping out discontinued participation contrary to the recommendations of the clinicians.)

2. Relapse rates were lower for patients having their first episode in PMFGs: 19% versus 44% ($p = .02$). Those same differences were seen in more medication-compliant cases (> 50% compliance: 23% in PMFGs vs. 39% in PSFTs; $p = .06$).

3. The nearly constant relapse rate for each modality meant that the difference in relapse rates between modalities increased over time.

4. Only 71% of relapses required rehospitalization, regardless of treatment type.

5. Over the two years, PMFGs generated significantly (31%) fewer total relapse episodes (PMFG, 38; PSFT, 60).

6. The first-year hospitalization rate was essentially unchanged from

the rate prior to admission to the study, regardless of modality. During the second year, this rate declined dramatically to an end point less than one-third the pretreatment rate ($p < .05$). Of the total sample, 15% had more than one relapse and were therefore considered treatment failures.

7. The 22 cases who entered the program while still symptomatic (BPRS per-item score > 3) showed significant improvement in *positive* symptoms at 2 years, reaching a mean BPRS score of 1.83 ($p < .001$), all but identical to the 1.74 score of the rest of the sample. (Scores under 2.00 are all but asymptomatic.) PMFG patients had fewer *negative* symptoms than PSFT patients at the beginning of the program. Over 2 years, negative symptoms in the PSFT cohort improved, while the PMFG cohort remained at the lower level throughout the study, yielding identical scores at 2 years (2.12 for both modalities). Negative symptoms for the total sample demonstrated a trend toward improvement ($p < .09$).

8. Mean PMFG drug dosage over 2 years *decreased*, while PSFT dosage *increased* ($p = .12$). Compliance was maintained at a high level for 2 years: PMFG cases exceeded 90%, and none of the patients who completed 2 years of treatment were totally noncompliant with medication. These levels of compliance are much better than those reported in the drug maintenance literature, in which there is a noncompliance range of 10–76%, with a median of about 46%.[294]

Because patients were experiencing long periods of remission and reduced family stress, work became one of the prime targets of clinical effort during the second year of treatment, once clinical stability was achieved. Employment rates increased significantly for the entire sample, from 17% baseline to 31% at 2 years. The rate in PMFGs—34%—represented an increase of 18%, compared to a 7% increase in PSFTs ($p = .08$).

The lower relapse rates in the multifamily groups are promising in view of the lower potential cost of that format. The PMFG approach is designed to require exactly one-half the staff time per patient of the PSFT format: 1 hour per month per patient for PMFG, compared to 2 hours for PSFT. Conservatively assuming a $350/day cost for state-operated inpatient hospitalization and comparing the rehospitalization rates during the prestudy to the 18- to 24-month periods, we derived a 1:34 cost–benefit ratio for PMFG and a 1:17 ratio for PSFT: [(.34 − .17 hospitalization/patient/6 months) × (68.5 mean days/admission) × $350]/$120 = 34. For every dollar spent on PMFG or PSFT treatment, $34 or $17, respectively, were saved in hospitalization costs during that period.

Discussion

The principal finding of these studies was that PMFG treatment extended remission and enhanced functioning more effectively than its single-family and nonpsychoeducational counterparts, while demonstrating consistent statistical trends toward greater positive symptom reduction, medication compliance, dosage reduction, and employment. These results occurred at 7 different public hospitals and 11 different public outpatient services, using over 40 different publicly employed therapists among a variety of socioeconomic, cultural, and ethnic groups in rural, large city, suburban, and smaller city environments. *In the end, 85% of all cases experienced substantial reduction in the risk for relapse.* The most dramatic advantage for MFGs occurred in the following conditions:

- At higher levels of psychiatric symptoms at the time of hospital discharge.
- In families with high expressed emotion.
- In Caucasian, or nonminority, cases.
- During the first episode.
- Under conditions of full compliance with either pharmacological or family treatment.

THE FAMILY-AIDED ASSERTIVE COMMUNITY TREATMENT OUTCOME TRIALS: EFFECTS ON CLINICAL, FUNCTIONAL, AND FAMILY WELL-BEING

In contrast, 15% of the cases in both of these studies continued relapsing at their prior rates. They were predominately younger men, without long institutional histories and with substance abuse and medication, and/or treatment compliance problems. Therefore, in 1987 we decided to integrate PMFGs with assertive community treatment (ACT), because the latter had been shown to be particularly effective in improving the clinical and life status of patients who were similar to our prior treatment failures. Systematic and ongoing psychoeducational family intervention integrated with ACT might combine the benefits of both interventions and eliminate their inherent deficiencies, especially for the high-risk patient. As described in Chapter 10, this approach was termed Family-aided Assertive Community Treatment, or FACT.[295, 296] Two studies exploring the effectiveness of the combined model are described here: one comparative and the other controlled. The first study focused on improving outcome for this less-treatment-responsive subpopulation.[296] The second, based on the unexpected results of the first, evaluated employment outcomes.[297]

Design and Methods

Sixty-eight persons ages 18–45, meeting DSM-III-R criteria for schizophrenia, schizoaffective, or schizophreniform disorder, and their families were randomly assigned to ACT combined with either of two levels of family intervention: psychoeducational multifamily group treatment (PMFG) or crisis family intervention (CFI). Participants were selected during an acute psychotic episode. Importantly, they were required to have at least one complicating factor: (1) lack of consistent participation in pharmacological or psychosocial treatment, (2) history of violence and/or suicidality, (3) frequent hospitalizations and/or emergency treatments, (4) arrests or criminal convictions, (5) homelessness, (6) unwanted pregnancy, and (7) moderate to severe substance abuse. The subjects' mean age was 30, 65% were male, 84% had never been married, and the modal subject was a high school graduate (31%; 29% of subjects had some college). Of study participants, 47% lived with their parents. Prior to the study, they averaged just over one hospitalization per year. The study was conducted at three mental health centers in urban, suburban, and rural areas of New York State.

Families and patients in the multifamily group cohort participated in group-based problem-solving sessions, as described in Chapter 9. After an initial psychoeducational workshop for family members only, multifamily groups comprising 6 patients and their families met biweekly with 2 ACT team members for 2 years. In CFI, family–ACT team coordination occurred only at times of crisis, without the input of other patients' families. To control for differences among treatment clinicians, CFI cases received treatment from the same ACT teams that performed the multifamily group treatment, and clinicians were instructed and supervised to provide equal effort to the two cohorts. Outcome evaluation over 2 years of treatment focused on several domains: rehospitalization in association with symptomatic relapse, employment, and family burden and well-being.

Results

The PMFG treatment resulted in higher employment activity. We found a higher rate in all forms of employment over 2 years (32% for PMFGs vs. 19% for CFIs; $p < .07$) in sheltered work (18% vs. 6%; $p < .05$) and average rates of employment (all forms) in the 4- to 20-month period (33% vs. 19%; $p < .05$). After achieving peak levels at 16 and 20 months, employment decreased somewhat in both cohorts at 24 months. Symptomatology and medication compliance had no effect on employment outcomes.

While there were no differences between PMFG and CFI cases with regard to hospitalization rates or changes in symptoms, significant improvements were demonstrated for the sample as a whole. The hospitalization rate decreased across the 2 years: In the final 6 months, it was only 38% of the mean pretreatment rate. Positive, negative, and general symptoms also[298] decreased from baseline to 2 years ($p < .001$). Remarkably, there was a *reduction* in chlorpromazine equivalents (CPZEs) from 975 mg at intake to 696 mg 2 years later ($p < .05$) and an *increase* in median medication compliance from the intake level of 75–90% to the 2-year rating of 100% ($p < .001$). There were significant improvements in family ratings of objective burden, subjective burden, dissatisfaction with the patient, and ratings of patient friction with others (see Table 4.1). Other family measures— avoidance and rejection of the patient, ratings of patient contact with the extended family, patient interpersonal contact with nonfamily persons, and patient well-being—improved, though nonsignificantly.

Discussion

The more intensive (PMFG) type of family involvement achieved greater employment than its episodic (CFI) counterpart; the nearly 40% rate is clearly higher than this sample's previous level and markedly higher than

TABLE 4.1. Effects of FACT and CFI on Family Status: Scores for Entire Sample over 2 Years

Family ratings of burden and patient adjustment (SAS-III)	Baseline ratings (SD)	Ratings at 2 years (SD)	t tests of changes
Objective burden	1.87 (0.49)	1.56 (0.45)	$t_{(43)} = 3.54$, $p = .001$
Subjective burden	3.21 (0.71)	2.54 (0.77)	$t_{(37)} = 4.87$, $p < .001$
Dissatisfaction	3.91 (1.26)	3.21 (1.41)	$t_{(45)} = 3.25$, $p < .01$
Friction	2.01 (0.96)	1.69 (0.89)	$t_{(45)} = 2.22$, $p < .05$
Avoidance	1.95 (0.92)	1.74 (0.94)	$t_{(45)} = 1.33$, NS
Rejection	3.35 (0.78)	3.14 (0.86)	$t_{(43)} = 1.66$, NS
Extended family	2.28 (0.99)	2.07 (0.88)	$t_{(37)} = 1.10$, NS
Overprotection	3.45 (0.66)	3.23 (0.83)	$t_{(42)} = 1.93$, $p = .06$
Interpersonal contact	3.46 (1.08)	3.33 (1.19)	$t_{(38)} = 0.74$, NS
Well-being	2.37 (1.26)	2.31 (1.18)	$t_{(41)} = 0.29$, NS

expected rates (about 10%).[299, 300] In the family domain, the improvements in the families' burden and satisfaction with their ill relatives' functional status contrast with earlier reports by Test and Stein[301] and Hoult and colleagues[302] that found only transitory or no differences in burden compared to traditional care over time. They are consistent with reductions in family burden observed in at least one other trial of family intervention.[303]

FACT AS VOCATIONAL REHABILITATION: COMPETITIVE JOBS AS GOAL AND OUTCOME

Because of the employment results demonstrated in the FACT study, the same approach to rehabilitation was used in the next study. It was designed to provide focused support and training in work-related problem-solving skills, carried out in the context of an expanded and rehabilitation-oriented family and social support system, as described in Chapter 10 in the section on employment intervention. The goal of this combined treatment and rehabilitation approach was competitive employment.

Design and Methods

The study was designed to compare directly vocational and clinical outcomes in FACT with those in conventional vocational rehabilitation (CVR) and to assess clinical outcomes and their relationship to work outcomes. Subjects were randomly assigned to FACT or CVR, after which ACT and the multifamily groups commenced in the FACT-assigned cohort. The principal differences between experimental conditions were that, in CVR, (1) there were no multifamily groups and no vocational specialists working closely with the clinicians; (2) all vocational rehabilitation was initiated by referral to the state-operated vocational rehabilitation agency; and (3) vocational rehabilitation staff, even if employed at site-affiliated rehabilitation services, worked on the basis of referral from the CVR clinicians and case managers. The study was carried out in two typical community mental health centers (CMHCs) that had close ties to excellent vocational rehabilitation services, one in a Westchester County suburb of New York City and the other in rural Ulster County, NY.

To be eligible for the study, a person had to be between 18 and 55 years of age, have a diagnosis in either the schizophrenia (e.g., schizophrenic, schizoaffective, schizophreniform disorders) or the mood disorder spectrum (e.g., major depressive, bipolar disorders); not have been employed competitively for the past 6 months, although stating a desire to work; and have an available family member. Sixty-nine patients were admitted to the study. They were predominately male, with a schizophrenic disorder and a long and chronic course, unemployed for over a year, not living with family, and possessed a lower level of acuity and substance abuse than many samples in other clinical trials. Prior employment was entered as a covariable in all analyses of employment outcomes, to control for potential bias. Employment outcome was documented every 3 months and reported as a cumulative employment rate over 18 months of treatment and rehabilitation in four categories: unemployed, sheltered work, unpaid work, and competitive work.

The FACT teams consisted of a senior clinician/team leader; two social workers or psychiatric nurses, with prior experience treating the study population; one vocational specialist trained in supported employment concepts and methods; and a psychiatrist. The staff to patient ratio was 1:8. The role of the clinicians was to implement solutions developed in the multifamily group, especially those oriented toward finding or avoiding the loss of a job. The groups included 7 or 8 cases, met biweekly for 1½ hours, and were led by two members of the FACT team. The CVR was implemented by master's-level clinicians who worked in the same mental health centers as the FACT teams. The CVR clinicians made referrals to the state-operated vocational rehabilitation service and assisted subjects in the assessment, training, and placement phases. They also followed up when crises or dropout interceded, provided family crisis support, and carried out some of the research assessment and tracking procedures. The case loads varied from 1:23 at Ulster County to 1:13 at Westchester County.

Results

By the end of the study, there were dramatically fewer unemployed FACT subjects (16.2% of the FACT cohort vs. 43.3% of the CVR cohort). More FACT subjects obtained competitive jobs: 28% of the FACT cohort held a competitive job compared to 10% of cohorts in CVR. Throughout the study, FACT subjects were significantly more likely to be employed than CVR subjects ($p < .01$). There was a slow and steady increase in competitive employment, until at 12 months it peaked at 37% in FACT compared to 8% in CVR subjects ($p < .01$; see Figure 4.3), after which it declined to 27% in FACT subjects ($p < .05$). By contrast, CVR competitive employment remained at essentially the same level throughout the study, ending at 8.0%, below its baseline level. There were 26 competitive jobs held by 17 FACT subjects, while 8 such jobs were held by 6 CVR subjects. The FACT and CVR cohorts had similar rates of sheltered and unpaid work.

The difference in amount of employment was not due to a "revolving door" effect, in which subjects were continually fired and getting new jobs. Job duration for competitive jobs between FACT and CVR subjects was similar: 6.9 months for FACT subjects and 6.0 months for CVR subjects. There was a trend toward FACT subjects having greater total time employed in study (10.4 mo. vs. 7.0 mo.; $p < 0.10$). For those with any competitive employment, FACT subjects averaged $1,448 compared to $320 for CVR subjects ($p = .038$), and FACT subjects received higher hourly wages ($6.34 vs. $3.64; $p = .055$).

Clinically, FACT and CVR were equally effective treatments as indicated by symptoms, rehospitalization, and medication compliance outcomes. For the schizophrenic subsample, there were significant reductions in negative symptoms ($p < .05$) and general psychopathology ($p < .05$), indicating improvement or no change, respectively, for FACT and worsening for CVR. As an increasing number of subjects became employed, the rate of hospitalization did *not* rise.

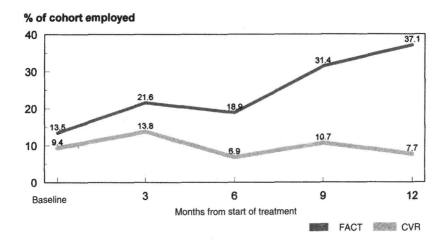

FIGURE 4.3. Competitive employment outcome in family-aided assertive community treatment and conventional vocational rehabilitation; 12 months: $F(1,56) = 9.21$, $p = .004$; 18 months: $F(1,56) = 5.11$, $p = .028$.

Qualitative Outcomes

Focus groups were held at the completion of the protocol for FACT subjects, families and clinicians. There were four structured questions:

- What were your goals? What were your goals for your participating family member(s)?
- Has the program helped you to reach these goals?
- Were there any obstacles to accomplishing your goals?
- What would you change about the program?

The themes that emerged from the "goals" questions for subjects included continuing education, developing a network, enjoying less formal bureaucracy (than previously experienced in the state vocational rehabilitation program), accessing clinical services, and "pleasing the family." Some subjects wanted to have their families put less pressure on them to work. Families' goals were less varied: They hoped that their ill relative would find work and get rehabilitation. They were, in general, quite sophisticated about the service system and what was and was not possible. They hoped that the ill family member would get to meet people, talk more, and just "hang out" more with other people. They hoped for more autonomy and expected greater education, guidance, and support for themselves.

The participants described the clinicians as both helpful and professional. Clinicians were perceived as encouraging, available, less concerned about medications, helpful to subjects in getting and keeping a job, and not "psychoanalytic." Patients appreciated meeting in the community (e.g., at a restaurant for lunch). They appreciated that the staff maintained an appropriate boundary between themselves and family members. Patients found that employment helped their lives and their state of mind, perhaps reflecting the modest decrease in negative symptoms in FACT. They praised the problem-solving aspects of the multifamily groups as useful, and they liked the team approach.

Families cited the staff, emphasizing their caring, knowledgeable, and nonjudgmental approach. They appreciated the continuity of care and the team's support for their attempts to set limits. They appreciated the multifamily group component, citing the relaxed atmosphere, the sharing, and decreased isolation. Several claimed that problem solving in the multifamily group was "the best part of the whole approach." They found "work" as the topic for problem solving heartening, though somewhat difficult.

Discussion

The results of this project are particularly encouraging: 84% of the FACT sample achieved some form of employment and 46% held a competitive position at one time or another, with more time spent employed and higher total earnings (up to four times greater) than for CVR. Given that the sample was all but unemployed at baseline, these outcomes represent a significant advance for a population often thought to be incapable of working at any level in the mainstream job market. This project demonstrated that there is little risk of relapse consequent to competitive employment if there is ongoing clinical, family, and rehabilitative support. Family members were crucial in this process, providing early warnings of relapse and buffering the stress for brief periods when subjects were getting a job. The principle implication of this study is that FACT, with supported employment specialists, achieves levels of competitive employment that are far superior to those achieved by a typical, publicly operated vocational rehabilitation service system.

CLINICAL AND THEORETICAL IMPLICATIONS OF MULTIFAMILY GROUP EFFECTS

These four studies, supported by previous research, lead to the following conclusions:

- Family intervention of this type—psychoeducation and family behavioral management—is vastly more effective than individual treatment and/or medication alone.
- In two studies with a total sample of over 200 patients at six sites, the multifamily group consistently yields lower morbidity and better vocational outcomes than single-family psychoeducation, when the only comparison is the treatment format.
- Multifamily group approaches are specifically more effective than single-family approaches for first-episode and high-risk patients, poor responders to medication, or patients with highly stressed families.
- Multifamily groups and psychoeducation result in higher rates of employment than minimal, crisis-oriented, single-family support, even when a rich and clinically sophisticated treatment system, ACT, is provided to both types.

- The multifamily group approach, when enhanced with vocational specialists as group leaders and a team working within the ACT framework, is markedly more effective in helping persons with major mental illnesses find and keep jobs than the vocational rehabilitation system of a large state.
- The benefits of the multifamily treatment increase with time, up to 4 or more years.

Patients entered these studies with greater, and perhaps more typical, morbidity than that in earlier outcome trials. Indeed, patients with high levels of positive symptoms and poor medication response were specifically protected from relapse by multifamily groups, experiencing a 7% clinical relapse rate. The same effect emerged for patients whose family members had high expressed emotion ratings.

The fact that patients discharged with relatively high levels of symptoms improved over the course of the study suggests that there is a long-term, symptom-stabilizing effect for multifamily intervention. The psychoeducational strategy appears to reduce the risk of early relapse for approximately the first year. The advantages of the multifamily group become substantial by the end of the first year; the best results, in clinical and vocational terms, occur in the second year. The multifamily group effect becomes progressively more protective during a lengthy period of community-based rehabilitation. While the psychoeducational and multifamily group effects appear to occur in sequence, there is significant overlap; the difference in relapse rate is apparent from the very beginning. It is particularly interesting that multifamily groups lacking any of the key elements of psychoeducation or behavioral management (FDMFG in the Bergen County study) achieved the same outcomes as the groups with more illness- and education-oriented techniques, and better outcomes than single-family psychoeducation. Spontaneous interaction between families, emerging after 4–6 months, preceded the development of differences in efficacy.

These results can be achieved in ordinary clinical and rehabilitative service settings. The sites for all these studies were publicly operated, or publicly funded, private, nonprofit clinical agencies, with inadequate resources, severely ill patients, and severe budgetary restrictions on their staff. The clinicians who led groups and carried out the treatments and rehabilitation work were (and for the most part, still are) permanent employees of the agencies. Thus, it is completely feasible to use these treatments in settings where they are most likely to be needed. There is little evidence that these outcomes were solely the result of exceptional therapists.

In the FACT/CVR studies, the reductions in burden and the very low rates of rehospitalization support both minimal and full family involvement when combined with ACT, while the employment outcome supports the higher intensity but still cost-effective multifamily group version. This supports the theory that stress reduction in the family milieu generates a degree of stress resistance that allows more successful functional adaptation. The employment study also indicated that in rehabilitating people with schizophrenic disorders, the FACT model is equally, if not more, effective than rehabilitation for mood disorders.

Differences in Outcome with Other Family Intervention Studies

Dyck and his colleagues at Washington State University have replicated these findings and demonstrated other domains of improved functioning in 63 outpatients randomly assigned to PMFGs or to standard care at a large community mental health center in Spokane.[304] They found lower rates of relapse in the PMFG subsample. Their most striking finding, however, was that negative symptoms declined, whereas they tended to increase in the control group. Negative symptom outcomes were not associated with atypical antipsychotic medication use. This study also demonstrated salutary effects on relatives' physical health. At baseline, 49% of the caregivers had visited their physicians more than one time. After the intervention, 31% of the caregivers from the standard care group and 23% of the caregivers from the PMFG group visited their physicians more than once. A preliminary, linear, stepwise regression analysis showed that treatment group, illness onset, and number of prior-year doctor visits predicted the number of postbaseline doctor visits ($p < .05$).

The most important comparisons with these studies are the studies by Leff and colleagues[305] and Hogarty and colleagues.[244] Leff and his colleagues in London did not observe a difference between a relatives' group and home-based, single-family behavioral management; 2-year relapse rates were 33% and 36%, respectively. The relatives' groups experienced a 50% nonengagement and dropout rate. However, the following points were noted in the PMFG groups, as opposed to the British relatives' group approach:

- The group leaders were also the primary therapists for the patients.
- There were at least three separate single-family and single-patient engagement sessions before the multifamily group commenced.
- Patients in multifamily groups attended the meetings.

We believe that these features are responsible for the observed lower family dropout and patient relapse rates. Patients, in our experience, need to attend the multifamily group to benefit from its social and vocational rehabilitation effects.

In the Hogarty and colleagues single-family treatment study, relapse rates *increased* during the second year.[244] This was attributed to the impending termination of cases. The study reported here found *decreasing* rates. This difference in outcome is best attributed to the promise and reality of continuity of care after the study. This protocol offered the same treatment in the same clinic, with the same therapist, after the data collection period ended.

Some of the same problems arise in evaluating an important study sponsored by the National Institute of Mental Health: the Treatment Strategies in Schizophrenia Study.[306] Here, the experimental conditions involved multifamily groups for both cohorts, but without the active, problem-solving component. One half of the sample received Falloon's intensive behavioral family management in a single-family format, in addition to attending a multifamily group, for the first 9 months of the treatment. At 2 years, there were no differences in relapse rates, although both cohorts had the same rates seen in our own and others' family-based outcomes studies. Also, this study excluded patients if they did not stabilize early on medication. Recall that poor medication responders are the subgroup that specifically appears to be better treated by multifamily groups. The parsimonious explanation for similar outcomes in the two experimental conditions is that a multifamily group effect increased with time and superseded the early effects achieved by the additional, more intensive intervention. That interpretation confirms a multifamily group effect beyond that for family intervention alone.

The four studies described in this chapter recruited patients without regard to the expressed emotion status of their relatives. This is an important difference when comparing outcome to other recent and similar studies. One would expect that this sample was at less risk simply because it presumably had a mixed, and presumably lower, level of EE than other studies of this type. However, the New York sample had higher rates of prestudy hospitalization and involuntary admission than the samples recruited by Hogarty (e.g., approximately 0.47 hospitalizations per year vs. 0.61 in this sample). These factors suggest that in more naturalistic settings, patient morbidity, often the result of medication noncompliance, can counterbalance a presumably lower average level of expressed emotion. Again, this is the very subgroup that appears to be treated more effectively by multifamily groups.

A number of studies have measured the effects of the educational component alone.[307–312] There is widespread use of education as the sole intervention offered to families, especially via programs sponsored by chapters of the National Alliance for the Mentally Ill (NAMI). The hope has been that providing education, without assisting families to implement coping skills, would nevertheless be effective. To date, all studies have confirmed that there are no persisting clinical effects, and weak and/or transitory effects on family well-being. The psychoeducational approach and our multifamily group variant are specifically intended to help families assist in the treatment and rehabilitation effort, with the clear understanding that such effort will only be successful if they themselves are supported and achieve improved well-being. *Education is necessary but not sufficient for that end.* It has also become clear from a clinical perspective that social support, recently observed to be a significant predictor of outcome, requires much longer to develop than is possible in an 8- to 12-week course, especially when little interaction among participating family members is fostered. The implication is that longer term work, extending for at least 1 year, appears to be necessary to achieve these effects.

It is unfortunate that the psychoeducational and educational strategies have been cast as competitive. There is no empirical basis for mounting large-scale, education-only programs. Furthermore, they represent a significant lost opportunity, because most of the effort required to run a psychoeducational multifamily group for 2 years is expended during case finding, engagement, setting up, and conducting the educational workshop. That same effort is required for an education-only program, but it does not yield the clinical and rehabilitative outcomes seen in PMFGs.

CONCLUSIONS

From the design of the first two studies, it is possible to derive a theoretical understanding for the superior outcomes in the multifamily format. Because the treatment strategies were similar, one is forced to look to the difference in the number of participants. In the single-family approach, the sessions usually included no more than two or three people, whereas the multifamily groups routinely involved at least 10 persons, and often more, with the larger number of relationships within the group being nonfamilial. Furthermore, because all cases were randomly assigned, without regard to any characteristic other than age and diagnosis of the patient, the groups were similar in ethnic, racial, and economic characteristics.

The most powerful and plausible explanation is that the multifamily group expands the patient's and family's social network. That argument is consistent with the studies reviewed in Chapter 2, and the processes described in Chapter 3 and observed in most multifamily groups over the past three decades. The studies demonstrate an association between the size and density of the patient's social network and a variety of outcomes, especially relapse and rehospitalization,[132, 141, 142, 144, 145, 150] and that extended networks usually diminish in size and capacity for support as the patient's illness progresses to chronicity.[144, 145] Thus, a multifamily group may fill a specific void in the family's and patient's social support system.[266] A network expansion hypothesis is consistent with clinicians' reports that relatives and patients gradually become more open, cooperative, and personally involved across family boundaries as the groups continue to meet. As that happens, intrafamily interaction in the group diminishes.

The effects of multifamily groups add to those of psychoeducation and medication to comprise a multilevel intervention affecting biological, psychological, family, and social systems. The present research experience with family intervention, including these studies, provides unusually consistent evidence for its efficacy and feasibility for the younger, community-based, relapse-prone patient suffering from schizophrenia.

Part II

The Practice of Multifamily Group Treatment in Schizophrenia

A Psychoeducational Approach to Developing a Healing Social Network

Chapter 5

An Overview
of Psychoeducational
Multifamily Group Treatment

The ultimate goal of the multifamily group model is to help the patient with schizophrenia attain full symptomatic recovery and achieve as rich and full participation in the usual life of the community as possible. The short-term goal is to prevent relapse and help the patient recover the functional losses that follow psychotic episodes. Multifamily group treatment engages the members of the family and their social support network as partners in the patient's treatment and rehabilitation. The family is essential to a reliable and comprehensive recovery effort. A key intermediate outcome of treatment is that family and patient develop individualized coping skills to manage symptoms, vulnerability, and disability. Improvement in families' psychological well-being and physical health is another critical outcome.

In these treatment groups, several families are brought together to form a mini-organization, led by professional clinicians, that meets regularly over an extended course of treatment and rehabilitation, with the participation of the patient. The approach builds upon the effects of antipsychotic medication and assumes that other treatment and rehabilitation resources are used when indicated. The multifamily group is the primary vehicle for case management for most of those participating and will be for many the only treatment other than medication. It provides patients and families with the following:

- An alliance with knowledgeable and empathic professionals
- Information about schizophrenia
- Guidelines for managing the illness itself
- Practice in solving problems created by the illness

The multifamily group format improves outcomes by reducing stigma and increasing social network size and support, allowing families to benefit from each others' experiences in solving specific problems and helping them to exploit shared opportunities that promote rehabilitation and recovery. The principal theoretical foundation is that almost all types of severe illnesses have a better course if the afflicted person has a large and knowledgeable social support system.[138] This is a restatement of the conclusions of literally hundreds of studies of social networks conducted over the past three decades (see Chapter 2). To put it more simply, this model follows the old dicta that "Misery loves company" and "There is power in numbers."

Multifamily groups are rooted in clinical and/or rehabilitation systems that have formal links to the health system. In that regard, they differ from self-help and advocacy groups. Groups involve clinicians, here referred to as family clinicians, key family members, any case managers involved with the individual, and friends who have chosen to stand by the patient. The multifamily group is a long-term effort that merges treatment, rehabilitation, and recovery. It organizes an illness-oriented social support network of individuals with common experiences but widely diverse personal characteristics and previous histories. The greatest relief of family burden will come from the extended remission of their loved one and from their maximum participation in the community. Reciprocally, relief of family burden is considered essential to achieving clinical goals for the patient.

Two unusual assumptions underlie the psychoeducational approaches:

- The family is functioning normally, until clearly proven otherwise.
- Better outcome for the ill member is most likely when the family makes compensatory adjustments in its daily life. These adjustments are dictated by the specific characteristics of the disorder itself, not by any model of normative family functioning.

Psychoeducation also assumes that these disorders tend to elicit responses that are self-defeating, though understandable and usually culturally appropriate. Families vary tremendously; therefore, the clinician practicing family psychoeducation can expect to encounter both well-functioning *and* highly dysfunctional families in roughly the same proportion as in the general population

The family needs to possess all the relevant and available knowledge about the illness; the treatment system should be a crucial source of that information. Psychoeducation assumes that the coping skills that are specific to the psychiatric disorder are counterintuitive and need to be taught: To expect families to understand spontaneously such a mystifying condition, and to know what to do about it, is unrealistic. Some families have developed, through painful trial and error, methods of dealing with positive and negative symptoms, functional disabilities, and the desperation of their ill relatives. Most families need to have access to each other via multifamily group contact, and indirectly, through professionals and leaders of the family self-help movement, in order develop effective means of coping with the day-to-day challenges of managing schizophrenia at home.

This chapter presents the basic structure of the clinical approach. The reader will hopefully understand how this approach strives not only to alleviate the patient's suffering and lessen the burden on the family, but also to yield effects on many of the psychobiological aspects of the disorder, especially vulnerability to stress and cognitive deficits.

BIOSOCIAL THEORY: A FOUNDATION FOR PSYCHOEDUCATIONAL MULTIFAMILY GROUPS

This treatment approach revolves around a central principle that we have found to encompass much current research and conceptual development about schizophrenia. It is termed the biosocial hypothesis:

> *The state of the individual with schizophrenia is determined by a continuing interaction of specific biological dysfunctions of the brain with social processes.*

The corollary to this hypothesis is that optimal outcome can occur only if the biological and social determinants are addressed together. Thus, multifamily group treatment comprehensively combines biological, psychological, family, community, and organizational interventions that are feasible in ordinary clinical settings. When applied to schizophrenia, the approach also assumes that modifying the social environment will be more effective than attempting to alter the internal psychological dynamics of a person with schizophrenia. Thus, effort is expended (1) in the biological realm, by providing and assuring compliance with a regimen of antipsychotic medication; (2) in the family realm, by training family members in coping skills that compensate for the inherent deficits of the disorder; (3) in the social realm, by organizing a social support system in the form of a multifamily group. The individual with the disorder will participate more and more in treatment and may profit increasingly from individual supportive therapy and rehabilitation. In one sense, drug and family interventions lay the foundations for individual therapy and rehabilitation that should be based on the person and his or her own hopes, preferences, and active participation.

Throughout the course of treatment and rehabilitation, the objective is to create a balance between protection from stress and stimulation, and the most rapid progression toward the goals of the individual patient and his or her family. Preventing relapse is a high priority, perhaps the highest, because continuing remission is essential to functional improvement and a more satisfying life. This strategy will necessitate treading a relatively narrow path between, on one side, excessive demands and overwhelming stimulation and, on the other, inadequate expectations, social rejection, and withdrawal and paralysis of will and action. The optimal degree of demand and stress will differ, sometimes dramatically, between individuals, and across time in a given individual. This approach is based on knowledge of the nature of prefrontal cortical deficits from studies on arousal and attention, as well as the variety of effects of antipsychotic drugs on brain and personal functioning. As Anderson and her colleagues described it, the goal is to construct an environment that has barriers to stimulation, especially at times and in places in which the ambient stimulus loads are high.[108] Early in the course of recovery, the goal is to create a specialized, somewhat simplified environment in which life is simpler, calmer, more benign, and of a slower pace than usual. Clinicians and family members collaborate to create asylum (i.e., protection from the dangers of everyday life and partial relief from normal performance expectations) for the patient in the community for as long as necessary to achieve remission and take initial steps toward regaining a role in the that same community.

Psychophysiological Dysfunction

Treatment of dysfunctions of arousal and attention begins with, but goes well beyond, using antipsychotic medication. All antipsychotic medications have significantly beneficial effects on the regulation of attention and arousal. They greatly improve resilience to environmental stimuli. However, schizophrenia leaves its sufferers, even when medicated, especially sensitive to intense, negative, and complex social interactions. In order to add to the effects of medication, intervention should be directed to the social domain. For example, one of the insights provided by expressed emotion research is that a narrow range of social interaction promotes stability and recovery. Thus, critical comments appear to be disruptive because they provoke arousal and activation of the limbic cortex, while the prefrontal cortical deficit means that more fine-grained, tactful responses in the cognitive domain are less likely to be mustered. The result is that criticism will tend to lead to destabilization and to symptom emergence. If we translate that perspective into a mode of interaction for families, friends, and treatment personnel, it means that direct requests for a change in behavior and positive reinforcement are more likely to succeed in actually changing patients' behavior than outright criticism. Interpersonal conflict in the social environment, even if it does not directly involve the vulnerable person, can quickly lead to decompensation.

Another insight from expressed emotion research is that there is an optimal interpersonal distance, one that is neither too close nor too remote. On one hand, schizophrenia results in an intolerance of sustained intimacy. On the other hand, too much social withdrawal can lead to deterioration due to insufficient interruption of delusional thinking and hallucinations. Prolonged withdrawal can lead to loss of social skills and demoralization. To achieve the most emotionally balanced, least disrupted state, families and others need to maintain contact and also allow the individual to regulate interpersonal distance. The degree of tolerance and the level of interest will vary over time. Family members need to understand this vulnerability and develop an ability to allow their loved one to withdraw as needed. Conversely, they also need to continue attempting to keep in contact, inviting involvement often enough to prevent regression, sensory isolation, and loss of social skills. The psychoeducational approach helps families to learn to adjust their relationship with their affected member to achieve an optimal mental state, thereby protecting the patient against relapse while also promoting as much social involvement as possible.

The degree of interpersonal warmth expressed by relatives has been found to predict clinical outcomes.[269] Like interpersonal distance, there is an optimal degree of affection and simple friendliness that buffers against other environmental stresses. At the same time, excessive enthusiasm and prolonged, intense emotional interaction appear to be destabilizing. This approach helps families to find the best balance between emotional restraint and emotional expressiveness. Similarly, schizophrenia imposes limits on its victims' tolerance for performance demands in work or school. Each person with schizophrenia has a maximum level of pressure to perform, beyond which performance deteriorates and symptoms reemerge. The challenge for clinicians attempting to guide rehabilitation is that this threshold point is different for each individual and different over time. The only way to know what is tolerable is to attempt small, careful steps toward more ambitious tasks and to then assess the effect on the patient's mental status and general emotional stability, as described by Anderson and her colleagues.[108]

Cognitive Dysfunction

Other social and interactional strategies are suggested by knowledge about prefrontal cortical deficits. Certainly, flexibly adjusting performance expectations makes sense given the difficulties some individuals have with processing complex, multilevel information. Decreased processing speed can account for much of this problem. As is implicit in the model developed by Weinberger, the greater the prefrontal dysfunction, the greater the vulnerability to stimulus overload and excessive arousal.[60] Thus, everything from conversational speed and complexity, to homework difficulty, to task assignment at work will need to be adjusted to match the current degree of deficit. Again, this will change over time, often for the better, especially as medications with fewer cognitive-impairing side effects are used. When prefrontal deficits are more pronounced, the individual will have less initiative and motivation. The family education is designed to help family members match their interaction and expectations to the patient's current level of deficit. Later, the problem-solving approach assists in refining day-to-day social interactions and rehabilitation planning to match the current cognitive capacity of the affected member. In more recent adaptations of this approach (see Chapter 10), results of formal cognitive tests are shared with family members to help them understand strengths and disabilities in the areas of memory, attention/distractibility, planning, and sequencing ability and motivation.

Accommodating cognitive impairments implies that communication, especially in the early posthospital period, should be clear, straightforward, concrete, and moderately specific. During the postepisode period, communication may need to be simpler than usual. There is abundant evidence from the expressed emotion literature that positive comments and a calm, supportive tone are crucial in getting through to, and helping to stabilize, an ill relative. Low-expressed emotion families tend to be markedly low-key, tentative, flexible, and nonpressuring in their communications to the patient, often waiting for the patient to take the initiative in conversation. Anderson has recommended acknowledging the statements of others directly and taking responsibility for one's own statements, purely from a practical point of view: Individuals with attentional and information-processing dysfunction will find it easier to track conversation if it is clear who is saying what and why.[108]

Life Events

The psychophysiological and cognitive aspects of schizophrenia produce a vulnerability to rapid change and stressful life events. Life events research suggests that there are a maximum number of events per unit of time that can be managed; beyond that threshold, symptoms and even relapse follow.[314-317] Families are trained to recognize when too many things are happening at once, to attempt to protect their affected member from rapid change, and to act quickly if the threshold has been exceeded. Stressful family events, even if they are perceived by most members as pleasant or exciting, are prepared for and scheduled when few other events or stresses are likely to occur. The family clinicians often confer with the psychiatrist to adjust drug dosages upward to prevent symptom reemergence.

Leaving home for college, the military, or just a getaway is planned very carefully and may be discouraged if there is symptomatic evidence that it will only produce relapse. One implication of prefrontal deficit is that the ability to organize one's affairs independently, as is necessary when away from family members, is impaired. The subtle, everyday cues that assist adults with schizophrenia to function are like an external ego that compensates for prefrontal deficiency. These cues and reminders serve as an external set of guideposts and limits that affect both trivial and major decisions, from remembering where one placed the keys to selecting a residence and applying for a job. Many life events involve loss of contact with familiar others, often leading to functional collapse. Those losses also disrupt the subliminal and minor cues that keep the vulnerable individual organized and protected. At the same time, entering a new social and geographic context is simply stressful at the emotional and physiological level. The combination of cognitive demand, anxiety, loneliness, and sensory stimulation in a new situation is often overwhelming, unless the move is carried out gradually and carefully. Family members can be extremely helpful in making necessary transitions, if they have the knowledge and skills to act constructively. The psychoeducational approach is designed to help families develop exactly those skills.

DEFICITS, BELIEFS, AND HOPE FOR RECOVERY

It is important to emphasize that attention to deficits enables recovery but does not justify hopelessness, inaction, and rejection. These deficits are not absolute barriers to achieving community integration and a modicum of satisfaction with life. Schizophrenia is a serious disorder with many cognitive impairments, but it is not dementia, and it definitely is not mental retardation. With psychosocial and psychopharmacological treatment and rehabilitation, those deficits can be overcome to a surprising degree. Attention to stress and stimulation, to specific cognitive demands, and to the pacing of change are means to promote functional recovery, an end that, in this approach, is achieved remarkably often. However, there is a kind of devil's pact that imbues the work with families and those affected by the illness:

> The more that the partial disabilities of schizophrenia are acknowledged, respected, and accommodated, the less they impede the path to recovery.

The implications of this principle extend to complying with medication, waiting for negative symptoms to subside, using results of cognitive testing creatively, abstaining from alcohol and drugs, forestalling leaving home, and deliberately cultivating and maintaining a supportive social network. If progress is slower and more carefully planned, it is much more likely to occur. When the specific impairments of the disorder are not understood or accommodated, relapse and deterioration usually follow. Unfortunately, in the absence of medication and more deliberate pacing and protection from stress, poor outcome and nearly total disability and deterioration are the rule. This general paradigm, though somewhat paradoxical and counterintuitive, is stressed to family members and the individual throughout this treatment and rehabilitation process. It is perhaps the core principle of psychoeducation, but it is initially a difficult one for most families and nearly all affected individuals to accept and put into use. It has been surprising to see how difficult it is for experienced and knowledgeable professional clinicians using this approach to adopt and work from this basic concept.

COURSE OF RECOVERY AND TREATMENT

Recovery from a psychotic episode of schizophrenia takes a similar course across individuals. The process starts with subtle, prodromal signs and symptoms, goes through medication-induced remission of positive symptoms, and then through predominance of, and sometimes diminution of, negative symptoms. This last stage is a consequence of both the episode itself and the side effects of medication. In most cases, it is an inherent phase of a full recovery process. This process is heavily determined by not only the major biological and psychological upheavals that occur in a psychotic episode but also the psychosocial characteristics and responses of those who interact with the patient most frequently after the acute phase resolves.

One way to conceive of this process is by analogy with another kind of major functional and medical cataclysm, a myocardial infarction (heart attack). In that instance, catastrophic biological processes thrust the person onto the health system and the support of relatives and friends. As the person is treated and begins to recover, those who make up the immediate social support system, both in the hospital and at home, must make major allowances for the person's slow and gradual recovery from an assault to an important organ. As that recovery occurs, the individual slowly begins to regain some of the functions, capacity, and resilience lost during the attack. Then, the best approach is to reverse directions gradually, to begin to remove some of the precautions, protections, and allowances, and to impose carefully and gradually some stresses to stimulate the healing heart. This gradually increasing demand helps the individual to grow reparative tissue and to increase the vital capacity of the undamaged tissue. This is the biological foundation of the rehabilitation process. Eventually, usually more than a year later, expectations are likely to be higher than the premorbid level, especially for exercise, smoking cessation, stress reduction, and dietary restraint.

In this approach to schizophrenia, the optimal course of recovery is seen to be similar. Immediately after the psychosis, rest and recuperation, with protection from stress and expectations, are critically important. These may be continued for several months, if necessary, until there are indications that a natural recovery is beginning to occur. Then, in small and careful steps, the patient's expectations are raised, with assistance from professionals, families, and friends, to begin to rejoin the life of the community. After roughly a year, the rehabilitation process is fostered more intensively, especially after the individual shows some signs of tolerance for increased demands and spontaneous interest in meeting them.

The risk for relapse is proportional to the level of positive and negative symptoms combined.[18, 19]

In Figure 5.1, relapse risk, indicated by the dotted arching line over the course of symptoms, is a value that declines gradually as negative symp-

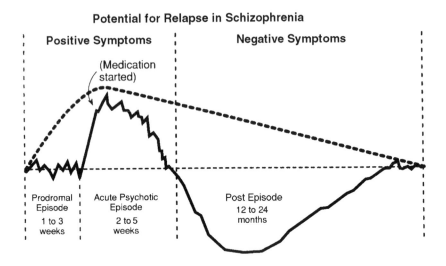

FIGURE 5.1. Course of recovery from acute episodes of schizophrenia.

toms decrease. It is surprising to many clinicians and families, but negative symptom levels are at least as predictive of risk for relapse as positive symptoms.[17]

SOCIAL STRUCTURE OF THE FAMILY AND TREATMENT

The family with a mentally ill member needs to have a sufficiently clear hierarchy, so that necessary rules can be established and respected, and the caretaking functions of the well members of the family will be carried out. A clear structure tends to allay tension; prevent nagging, criticism and excessive interaction; and induce clarity and predictability in family life. Structure and limit setting become very important with regard to medication compliance: Parents may decide that the patient's use of medication as prescribed is necessary for the *family's* well-being and require its continuation, even if the patient does not agree. The same is true for dealing with violence and bizarre behavior: Setting limits will often be the only way to extinguish these behaviors and to preserve a semblance of normality at home. Family relationships in which the caretakers are clearly and benignly in charge and backed by the clinical team constitute the calmer, more therapeutic social environment. This principle extends to nonfamily environments as well, as described in Chapter 11.

The family is part of the treatment and rehabilitation team. Thus, psychoeducational treatment puts family and professional caretakers on the same level, with each group having distinct areas of expertise and responsibility. The family is *not* the object of therapy. The object of treatment is schizophrenia or another disorder, with the affected person as a potential collaborator in that treatment. This is usual for medical disorders, though that social organization is unusual as treatment of a psychiatric disorder. Family members facilitate treatment, participate in its planning, and create optimal environmental conditions for remission and rehabilitation, but are neither treated themselves, nor are they the therapists. In many important ways, they carry out crucial aspects of treatment and rehabilitation, but largely as an extension of the clinicians. Some aspects of the effort are designed to meet their needs and to protect them from the burdens of the illness, and from the burdens of the treatment and rehabilitation process itself in some instances. Family members are not assumed to be experts on schizophrenia, but their expertise and experience regarding the previous history and the current state of the affected person are considered crucial and indispensable to optimal clinical and functional outcomes. The social unit for treatment is thus a three-sided partnership, involving the clinicians, family members, and a patient. Each plays a unique and irreducible role in achieving recovery.

TECHNIQUES SPECIFIC TO MULTIFAMILY GROUPS

The four types of intervention delineated here are the foundation for implementing the psychoeducational approach within the multifamily group context. The overall strategy is to maximize the impact of psychoeducational strategies by exploiting the unique social structure of the multifamily group. Thus, putting into practice the family management guidelines, doing problem solving, working on social and vocational rehabilitation, enhancing interpersonal boundaries, and beginning the social-network building process are interactions involving as many members of the group and as many different families as possible. The emphasis in the following descriptions is on the direction, the interpersonal vectors, of interaction rather than the verbal content, because it is the social structure that is so critically important to efficacy.

Self-Triangulation

This technique involves serial individual and family interviewing. The clinicians interact with specific individuals within a family or focus on one family, as if in a single-family context. They intentionally interpose themselves between the members of different families, directing interaction through themselves and inhibiting interaction between families or individuals.

This form of intervention has several uses. Primarily, it establishes a clear social structure by emphasizing the leadership role. The clinicians allay uncertainty about what family members are supposed to do by setting a clear direction, and initiating and controlling interaction. The leaders use this approach at times when the families would be most likely to expect strong leadership, and when the leaders' role lends authority to advice and suggestions based on family management principles. Especially during the beginning meetings of the group, this method builds cohesion in the group and allays anxiety. Specific applications of value in the psychoeducational multifamily group model include the following.

Relating a Problem to a Family Management Guideline

The clinicians will need to use leader–family member intervention to link problems presented by a family with the appropriate family management guideline. This kind of move will be necessary in the early phases of the group, before families have begun to utilize fully the problem-solving model. The directive, authoritative mode is used primarily for teaching group members to determine which guideline is most relevant and how to implement it. Most families members appreciate this approach given that the guidelines are based on clinically and empirically derived principles, the usual domain of professionals.

Eliciting Interactional Information

It is essential in successful problem solving to elicit specific information about the problems families present in the psychoeducational multifamily group. The leaders will usually need to take the initiative in defining the problem in limited, specific, and behavioral terms. As will be seen in Chapter 9, this is one of the most demanding aspects of the approach, requiring skills, knowledge, and comfort with behavioral methods.

Directing Problem-Solving Sequences

Active involvement in guiding structured problem solving is a legitimate use of this type of intervention early in the group or at points of unusual difficulty. Deliberate problem solving comes naturally to few families, with or without schizophrenia. Therefore, in the first several attempts to use this approach, the leaders remain central, tracking and guiding the sequence, making explicit what step is in focus and when the process seems complete. Wherever possible, the leaders should avoid the temptation to provide the "definitive" solution to a particular dilemma, but rather should contribute ideas alongside those of group members. In some groups, the leaders will find that they need to continue directing the problem solving for an extended period of time, while in others, the families quickly learn and apply the method, both within and outside the group.

Blocking Interruption

A primary therapeutic intervention in any multifamily group is blocking interruption of one group member by another, especially the interruption of the patient by a well member of his or her family. Negative consequences may follow from some members' habit of habitually interrupting their relatives. Experience has taught that simply insisting that everyone be allowed to complete their comments without interruption seems to reverse the expectation and, gradually, the actuality that the members with schizophrenia are incompetent in a social situation. Here, remarkable progress can be seen simply through consistent validation of the patients' potential for more active and appropriate social participation.

Addressing Poor Attendance

It is the leaders' responsibility to ensure the maximum effectiveness of the group by intervening when poor attendance by a family, or crucial members of a family, threatens its viability. Although progress in a psychoeducational multifamily group seems not to be critically affected by less-than-perfect attendance, families who consistently miss more than half of the meetings are likely to make little headway. Also, a spouse or parent who misses more than half of the sessions can block progress. Furthermore, it is absolutely necessary that the key relatives, at minimum, those living on a day-to-day basis with the patient, attend the educational workshop. Guided by these rules of thumb, the leaders will need to contact families, by telephone or home visit, that consistently miss sessions, try to identify any dissatisfaction that may be a barrier to attendance, and emphasize the therapeutic importance of full attendance in the group to achieve a result.

Controlling Extreme Affect, Negativity, and Violence

Very rarely, individual families will become involved in extreme disagreements, with strong expressions of feeling and criticism. Sometimes a family may be so critical that symptomatic exacerbation in the patient is provoked. The leaders carry the final responsibility for group interaction and the well-being of all its members; they must intervene directly and quickly when indicated. The usual methods are to ask an involved member to take a time-out, either in the room or outside, or to change the topic and return to it after negative feelings have subsided.

Group Interpretation

The clinicians occasionally take a complementary position to the entire group in order to lay ground rules, to share personal reactions, to point out commonalities in the families or in subgroups (mothers, parents, etc.), to set group themes and, very infrequently, to make conventional group interpretations.

The main function of this type of intervention is to validate the group as a group or, more specifically, to validate the families' contributions to each other and to the group as whole as being therapeutic for the patients. The group is explicitly defined as the instrument of change and improvement. Thus, these group-oriented techniques serve as the technical bridge between leader-centered/educational and group-centered/problem-solving processes. Experience suggests that group-dynamic interpretations are to be avoided, especially those having to do with group member-to-leader transference.

Setting and Eliciting Themes

A primary task for the leaders is to reflect to the families the shared feelings, issues, problems or problem solutions that emerge in the discussion. Whenever it is meaningful, leaders should define these factors as experiences common to many families with a schizophrenic member, emphasizing that each family is involved in a struggle shared by other families. That reality can then be linked to families' inherent expertise and value as collaborators with each other, and with professionals, to achieve the highest level of recovery possible for the patients.

As themes emerge in the group, the leaders validate them and may offer solutions based on guidelines or clinical practice and experience. Redefinition of an emergent theme will often enhance the focus on problem solving, because it will seem relevant to most of the group's members. Common examples have to do with anxiety, confusion, despair, and conflict, as well as clinical management issues such as medication side effects, life events, and substance abuse. As much as possible, these problematic affects and interactions are redefined as being nearly universal responses to the disorganizing influence of schizophrenia on patients and families alike. That theme is then generalized to all families and, in a limited way, to the clinicians.

Praise for Interfamily Assistance

One of the key uses for a group interpretation is to recognize and reward efforts of family members to provide emotional support and to help one another think through solutions. The leaders should make a point of acknowledging all attempts to provide assistance, even if they are not fully accepted or immediately successful. The rationale for this intervention is the time-proven value of positive reinforcement in shaping individual and group behavior: It is one of the simplest methods of encouraging further interfamily interaction and participation in creative problem solving.

Handling Intragroup Social Conversation

As opposed to dynamically oriented group therapy, random discussion of everyday topics (i.e., grousing, joking, general socializing) is considered neither defensive nor diversionary in a psychoeducational multifamily group. As we will see in Chapter 9, a significant portion of the session may be given over to this kind of interaction as long as it is across family boundaries. The value of more naturalistic socializing is that it forms the basis for the group to become a social network. Thus, interaction that is not patient- and illness-focused needs to be encouraged, so that the members of the group experience each other as peers and friends. Most sessions of a multifamily group begin with general socializing, which seems to foster better concentration on therapeutic work later in the meeting. The leaders should validate such interaction and explicitly encourage it at appropriate times.

Also, leaders should feel free to join in the discussion, particularly if the topic is relatively neutral and does not involve disclosure of any sensitive personal information.

Cross-Family Linkage

While this technique is less varied in form than others described here, it is crucial for accomplishing the core tasks of the psychoeducational multi family group: application of the guidelines, problem solving, and social/ vocational rehabilitation. This technique fosters therapeutic interaction between families, work that appears to be more effective than efforts by professionals trained in the single-family psychoeducational approaches. It is often more congenial to families than professional intervention, perhaps because the families in the group know that the other families have had the same sorts of experiences: Their supportive comments and suggestions come with a built-in credibility.

In essence, the clinicians use their relationships with family members, built up during the engagement phase and early group meetings, to promote relationships across family boundaries. As in a natural network, these efforts are not intended to be transferential but rather are real social bonds in which there is sanction for sharing, open feedback, and a creative search for solutions and opportunities among participating families. The aim is the creation of a task-oriented social network, in which structured problem solving and individualized application of the family management guidelines constitute the overt vehicle for both cross-family linkage and managing the patient's illness.

The most common context in which this intervention is used is within the problem-solving approach. This approach, described in Chapter 9, is a variant of this process, a more structured and behavioral way of both developing and capitalizing on interfamily relationships. For instance, a question or issue is raised by a member of a specific family—let us call it the index family—with the expectation that one of the clinicians will answer or deal with it. Another applicable situation occurs when the index family members are discussing a problem among themselves, implicitly expecting the clinicians to intercede with a suggestion or a process intervention. Yet another use of this approach occurs when members of two families are discussing an issue but not making any progress toward an acceptable solution.

A specific sequence of maneuvers constitutes the usual technique in these situations. First, for a brief period, the clinician may discuss the problem with the index family to clarify it and to make sure everyone has contributed to a specific and behavioral definition of the problem. Then, the clinician turns to the other clinician or members of other families and briefly discusses the situation in the index family. Some discussion between clinician and member(s) of the other families can then proceed, focusing on the index family's various options or other ways of understanding their interaction. The next step involves asking specific members of the group to share their suggestions with the index family directly. The clinician may ask them to describe their thoughts in more detail, especially when the previous discussion has involved considerations of alternatives or complex observations, or lengthy descriptions of the other families' solutions to similar problems.

The next step is to encourage a full discussion between two families, or with members of several families, as to what might be helpful. In general, these directive interventions should be short and to the point, with the implication that the clinicians are not likely to intervene to make further suggestions. One of the leaders should make a concluding comment if the index family does not acknowledge the other families' input, or if the discussion ends before the index family has developed a prospective plan. Here, members of the index family discuss group members' ideas. If members of the index family ask for professional guidance, defer to other families, and save any indicated additions until later, after the groundwork has been laid by those families. During the subsequent interfamily discussion, the clinicians need to assume a more reflective stance, encouraging families to continue, keeping the discussion on track and, if necessary, intervening to structure a problem-solving sequence. The clinicians summarize the input from other families, assist the index family in choosing among the suggestions, and develop a detailed, concrete plan to apply them.

Cross-Parenting

This type of cross-family linkage seems to be of therapeutic value to the social functioning of patients within and, over time, outside the group. The relative in one family engages the ill member of another family in either unstructured socializing or focused discussion of a problem affecting the ill member. This most often occurs spontaneously, but it can be deliberately planned when a relative is known to manifest a particular style in coping and problem-solving that differs dramatically from that used by a particular patient's relatives. Even when the content of the "cross-parent's" comments is quite similar to what the actual parent may have been saying, the style is usually one of symmetrical joining and friendly advice, without overt or covert exasperation or criticism. In some instances, the cross-parent may have vital information that is not available to the patient's own relatives or even to the clinicians. This frequently happens with regard to job openings or other subjects pertaining to concrete, occupational issues raised during the social/vocational rehabilitation phase.

Another important use for cross-parenting linkage is to help a relative who is unable to accept the seriousness and reality of his or her own patient relative's illness. As noted earlier, a conversation with another family's ill member will usually convince the most denying parents, siblings, or spouses that their ill family member is not lazy, malingering, or exaggerating his or her mental disorder. The technique here is nonspecific and involves framing the issue as an understanding of the effects of the illness, gentle encouragement of the two individuals to interact, some urging, if the patient is unusually recalcitrant and, if necessary, intervening to help the other family's members listen. Blocking the relatives' interruptions of the patient is sometimes needed, since they may want to speak for the patient or interpret what they think he or she means.

Interfamily Management

Once family members have developed relationships across family boundaries, the clinicians use a nonspecific technique to regulate and enhance the group process. In essence, the clinicians use this approach in mature groups to guide and facilitate interfamily conversation, group-based problem solving, and social network development. The position adopted is nonhierarchical, more detached, collegial, and unobtrusive. The specific objective is to enhance and reinforce interfamily contacts and thereby promote the process of quasi-natural social network development. There are several identifiable applications for this approach:

1. Reinforcing, primarily through praise, families' support or constructive confrontation with each other.
2. Regulating group tone, or even the overall direction of interaction, with reminders of guidelines, comments about dropped subjects of importance, and hints to follow up on previous problem-solving efforts.
3. Expanding a conversation between members of two families to include others.
4. Disagreeing, in rare situations, with the general direction of a problem-solving process and suggesting alternatives.

5. Concluding, summarizing, or modifying cross-family interventions when family members have successfully engaged one another across family lines in mutual problem solving.

THE STAGES OF TREATMENT IN PSYCHOEDUCATION

There are four major stages in the treatment program:

1. Joining with individual patients and families.
2. Conducting an educational workshop for families.
3. Preventing relapse through the use of problem-solving groups attended by both patients and families.
4. Pursuing vocational and social rehabilitation in the same multifamily groups.[108]

In the joining process, the primary aim is to build an alliance with the patient and his or her significant relatives (see Chapter 6). The clinician, meeting with the family separately, conveys genuine interest in the family's experiences and expresses the desire to help both family and patient. The joining sessions should accomplish one major goal: the creation of a collaborative treatment system in which family members become engaged as partners and experts on the daily life of their ill relative. Next, the family clinicians conducts an educational workshop for the same families, preferably as a multifamily meeting of five to eight families, usually lasting most of a day, and usually on a weekend (see Chapter 7). This workshop is specifically oriented toward family members and friends of the patient; patients usually are not invited unless they are clinically recompensated and interested. The clinicians working with the families conduct the workshop, assisted by the psychiatrist(s) treating the patients. Brain function, medication effects, and symptoms and signs are explained, as are guidelines for the management of schizophrenia. The multifamily group convenes after this workshop, led by the same two clinicians, meeting biweekly and including the patient. In that format, the third and fourth stages are pursued using problem-solving methods as the main focus of the group process (see Chapters 8–9). The strategy of these groups is to help families to implement the workshop's family guidelines and conduct group problem solving. Initially, these meetings are intended to extend and to protect remission and, later, to foster functional improvements and an enhanced quality of life.

PHASE-ORIENTED TECHNIQUES

Community Reentry

A psychoeducational multifamily group usually assumes a long-term, closed-membership format, because that is the form that has consistently shown the greatest efficacy. Much of that effectiveness depends on the formation of a close-knit social network among the families in the group, a process that takes time and consistency of membership to evolve. This format also seems best suited to the chronic course of the illness. Because the psychoeducational multifamily group begins as an educational workshop, with a clear message that the illness may be prolonged and responds best to gradual, long-term efforts toward recovery, there is a natural congruence with a closed, low-intensity, and long-term group format.

Multifamily groups that are conducted with a relatively stable membership typically go through phases, much as do all persistent social networks. An effective psychoeducational multifamily group moves from one extreme (leader-centered) to the other (group-centered) over a 2- to 3-year course. That process is inherent to this type of group, but experience suggests that it is more effective to exaggerate these extremes in groups for patients with severe mental illness and their families. In the beginning, group process and content is markedly determined by the clinicians. By the last phase, the leaders' interventions become more dispensable and symmetrical; peer-like interactions with the group's members predominate.

For roughly the first year after the workshop, the emphasis is on achieving a stable recompensation of the patients. Generally, this involves reducing family tension, dealing with medication compliance, and avoiding or buffering stress. Leader–group member interactions (i.e., self-triangulation and group interpretation) predominate during the early sessions. The educational workshop involves this type of intervention. Discussion in the first group sessions focuses on sharing personal information and common experiences of having mental illness in the family. Methods of fostering recovery and explanations of the family guidelines are described. During the go-round phase of each group session, as spontaneous cross-family interaction begins to take place, the orientation becomes more group-centered. Group members' impatience with this leader-centered process, manifested by directing comments to one another or openly initiating more group discussion of the workshop content, guidelines, or common clinical problems, is a good indication that the group is sufficiently cohesive and able to benefit from a more intensive interfamily process.

Then the leaders gradually shift the process to individualized implementation of the family guidelines, using a problem-solving and group-centered leadership style, using whatever issues are of concern as a vehicle for teaching the problem-solving approach, which increasingly focuses on one family in the rotation. Other family members contribute possible solutions and "pros and cons" to the problem-solving process. Repeated discussion of the key family guidelines occurs in relation to almost all problems raised by families. The activity of the leaders shifts from initiating therapeutic work to facilitating, tracking, and reflecting it. At a deeper level, this process reinforces the natural tendency for relationships to develop across family boundaries, initiating a social network.

Of particular importance is ensuring that as many group members as possible contribute in one way or another to the problem-solving process and increasingly encouraging interaction across family boundaries, even if such interactions are briefly distracting. The patients contribute as equal partners in socializing and problem solving; this is accelerated when the clinicians consistently seek their input. Problem solving should be characterized predominately by the use of cross-family linkage techniques as a principal means of encouraging interaction between patients and members of other families. Also, specific kinds of interactions can be encouraged as subgroups begin to form. For instance, facilitating discussions of relatives' reactions to the ill members' progress in treatment, followed by the latter's descriptions of their own subjective experiences, is usually deeply moving and further builds morale while it begins to break down the barriers between families, and between patients and their own relatives. This type of sequential subgroup discussion gradually diminishes family boundaries and brings the group much closer to being a natural network.

Social and Vocational Rehabilitation

The second, major postworkshop phase, beginning at about 1 year and lasting from 6–18 months, focuses on patients' resumption of responsibility in the multifamily group. Their own families, and the other families in the group, collaborate in the effort to enhance the disabled members' psychosocial functioning. The leaders explicitly frame this as a task for the group and gradually turn over much of the actual implementation, so that family members work with each other across family boundaries.

The dominant technique to be used throughout this phase is cross-family linkage within a problem-solving format. Cross-parenting interaction is more emphatically fostered to enhance the sense of maturity and competence in the patients. The goal is that the family and the psychoedu-cational multifamily group serve as a bridge of support and encouragement as the patient gradually emerges from the family environment into the more pressured, nonfamily world of work and social activity. In that regard the multifamily group functions as a proxy for the larger and less accommodating outer world, but it is similar enough in structure to the outer world that relevant social skills are learned and generalized.

A specific function that the psychoeducational multifamily group can serve in this phase is to reduce family members' residual overinvolvement, especially excessive protectiveness, and tendencies to avoid challenging the patient to take on a more independent role. The means for achieving this are relationship substitution and, in rare instances, direct confrontation across family boundaries, as described previously. If it becomes clear that family members are overcompensating and interfering with the rehabilitation process, leaders can encourage members of other families to work with the involved family to raise their expectations for the patient gradually, while validating the interfamily relationships that evolve in this process. As all members of the family develop more independence and appropriate degrees of autonomy, the leaders' task is to extend the process and to monitor the rate of change to see that it is done safely. The groups can absorb a remarkable amount of stress, because distancing within families can always be accompanied by developing closer cross-family relationships and activities enjoyed outside the family, often with other group members.

BASIC LOGISTICS: TYPICAL AND ATYPICAL VERSIONS

The Typical Application

This approach usually begins at the point of relapse and admission to a psychiatric hospital or an acute day treatment program. The family is contacted within a day of admission and seen for the first joining (engagement) session within 3 days. Under recent conditions, in which brief hospital stays are the rule, only part of the joining process is likely to be completed during the admission, and the educational workshop is almost always scheduled after most, if not all, the patients have been discharged. The patient is assumed to be at high risk for relapse after such a short period of recuperation, so the family clinician uses even greater caution than would occur if the admission were in the 30- to 45-day range. Fortunately, with atypical antipsychotic medications, many patients leave the hospital with fewer positive symptoms and are less likely to experience negative symptoms. The principle advantage of beginning work at the acute stage of the illness is that families are usually in dire need of support, information, and guidance. They are much more likely to appreciate the outreached hand of the family clinician and to develop the necessary alliance on the basis of the perceived relevance and usefulness of that relationship. If the offer of help arrives when it is most needed, the clinicians are much more likely to gain the trust and participation of family members.

The work usually begins at the time of an acute episode and continues for 2 or more years, with much of the rehabilitative and community integration interventions occurring after 9 to 12 months. Clearly, for patients who have had more frequent or numerous episodes and more severe positive and negative symptoms, the time needed to complete each phase increases as well. As will be seen, the final arbiter of therapeutic strategy is the overall clinical condition of the individual with a schizophrenic disorder, not adherence to a preordained timetable.

Beginning with Stable Outpatients

Occasionally, the work starts when the ill family member is an outpatient and may have already achieved a degree of stability. In such cases, the family clinician simply proceeds through the joining and educational phases as described, but he or she moves rather more quickly through the community reentry phase and into rehabilitation. It is important to remember that establishing these new relationships and achieving comfort and integration in the multifamily group is stressful in itself. So, even with clinical stability established, actual rehabilitation effort still begins several months into the process to allow for the destabilizing effects of the engagement process itself. In the end, clinical judgment prevails here as well.

When there is no crisis, it may be more difficult to engage some family members. The family clinician may need to spend more time in the joining phase and explore in more detail the ways in which the family and patient feel vulnerable and have specific issues that need to be addressed. The key is to find ways in which the psychoeducational process and the multifamily group may serve specific needs for them at that particular time. Often, this will require additional joining sessions, beyond the recommended three or four sessions. A good guide is to continue in the engagement phase, in single-family meetings, until an unequivocally positive working alliance has been developed.

Frequently, members of the family want their ill member to find employment. If they can accept the incremental approach used here, they can frequently be engaged and energized around that goal (see Chapters 9 and 10). If all the patients are well-stabilized and interested in work, it is strongly recommended that an employment specialist, occupational therapist, or vocational rehabilitation counselor join the group as a leader, perhaps allowing another leader to phase out. Once such a group is formed, it follows the process described in Chapter 10, "Family-Aided Assertive Community Treatment." With or without employment specialists, the focus of the group, especially the brainstorming and problem solving, shifts from clinical to rehabilitative emphases, and from problems to social/vocational opportunities and the next steps in recovery.

Substance Abuse

When the patient has a significant substance abuse problem in addition to a major psychiatric disorder, a number of modifications come into play. Substance abuse interferes with all other attempts to treat symptoms, achieve clinical stability, and enter into a rehabilitation process. For that reason, the focus remains on substance abuse throughout all phases of the treatment effort, or until the substance abuse reaches subclinical levels. During the joining phase, there is an attempt to explore the patient's latent motivation to reduce or discontinue consumption of alcohol and illicit drugs. There is also an attempt to link achieving short- or longer term personal goals to decreasing consumption. In essence, the family clinicians frame almost every problem as related to substance abuse and every goal as difficult or impossible to achieve in its presence. Great care is taken to avoid a judgmental stance or tone. As in motivational methods,[318] the final choice is always left to the individual and the family.

If a number of the patients in a multifamily group share difficulties with substance abuse, extra material and emphasis added to the educational workshop are devoted to the functional and clinical interference that is inevitably produced by excessive alcohol and drug use. It is explained that alcohol is a depressant and depresses mood while also serving to increase arousal and, thereby, positive symptoms and risk for relapse. Few patients or family members are aware that there is a steadily increasing level of arousal that accompanies continued, heavy use of alcohol, and that arousal, when interpreted as anxiety, is one of the factors that drives people to heavier drinking. This is a vicious cycle and can lead not only to true physical dependence (i.e., addiction) but also to psychotic relapse in the process. Since there is usually discussion about dopamine and its role in schizophrenia and relapse, participants are told that cocaine and the other, more potent stimulants increase dopamine levels, in "crack" cocaine's case, massively and suddenly, with catastrophic results. Although marijuana in a very mild form may serve to reduce arousal, in the common, highly potent forms available, it is a powerful hallucinogen that predisposes to relapse and prevents remission of positive symptoms. Its effects on the prefrontal cortex are very similar to what occurs naturally in schizophrenia and major depression; that is, it greatly impairs motivation, intellectual and social functioning, and judgment. Because "designer" drugs, especially phencyclidine or "Angel Dust," contain psychotogenic substances, as well as often being simply poisonous, they are to be avoided absolutely. Everyone is reminded that substance abuse is a nearly absolute barrier to vocational rehabilitation, especially if the goal is competitive employment.

Tobacco is reviewed as well. Though there is some evidence that pure nicotine may improve some forms of cognitive impairment, when used chronically, it raises arousal and directly counteracts the therapeutic effects of antipsychotic medication. The result is either higher risk for relapse, with persistent psychotic symptoms, or the need for higher doses of medication, with all the resulting risks for intolerable side effects. Of course, tobacco carries a significant and deadly health risk and remains one of the most powerfully addictive drugs. Because most hospitals are now smoke-free, smoking puts patients at risk for experiencing nicotine withdrawal each time they are hospitalized, which only makes treating the psychosis that much more difficult.

During the ongoing multifamily group sessions, alcohol and drug consumption are explored at every meeting as part of the review of the previous weeks' events. The emphasis remains on substance abuse and its effects during every problem-solving focused on individuals for whom that is the key issue. This approach is similar to that used by Alcoholics Anonymous in that, until abstinence or major reduction occurs, there is little to be gained by focusing on any other issue. The goal is abstinence or, at least, clinically insignificant use, because many patients with schizophrenia are not fully addicted and some seem to be able to indulge in social consumption without negative effects. If occasional use leads again to heavy use, then abstinence is the only acceptable goal. In general, the same approach is used with individuals who are chronically noncompliant with medication on principle. If the noncompliance relates to side effects that have not been addressed, problem solving and routine clinical effort outside the group are focused on alleviating those side effects.

Conducting Multifamily Groups in Rural Settings

In some settings where there are great distances or travel difficulties, some variations have been developed that accommodate the distance barrier. Some groups have met monthly initially, but for 2 hours. That allows for two problem-solvings, usually with a refreshment break in the middle, yielding the same frequency of attention to each case as in the biweekly version. Leaders must conduct the groups with a bit more discipline and efficiency or negotiate a longer meeting time with participants. Two hours with a break appears to be the maximum time that individuals with a recent episode of schizophrenic psychosis can tolerate. In the initial stages, this approach also requires the leaders to be available for single-family sessions and crisis intervention.

The meeting site can be rotated to each family's home town. This equalizes the distance traveled over time and among participants. It also builds group cohesion and interfamily bonds, because all participants get to know their respective neighborhoods and sometimes their homes. A frequent site of groups meeting is various members' churches, which can also strengthen ties in the group. This rotation can be interspersed or supplemented with full, 45-minute sessions by telephone, usually on a monthly basis. The leaders can adopt methods used for centuries by circuit-riding clergy and judges.

Participation by Patients

Multifamily groups usually include patients. Experience with multifamily groups strongly suggests that to realize functional goals, the individual with the illness needs to be present. Paradoxically, many family members assert that before they experienced a multifamily group, they would have preferred not to have their ill relative present. On the other hand, families who have had relatives present throughout the process have been nearly universally emphatic about preferring to have them there. Regardless of preferences, it is nearly impossible to develop rehabilitation strategies in the absence of the person who will participate in that rehabilitation. For that reason alone, we have found it essential to include the person toward whom rehabilitation is directed at each step of the process. Problem solving is greatly facilitated by the presence of the person or persons who will carry out the solution. Therefore, patients are invited to participate in the group from the first session after the educational workshop, and every session thereafter.

Patients who have no family participate in the group as single individuals. The usual guideline for assembling a group is that no more than one-third of the cases in the group should be without a key relative or close friend that attends the group regularly. Clearly, during the engagement phase, every effort should be made to contact relatives or friends who might participate as a "sponsor." However, a small number of persons without a sponsor can participate and benefit. In most multifamily groups, this individual is, in a sense, adopted by other families' members, who often take a strong interest in his or her welfare and progress. As long as these individuals respond positively to the other group members, there is no noticeable difference in long-term outcome between those who have and do not have relatives in regular attendance.

GROUP MEMBERSHIP

Most multifamily groups function better as closed groups (i.e., with a fixed membership). This greatly promotes developing relationships among the members of the various families, a key therapeutic element of the approach. The families that attend the educational workshop comprise the regular and ongoing membership of the multifamily group. However, over time, and with attrition, the advantages of the closed group format may be outweighed by the disadvantages, especially if members have come to appreciate the assistance and lively process generated by a larger group. In that case, it is best to introduce one or two new families after they have completed the engagement and educational phases. During the first session with the new members, the group needs to be devoted to the introductory process outlined in Chapter 8. It is necessary to familiarize everyone with the patient's stage of recovery, in order that they may accommodate to the discrepancies between new and more experienced members in recovery. Many families find it gratifying to help the new members adjust to the group's approaches to relapse prevention, to gradual rehabilitation, and to the usual group process.

It is not uncommon to combine groups that have been meeting for more than 2 years if, by attrition, any one group has fewer than four cases on a regular basis. Again, when combining groups, it is important to attend both to introductions and to the issues faced and addressed by the remaining members. Usually, one leader from each group becomes the co-leader of the new group, or all four leaders rotate their participation.

ROLES OF OTHER CLINICIANS AND SERVICES

As patients reenter the community after discharge from the hospital, many mental health services refer them to day treatment programs, residential treatment programs, vocational rehabilitation, social skills training, and other ancillary treatment services. This often puts the family clinicians in the uncomfortable position of balancing the stresses and pressures that these programs create with the relapse prevention and gradual rehabilitation strategies of family psychoeducation. On the one hand, experience has shown that achieving good outcome requires that clinicians intercede on their patients' behalf. On the other hand, many program directors and supervisors resist attempts to alter their usual procedures, especially if they are encountering family psychoeducational approaches for the first time.

The role of the clinicians in these situations is that of educator, arbitrator, and patient advocate. However, we have found that it is important to use some of the basic principles of the psychoeducation approach in conducting this kind of advocacy. It is far preferable to spend time with the key program personnel to educate them about the modern psychophysiological basis for psychological and social interventions than to confront them directly or challenge their assumptions. The usual approach has been to ask the staff to try a more gradual, protective approach in a single case, to judge for themselves the efficacy of these kinds of methods. It is sometimes framed as a field trial of the new approach, to allow the staff to better understand and to evaluate it for themselves. Program directors are often alienated from family members or fear that the families will be critical of their program. If possible, it is desirable that family members support the program staff's attempts to be more flexible.

Many residential programs require that all residents be away from the house for at least 8 hours per day to attend a full-time program. In contrast, the psychoeducational approach suggests that patients, upon discharge from a hospital, have the option of resting for several hours a day and be required to participate only in partial hospital or rehabilitation programs for a few hours per day, perhaps on alternating days. This schedule would be gradually increased to full-time patient participation, but over the course of several weeks or months, and only at a rate that the patient can tolerate. That kind of schedule may require renegotiation of contractual agreements in the home, so it is important to help program directors and residential operators justify changes in scheduling and requirements to their funders and regulators, and support the staff as they attempt to implement changes and evaluate the results.

As the program's leaders and staff begin to understand and appreciate the value of partnership with families, the clinical–ideological issues tend to drop to the side. The program staff begin to notice that the patients who are approached in this more flexible and incremental manner tend to have fewer crises and provoke fewer incidents. If the staff are in a position to follow the patient for more than 6 to 8 months, they are often gratified to see substantial improvement in the outcome of their work. After one or two cases have gone well, our experience has been that program staff will adopt the strategies willingly. Of course, that greatly facilitates the integration of the various elements of the treatment system and allows the multifamily group to become a team that coordinates the various contributions of all the involved parties. The effort to coordinate all elements of the treatment and rehabilitation of a given patient via the multifamily group has been one of the determining influences that led to the creation of Family-aided Assertive Community Treatment (see Chapter 10).

THERAPEUTIC STYLE AND GROUP CLIMATE

The optimal tone for therapists to adopt in psychoeducational multifamily groups is rooted in concepts regarding cognitive deficits and arousal dyscontrol. These deficits may be shared in a subclinical form by some family members. A major modification of conventional multifamily therapy technique is the educative mode used extensively in the workshop and in the beginning months of the group. In this period, the clinicians adopt a much more directive, expert role than that used in most other therapies.

In addition, the leaders should adopt a warm, low-key, deliberate, and business-like approach that may at times, at least from the perspective of psychodynamic or family therapies, border on tediousness. However, quiet confidence, coupled with a willingness and ability to lead the group unobtrusively, will set an optimistic and nonprovocative tone, providing for the families an example of an optimal, low-intensity style. Furthermore, this deliberately calm approach is necessitated by the fact that a multifamily group tends to become overly intense, especially in the beginning, in ways that are similar to the high expressed emotion that characterizes some high-risk families.

Some interfamily intensity can be constructive, but at a later stage, and under carefully controlled conditions (e.g., in cross-family suggestions and, occasionally, in constructive challenges). A gradual increase in intensity is seen as therapeutic, because it helps the patient become tolerant of somewhat higher degrees of emotional activation. Even then, the group leaders need to remain calm and in control to avoid overstimulating patients or offending family members. Group leaders should create a group tone that is low in complexity, intensity, challenge, and rapid change, especially in the early meetings. Furthermore, by acknowledging and validating the relatives' and the patients' experiences, a warm, accepting, nonjudgmental, understanding approach can be established as a model for family interaction. It is important that the therapists also acknowledge and allow for the cognitive and social skills deficits of the patients, without appearing to condescend. Whenever possible, humor and lightness of mood should prevail. During the rehabilitation phase, a more focused, optimistic therapeutic style should be adopted in the attempt to achieve the previously delayed goal of reestablishing the patients as participants in the outer community. This involves continuing the supportive and accepting tone adopted earlier, now expanded, with a clear sense that, if carefully done, increasing responsibilities, and pursuit of goals and hopes, is not only possible but is actually the core intent of the group, a product of concerted work by patients, professionals, and relatives alike.

THE SOCIAL AND PERSONAL STANCE
OF MULTIFAMILY GROUP LEADERS

Because schizophrenia and other psychotic disorders are conceived primarily as brain disorders, a more direct and open relationship with family members and patients is indicated than that usually encountered in psychotherapy. The closest analogy, again is with general medical practice. Good family physicians see families as crucial allies in conducting a successful assessment and treatment, and most of them appreciate the value of family members in maintaining hope and morale in the healing patient. The relationship is seen as a partnership, in which therapeutic neutrality and a reserved interpersonal style would be considered rude, perhaps even arrogant, and not supportive or validating.

Clinicians, families, and patients bring unique expertise that is complementary, indispensable, and interdependent. For that reason, clinicians are expected to socialize during the group meetings and to share appropriate personal information with clients to a greater extent than before. The clinician's role is to communicate empathy and understanding, to provide information, to make specific suggestions, to be actively helpful, and to lead families in a formal problem-solving process.

Clinicians must be willing to share some aspects of their lives in the socializing periods that are a key feature of this approach. Communication between clinicians and family members is more typical of social or work settings than of therapy sessions. Family members are treated as partners— respectfully, empathically, and sympathetically. It is assumed that what they say about their experience and observations of the illness is honest, accurate, and valid, given the circumstances. Second-guessing their "real" motivation and looking for signs of hidden interactional dysfunction are not considered useful and are never used in interpretations or confrontations. Humor is used abundantly; opinions about movies, books, current events, and recipes are shared freely. No one is ridiculed, but in multifamily groups, patients may begin joking about their symptoms, seeing themselves as "special" rather than stigmatized. This will only happen if the clinicians model a matter-of-fact approach that takes psychosis seriously, without considering it shameful or unmanageable. As the groups mature, some meetings are entirely social, such as at holidays and patients' birthdays. Here again, it is incumbent on clinicians to join in, in a symmetrical, socially appropriate manner, not in the reserved, hierarchical style required of psychotherapy. Families rarely abuse this shift of style and, in fact, develop great loyalty to clinicians who can master this mode of interacting. If for no other reason, this style should be adopted to make the long process of recovery more humanly pleasant and enjoyable.

At the practical level, family clinicians serve as the family's ombudsmen, intervening when necessary to wrest needed services from other clinicians, programs, agencies, and bureaucracies. To paraphrase Carol Anderson, "If you don't know what else to do, do something useful."[108] This is crucial in engaging families and holding them in the process. Often, the smallest gesture, not necessarily a major victory, is enough to convince family members that these particular professionals clearly care about their needs, hear their pleas, and are willing to try to obtain assistance. This effort may include anything from acting as liaison to the psychiatrist, to opening a Medicaid account, to finding an item of clothing lost on an inpatient unit. It means doing what seems to be needed at the time rather than following procedures literally or strictly conforming to a job description. While this inevitably involves a small degree of extra effort, it solidifies the clinician–family relationship, which then tends to provide a surprising depth of support to the clinician over time.

Chapter 6

Joining with Families and Patients

WILLIAM R. MCFARLANE, SUSAN GINGERICH,
SUSAN M. DEAKINS, EDWARD DUNNE,
BONNIE T. HOREN, AND MARGARET NEWMARK

"Joining" means to connect, build rapport, convey empathy, and establish a collegial alliance. In the psychoeducational multifamily group joining with patients and their families is the first stage of treatment. There are several necessary technical aspects to joining, but it is an essentially emotional and social intervention, designed to create a bond between family members and family clinicians. In addition, that bond is established as strongly, and as equally as possible, with the patient. Many practitioners have commented that building a collaborative, respectful, and symmetrical relationship is one of the four key elements of multifamily psychoeducation, along with the educational, problem-solving and social network-building interventions. Joining continues throughout the families' involvement in treatment, but it is especially important in the beginning. The joining process described here is based on the approach developed by Anderson, Reiss, and Hogarty.[108]

Most families begin treatment when the patient has just experienced a crisis, an exacerbation of symptoms, or a hospitalization. It is best to meet separately with the patient and family at this time, because the patient is in the early phases of stabilization and the social demands of lengthy discussions are often too stimulating for the patient. Separate meetings with the patient and the family begin as soon as possible after a crisis or hospitalization. This prompt attention is reassuring to both family and patient. The goal is to establish the clinician as an advocate for both the patient and the family. Although meetings with the patient are briefer, it is important for the clinician to begin engaging the patient, in order to establish that he or she is there as much to help the patient as the family.

Family clinicians establish a strong, friendly, working alliance with all members of the family who are available and even marginally concerned. The emotional tone of sessions, positive comments about the process or the clinicians, relative enthusiasm about continuing, gratitude about the support and information provided, good attendance and increasing interest of initially neutral or avoidant relatives indicate success in the joining process. Many clinicians judge the relationship by how *they* feel about the family, hoping to establish an emotional climate such that they enjoy meeting with family members, look forward to seeing them, and feel a sense of professional accomplishment and value in the quality of the relationship. The family clinician must be explicit about the bias of this approach in *favor* of the family, as would be logical given the biological basis for the disorder. As Anderson put it so incisively, we start with the assumption of least pathology in this work and use the approach itself to demonstrate any lingering family systemic dysfunction.[108]

While creating the family–professional alliance, the clinicians must also gain a comprehensive picture of the family's situation, stresses, problems, reactions, and responses to the illness. The same applies to their social and instrumental resources, coping skills, and previous less successful attempts at coping. It is even more important to assess and reflect back their strengths, as individuals and as a family. There are clinical goals as well: identifying prodromal symptoms, assessing specific precipitants for the particular patient, and, for outpatients, establishing the stage of recovery. The joining process is complete when the relatives, the patient, and the family clinicians have developed a contract that is agreeable to all.

There are at least three joining meetings with each family and each patient before the educational workshop. The two clinicians who will eventually lead the multifamily group divide the responsibility: Each joins with half of the patients and their families. These meetings should occur weekly, for 1 hour with families and about 30 minutes with patients. The joining sessions with families follow a clear sequence of important steps, described in order of occurrence.

SESSION 1

The clinician begins by making small talk with the family about such things as traffic, getting to the meeting, weather, and recent holidays. The goal is for the family and the clinician to become acquainted, apart from the illness; it also helps everyone relax. After 15 minutes of social talk, the clinician reviews the patient's present crisis, listening to learn who has been helpful during the crisis and what interventions have helped the situation. Crises that result in hospitalization of a family member are always difficult experiences, and the clinician needs to express his or her appreciation of this fact and offer appropriate assistance.

This first session is also used to begin the process of delineating each patient's prodromal symptoms and personal early warning signs. The clinician guides the family through a review of the prior weeks, with emphasis on any changes in the patient's behavior, thoughts, or feelings during that time. These changes, which may be either quite apparent or barely noticeable, constitute the prodromal symptoms for that particular patient. In most cases, patients have idiosyncratic behaviors that precede the more common prodromal symptoms. These may appear substantially before the more classic anxiety, insomnia, anorexia, and loss of sexual interest. These early signs are often visible only to the family, because the patient is often amnesic for much of the prodromal period. These signs can include slightly odd but not psychotic behaviors, such as reading the Bible, drinking milk, singing, wearing a handkerchief tied around the head, and so on, that are not in character for that individual.

The clinician carefully notes each specific early symptom; maintains this list for future reference, and distributes it to family members. Throughout the course of the treatment for both the family and the clinician, it will serve to evaluate the patient's condition. It is common for families to miss or underestimate the significance of certain early warning signs, so the clinician needs to help the family construct a more complete list in subsequent sessions.

A short list of the specific types of precipitants for episodes should be developed in a similar manner. Many patients deteriorate in response to idiosyncratic stimuli that, again, only the family may be able to identify. One patient began to withdraw and become more suspicious whenever his sister came home from graduate school to visit. Another responded symptomatically to large family gatherings, another to pressures to return to work, and still another only to loss of affectively or romantically laden relationships. It is useful to attempt to corroborate these responses with the patient and, when the psychosis has abated, to explore his or her own perspective on precipitants. A summary of the course of symptoms and the determination of whether dangerous behavior has ever accompanied the patient's psychosis completes the review of principal clinical observations.

Following the collection of information about early warning signs and precipitants, the clinician then describes the psychoeducational multifamily group: five to eight families will meet every other week for 1½ hours, for at least 1 and usually 2 or more years. The last 5 minutes are spent socializing, reinforcing the importance of normal daily life, and closing the session on a hopeful, positive note. By the end of the first session, the clinician should have established that he or she will treat all family members with respect and act as an advocate for the patient and family.

SESSION 2

The clinician socializes with the family for about 15 minutes at the beginning of the session. Then he or she asks about the family's experiences during past episodes of schizophrenia. This is a crucial aspect of the relationship-building and joining process. This is the first opportunity for many families to share with a professional what are often severely traumatic events. Family members can have reactions that run the gamut from anger and bitterness, to marked sadness and depression, to numbing and withdrawal. Some have learned to accept the illness for what it is and attempt to cope with it in a more dispassionate way. The usual reactions and responses, though more destabilizing to all concerned, are completely understandable in the light of the many complexities and devastations of schizophrenia. A well-known social worker, educator, and parent once described the onset of schizophrenia in a child as if the child had died and the family then lived with the body, hoping that the person they once knew would reinhabit it. In addressing the emotional burdens exacted by this illness, clinicians need only think about how they might react themselves.

It is useful to explore what the family members have understood as the causes for the psychosis and what other, more distant family members, friends, and neighbors have said or implied about causation. Families can be as devastated by their relative's and friend's responses as by the episodes themselves. Some family members have been openly blamed by people they previously trusted, only adding to their pain, sense of guilt, and increasing isolation. The mental health system may have been the cause of anger and resentment over inadequate services and professional attitudes. This needs to be acknowledged and contrasted with what the family clinicians are going to provide.

The clinician then explores the family's social network and resources. Drawing a genogram or a sociogram is useful in this session. Identify those who help in material ways and those who help in emotional ways. Similarly, differentiate between those who have stood by the family and those who have dropped away since the onset of the illness. It is useful to know if any of these now more-distant friends actually blame the family or have had any exposure to current educational and scientific information. Identify the patient's friends; they can play an invaluable role as the rehabilitation phase begins. They can serve as a bridge from the family to the nonfamily world and help to represent in the present the positive personal qualities that may have become obscured by symptoms. Friends and peer support groups can combat stigma and fear among other friends and open up more social opportunities for the patient. The session ends with 5 minutes of socializing.

SESSION 3

The session begins with 15 minutes of socializing. The clinician then finishes gathering information, paying special attention to work, school, and other institutional connections, as well as areas of personal strength and resources. If the patient is scheduled for discharge from the hospital, the clinician helps the family plan for this. It is important to agree on short- and long-term goals. The usual short-term goal is to stabilize the patient's symptoms and prevent relapse; increasing his or her social skills and working toward employment or higher education are typical long-term goals. Regardless, it is essential to survey the patient's and family members' preferences and hopes, and to negotiate goals that are important to them, and that will motivate effort and elicit hope.

The clinician prepares the family for the educational workshop, where they will meet the other group members for the first time, and for the regular meetings of the multifamily group that will follow. He or she inquires about the family members' experience with groups and whatever concerns they might have, including confidentiality, shyness, and feeling pressured to speak in group settings. Resistance to meeting with families of other ethnic groups or social classes may need to be aired. Some families may have secrets that they do not wish to have divulged, or they may be unusually isolated and fear simply having to interact and converse. In all these special situations, families can be assured that diversity is helpful and has not proven to be a barrier, and that they need only share and participate to the extent that they feel comfortable. The clinician briefly describes how the groups proceed and what other families have gained from such groups, particularly new and workable solutions to difficult problems of illness management. Extra meetings with the families should be scheduled if the educational workshop is to be held more than 2 or 3 weeks after the third joining session.

At least three meetings are set up separately with the patient. These meetings are shorter and less structured. If possible, they are carried out while the patient is in the hospital. The main goal is to allow the patient to become acquainted with the clinician and to see him or her as an interested, sympathetic person who will act as an advocate. It is essential to develop an alliance that will allow the person, who may have only partially remitted symptoms, feel safe and protected during the first sessions in the multifamily group. This alliance will serve as an emotional cushion should there be negative experiences in the first few sessions. Meetings with patients should also include several minutes of socializing. The clinician tells the patient that his or her family will be attending an educational workshop. As with the family, it is important to agree on short- and long-term goals. Again, the clinician is free to schedule as many additional sessions as needed.

GUIDING PROCESS IN JOINING SESSIONS

From the first meeting, the clinician is active in guiding the conversation. The clinician needs to be in control of the sessions and structure them from the beginning. Structure reduces the patient's and family's anxieties. Sometimes family members may quarrel or monopolize discussions, or make repetitive complaints. This kind of communication can be interrupted by acknowledging the person's frustration and worry about the illness.

The clinician keeps his or her manner positive, informal, and collegial. During joining sessions and throughout all the stages of treatment, the clinician needs to be confident in what he or she knows about the illness and also respectful of what the family knows and has experienced firsthand. If the clinician does not know the answer to a question, he or she acknowledges ignorance and assures the family that the information will be sought out. Part of joining is providing concrete help, such as obtaining information from the psychiatrist and being available to patients and families. This kind of involvement shows that the clinician will be acting as a colleague and can be trusted. Most families have felt blamed and criticized by the traditional assessment questions that search for failure and pathology. In this model, the clinician emphasizes successful coping and resources. It is essential that the clinician explicitly disavow any belief or suspicion that the family caused the illness. It can be assumed that nearly every family will harbor doubts and a sense of guilt and shame that they have done something to bring on this illness. Without an explicit acknowledgment, families will tend to assume that the clinicians hold them responsible, and they will nearly always drop out.

Families also need the opportunity to express their feelings of loss, frustration, anger, despair, hopelessness, and guilt. The clinician validates the expression of these feelings and may gently inquire about them without undue probing. When feelings of loss and latent grief are left unexpressed, they can form a barrier to a family's finding the energy and openness needed to learn new ways to cope. Clearly, it is better to explore the family's sense of loss in the absence of the patient, who often feels acutely his or her relatives' anguish and guilt. Some families may need to revisit these feelings privately with the clinician periodically, in order to stay focused on the work of treatment and rehabilitation. Eliciting reactions to the illness, validating almost any variety of emotional response, is one of the most supportive and potent aspects of the treatment. This validation quickly reduces family members' pent-up anger at themselves, the patient, and the mental health system, and probably helps to reduce tendencies toward critical attitudes and overinvolvement. Just as important, many families seem to need and appreciate what transpires when clinicians become advocates for the family. Some of them are moved to a new commitment of hope and effort by the example of the clinician making a few extra efforts to be helpful to the family.

Whenever relevant, the clinician shares information about schizophrenia with the family. As soon as possible, he or she expresses the belief that schizophrenia is an illness of the brain that is not caused by the family or the patient. It is often necessary to repeat this several times in the course of treatment, because so many families blame themselves. It is also helpful to emphasize that families will be able to prevent relapses and crises using the information that they will learn in the treatment program. Families appreciate this positive point of view about their contributions. The clinician also takes an interest in each member of the family, apart from his or her involvement with the illness. This principle is realized partly during joining through the socializing that is built into the beginning and end of each session and continued in the multifamily groups.

Whenever a crisis occurs during this period for either patient or family, the clinician must deal with it as soon as possible. It is highly desirable to arrange to be accessible to families on a 24-hour, 7-day per week basis, through an answering service, crisis team, or home number and personal answering machine. This does not have to serve as an emergency service—few clinicians can substitute for what an emergency service in a hospital or crisis service can provide. However, knowing that the clinician can be reached to consult and do some fine-tuning of a treatment plan greatly alleviates family anxieties and actually reduces the number and severity of crises. The privilege of this kind of accessibility is almost never abused. In fact, many families need to be encouraged to report prodromal symptoms and signs; that is, they often decide not to report, just to protect the clinician's privacy. But families need to understand that the group leaders are not prepared to provide emergency services, such as immediate intervention to prevent a suicide, or to treat sudden increases in symptoms or to control threatened or actual violence. However, early notification leads to a reduced total workload for everyone, and families may need to be persuaded of this reality. Discharge planning is often a crisis for families—being included and having their wishes honored rapidly builds morale in families, especially if the plan is also negotiated with, and acceptable to, the patient.

Because some families find that the multifamily group does not meet all their needs in the beginning of treatment, it is incumbent on clinicians to make themselves available in the first few weeks to months by telephone and in person for ad hoc sessions or consultations. This may be necessary to develop further the personal side of the alliance. Also, families will need to deal with a specific illness management issue in a single-family context, if they are unable to share it with the multifamily group. They may need special focus on what some of the guidelines mean, how to implement them, and how to evaluate the results. If they are multifamily group veterans, they may need single-family consultations to address specific issues that they perceive as not important enough to raise in the group, but that the clinicians assess to be potentially capable of destabilizing the affected member of the family. Over time, extra single-family sessions will need to be curtailed if they impede progress in addressing problems within the multifamily group.

Clinicians need supportive supervision, beginning with the preparation for contacting families. For many clinicians, the techniques described earlier are new. It can be stressful to learn new ways of forming alliances and conducting sessions. It can also be stressful to hear about the difficult experiences and emotional pain that the families have endured. Supervision can be very helpful in dealing with these stresses when it is conducted with the same positive, supportive, collegial tone that the clinician uses with patients.

Chapter 7

Educating Families

A Multifamily Workshop on Schizophrenia

WILLIAM R. MCFARLANE, SUSAN GINGERICH,
SUSAN M. DEAKINS, EDWARD DUNNE,
BONNIE T. HOREN, AND MARGARET NEWMARK

All of the family interventions that have been developed and empirically validated since 1978 have education as a core component. Education is one of the four essentials of psychoeducational multifamily group treatment, along with joining, problem solving, and social network expansion. While there is some variation among the educational approaches in the models of Anderson, Leff, Falloon, and the approach described here, the commonalities predominate. The principle involved in education of family, other caretakers, and patients themselves is clear-cut. Enough is now known about the underlying biological and social processes of schizophrenia, and even about its causation, that a reasonably coherent picture can be shared with, and absorbed by, the involved parties. Having a scientifically validated concept from which to work, families can not only be relieved of the burdens of guilt and anxiety but also go on to make major contributions to treatment and rehabilitation.

When no education or sharing of information occurs, the situation is dramatically different. Families will tend to be confused and adopt whatever concepts are current in their own families, culture, or community.

They will tend to act and filter experience on the basis of those concepts and beliefs, and often act in ways that they believe to be helpful and that make sense to them, but that actually interfere with recovery. Although that is unfortunate, it is completely predictable if they do not have information and guidance from professionals or others with legitimate expertise. Thus, there is a new ethical imperative: It is a professional responsibility to provide caretakers and concerned relatives with the information and guidance that they need to foster recovery and rehabilitation.

RATIONALE

Family education has many purposes and arises from several sources. One of the most powerful sources is work by Vaughn, in which she discovered that families with low expressed emotion tend to understand schizophrenia as an illness and, therefore, as something largely beyond their control.[319] They tend to take a more relaxed, *laissez-faire* approach, seeing the course of the illness and its very existence as something to be accepted and endured, often within a religious conceptual framework. By contrast, many families that manifest high expressed emotion do not see the condition as an illness. They tend to feel guilty and to work hard to correct the situation, with everything from excessive attention to anger and criticism, especially when their efforts and concern fail to achieve improvement. Many of them have been blamed by professionals, their own families, or neighbors and friends. In short, they, too, have been stigmatized. Vaughn concluded that the high-expressed emotion families are in a very real sense victims of lack of information, who also carry a deep and abiding concern for the patient and experience considerable psychic pain from being so helpless. A principal cause for that kind of agony is professionals' failure to inform, support, and guide the family. It was unfair to ask families to figure this all out on their own, because many of the most effective interpersonal and rehabilitative approaches are counterintuitive. The implications are clear: it is professionals' duty to help all families, especially those who are most exasperated, to understand the condition as a bona fide illness, one that required specific interpersonal and rehabilitative methods.

Another influential source has been the family advocacy movement, particularly as represented by the National Alliance for the Mentally Ill (NAMI). Beginning in the late 1970s, increasingly articulate and persuasive voices began to call for an end to keeping families excluded from treatment decisions and in the dark about their loved ones' diagnoses, treatment rationale, and longer term prospects. Information for families becomes indispensable if one is developing a collaborative relationship with the families of the patients for whom one is clinically responsible. The goal is to develop as full a shared base of knowledge from all parties as possible, and to base intelligent action on that entire base of information. The multifamily group takes this one step further by sharing information, ideas, and inspiration among several families at once. Thus, one purpose of the educational aspect of this approach is to empower families and, over time, patients with the illness.

For families to apply guidelines successfully and solve problems of illness management, they need to understand the physiology and psychology of schizophrenia at a basic level. Furthermore, once they do understand how the brain is working in health and illness, they can develop their own strategies to fit their particular circumstances. For instance, we emphasize to families the impairments in the general area of attention carried by many people with schizophrenia. That helps families to learn to modulate the way that they communicate, to look for cues of understanding, to reduce distracting noise, and to pace what they say carefully and simplify how they say it.

Ultimately, the goal is that families and patients know in no uncertain terms that they did not cause this disorder and that the professionals who are asking for their help do not hold any such beliefs. Education is offered as a rather elaborate demonstration that these professionals, at least, understand that families are not the root cause. This is crucial to joining. If families are fearful of the underlying beliefs of those engaging them in the treatment process, they will not commit fully to the effort and are likely to decline to participate or to drop out. On the positive side, once the educational effort is under way, families will often show abundant gratitude and relief that they are absolved. That gratitude accrues to the credibility of, and appreciation for, those doing the educating. That is why it is somewhat less important if families understand the fine details of brain structure or neurotransmission. One father, although his interpretation of ventricular enlargement was that his son had "water on the brain," was nevertheless effusive in his gratitude to the clinicians, because his own brother had convinced him that he had caused the illness through being neglectful (which was not the case). Clinicians are best positioned to interpret technical, scientific, and clinical knowledge, and to help families put this information into practice in a clinically effective way.

A more positive purpose of the education provided in the psychoeducational approach, especially as developed by Anderson and her colleagues,[108] is to instill hope and motivation. Most families come to this work with ambivalence: In first-episode cases, families are hoping that nothing serious is amiss, and in more chronic cases, they may have become discouraged, angry, and distrustful toward clinical services. The education described here invites families to attempt something different, to work alongside clinicians and to try deliberately to alter the course of illness. While many family members voice skepticism at first, the educational workshops usually convert that skepticism to expectancy, renewed hope, and at least enough commitment to continue into the next phase. The results of outcome trials are shared with families to make sure that they see what other families have been able to do and what these clinicians might be capable of achieving with their help. In settings in which these services have been available for a year or more, other families are available to provide assurance that the results are worth the effort. Families gain a sense of mastery and, in multifamily groups, a strong group identity centered around increasing evidence of their own effectiveness. As the patients improve, they begin to join in the process as partners. They become interested in the information and use the guidance to achieve their own rehabilitative goals. As they begin to use the principles, families gain further gratification and reassurance. In the end, much of this success reflects back to the clinicians, most of whom report that this work has substantially improved their professional lives. Over 1,500 families have attended these workshops; there has been no instance in which information has had a significant negative effect, and there are hundreds of examples of dramatically relieved and grateful families.

CONDUCTING A PSYCHOEDUCATIONAL WORKSHOP

The practical purposes of the educational aspect of this approach include helping families to understand the following:

- The seriousness of the disorder.
- The role of stress in precipitating episodes.
- Early signs of relapse.
- The more mysterious aspects of symptoms, especially the negative variety.
- The basics of brain function and dysfunction in schizophrenia.
- The ways in which psychiatric medications affect brain function and cause side effects.

- The usual ways that families are affected by severe mental illness in one of their members.
- Preferable and more effective coping strategies and illness management techniques.
- The causes and general prognosis of the illness.
- The psychoeducational treatment process itself.

Thus, the educational effort operates at several levels. It is organized to change the relationship between families and clinicians, patients and their families, and between families who begin as strangers to one another. However, it is also critical that families learn, through direct education or, later, through problem solving and application of Family Guidelines, how to cope with, and improve the outcome of, schizophrenia and other major mental illnesses. Those coping solutions are applications of general principles that follow from the biological nature of schizophrenia. However, those solutions must also be consistent with the style, unique history, and organization of a specific family and its ill member. Therein lies the challenge for clinicians, in that adaptation for each participant appears to be essential for success. The effective clinicians and multifamily group are those that can make the transitions from biological/pharmacological to psychological and social levels with ease and clarity. It is this characteristic blending of wisdom from all systems levels that makes this approach truly systemic. It means that the effort is both educational, in the narrow sense of the word, and also therapeutic, in that it is intended to change attitudes, reduce guilt and shame in family members, improve interaction in the family, create an optimal social environment for recovery, instill motivation and hope and in the multifamily group format, and create the conditions for families and patients to become a social network.

Anderson and her colleagues[108] have emphasized that the workshop seems to be most effective if certain themes are used as a framework for presenting information and guidance, and if the information is tailored as much as possible to the actual participants. North and her colleagues have extended this concept further by developing a polling method that allows presenters to develop each workshop specifically for those who will attend.[320] This contrasts with another approach being used by the Journey of Hope, a 12-session curriculum developed by Burland and colleagues[4] that uses the themes, basic information, and form of Anderson and colleagues' workshop but presents it in a classroom format like a course, with content predetermined and manualized. Thus far, there is little evidence as to which method is preferable, but given the ability of most experienced clinicians to focus intervention on the specific needs of individuals and their families, we have preferred the more tailored and flexible approach. It also tends to engage the creativity and skills of clinicians, which not only energizes them but also seems to engage the participating families in a mutual search for solid and relevant information that seems ultimately to increase their commitment to the process.

In our more recent experience, in which cases come with a variety of diagnoses, degrees of chronicity, and family experience, the premium on individualizing the educational material has only increased. Particularly in rural areas or other settings in which diagnoses and degree of chronicity will be more mixed than in urban areas, the more tailored curriculum will be more effective. Gathering requests for certain types of information can readily be done during the joining process or even at the beginning of the day, as part of the introductions. Fortunately, there is a great deal of information now available in the form of brochures, videotapes, and books that can be incorporated as needed. We have developed a videotape that reviews the psychobiology of schizophrenia specifically for lay audiences and paraprofessionals. The National Institute of Mental Health provides excellent material, as do several pharmaceutical manufacturers. Mueser and Gingerich's *Coping with Schizophrenia*[324] has been written specifically to complement psychoeducational work with families and nicely expands the information beyond that presentable within the limited time frame. Hatfield has done the same, more from the families' perspective, in *Family Education in Mental Illness*.[322] A classic contribution is Torrey's *Living with Schizophrenia*.[323]

Guidelines for Clinicians

The presenters are the leaders of the multifamily group. This arrangement challenges some clinicians to develop new skills in teaching and giving direct advice, both of which are forsworn in some psychotherapies. However, there is such great value in having the leaders, rather than educational specialists, present the material that a degree of transitory anxiety or awkwardness is more than worth the enhanced total effect. Family members are nearly universally interested in working with the key clinicians who work with their ill relative. Our experience is that families are remarkably forgiving about the content but very sensitive to implications of blame and the quality of interaction with the clinician/teachers. The presentations will need to be empathic and informative at the same time. The process is greatly enhanced if the clinicians use group leadership skills to elicit confirming comments and experiences from the audience in a manner that invites, but does not obligate, participants to respond.

Another implication of the education being done by clinicians is that they will need to keep current with developing knowledge. Over the past two decades, each year has seen at least one breakthrough that expands or even redefines our understanding of schizophrenia and opens new avenues for treatment. For instance, research on N-methyl-D-aspartate (NMDA) as a neurotransmitter and its role in the prefrontal cortex is developing rapidly and may change what we say about the fundamental mechanisms of symptoms, treatment, and course of illness. Potential causes for schizophrenia expand each year, with increasing likelihood that pre- and perinatal neurodevelopmental delay is their final common pathway. This information will not only help families but also could well reshape the way clinicians of all disciplines approach treatment and rehabilitation. Keeping abreast of the literature greatly increases the clinicians' credibility vis-à-vis the families and preserves their role as the representatives of the clinical system. On the negative side, it is less helpful if families become aware of new developments sooner than the clinicians. Integrating new information is not difficult, if the stage has been set during the joining and educational phases. Minor developments can be shared with participants during the go-round in the multifamily group, or miniworkshops can be substituted for the regular meeting of the group to review major new or accumulating developments. If the patients are clinically stable, it is usually best to include them in the educational process.

Thus, multifamily group leaders need to enhance their own knowledge but also should always be ready to recognize and share the limits of their knowledge. The field still does not know what it does not know about this remarkably complex illness, so ordinary clinicians need not hold themselves to a standard of omniscience. Families will accept those limits as long as they sense that the presenters are committed to their welfare and to a long-term effort to relieve their uncertainty and burdens. In many cases, collective acquisition of knowledge by all the participants will relieve the clinicians of the demand to know everything, while emphasizing the teamwork aspect of the ongoing multifamily group.

Practicalities and Procedures

After families have had at least three joining sessions, they attend an all-day educational workshop, commonly held on a weekend day. This workshop is modeled after the workshop described by Anderson and her colleagues.[108]

The purpose of the workshop is to provide information about the nature of schizophrenia and effective ways of managing the illness. The leaders present the information in an open, collegial manner, which should create an atmosphere in which families can comfortably ask questions and discover that their experiences and problems are similar and understandable. Because the workshop is conducted by the two multifamily group leaders, it is the first time families meet the other members of the group and the other family clinician. If some relatives, and even key family members, are reluctant to participate in the overall treatment process, every effort should be made to ensure that they attend the workshop. The psychiatrist who is treating the patients should present the material on the psychobiology of the illness. Staff whose professional disciplines are not represented by the leaders should be invited to contribute their expertise.

Some clinicians may feel apprehensive at first about organizing and presenting factual information clearly. It is helpful for clinicians to review the materials several times in advance of the workshop. Practicing presentations with colleagues increases confidence and provides an opportunity to receive comments on clarity, manner, rate of speech, and so on. Some clinicians find it useful to videotape or audiotape their practice presentations to see for themselves their strengths and areas in which they may want to improve. Anticipating the kinds of questions that families may ask and rehearsing responses also increases preparedness. Clinicians report that the more often they conduct workshops, the easier, and more manageable and enjoyable they become.

Clinicians attempt to create a classroom atmosphere, so that this first meeting of group members is as free of social tension as possible. Chairs are set up in rows facing the front, and the leaders use blackboards, charts, slides, or other audiovisual aids. Family members each receive a folder containing printed information, the Family Guidelines, diagrams, references, and other aids that can be followed throughout the day. Refreshments are supplied throughout the all-day workshop, including morning coffee, lunch, and afternoon tea. Only decaffeinated beverages are served, and there is no smoking in the meeting room. Refreshment breaks provide an informal setting for spontaneous socializing. The group leaders act as hosts and hostesses during these interludes; it is strongly recommended that they spend time during the breaks with families and other attendees, and not solely with their colleagues.

After coffee and a light snack, the leaders identify themselves and explain the day's agenda. They also provide a rationale for the workshop. For example, a leader might say:

"We want you to know as much as possible about this illness—what's known, and what's not known, as of now. Schizophrenia is a very complex and confusing illness. We have found that the more information people have, the more equipped they are to deal with problems that come up. We will also be discussing some guidelines for coping that have been shown to be effective.

"This workshop is only one step of our treatment program. After the workshop, we will be meeting together as a group of families, including patients, on a regular basis and we will continue to provide relevant information and assistance to you. We have found that working together with patients, families, and the treatment team in this program has resulted in fewer and less severe relapses for patients. We will answer as many questions as possible in this workshop today. If we cannot answer something, we will find someone who knows the information and get back to you."

A Curriculum

The leaders provide a detailed agenda, an example of which appears in Table 7.1.

The leaders then repeat their names and their position in the agency, and ask the rest of the group, including any other staff members attending, to give their names. There is a great deal of information to be covered in the workshop, so it is important to stick to the agenda of the day and to keep track of the time. Sometimes families ask good questions that may lead to long discussions. Because it is likely that questions will be answered by the content covered later in the day, clinicians may ask families to save certain detailed questions until after the appropriate section is presented. Discussions can also be continued either after the workshop or during a meeting of the multifamily group.

The leaders begin with a presentation of the biological information about the illness of schizophrenia. Chapters 1 and 2 contain most of the clinical and biological information needed for the presentation, while descriptions of the inner and outer experience of schizophrenia can be found in Anderson and colleagues' *Schizophrenia and the Family*.[108] The clinical and biological information and interpretation is much more effective when presented by the psychiatrist or nurse practitioner who is prescribing and managing the pharmacotherapy for most of the group's patients. In lieu of such a presenter, our videotape, *Explaining Schizophrenia*, can be used as a comprehensive description of the biological information, in lieu of a pre-

TABLE 7.1. Outline of the Survival Skills Workshop

9:00–9:15	Coffee and informal interaction
9:15–9:30	Formal introductions and explanation of the format for the day
9:30–10:30	Information about the phenomenology of the illness
	Information about the etiology, course, and outcome of the illness
	Biochemical theories
	Genetic theories
	Sociocultural theories
	Family theories
	The private experience of schizophrenia
	The public experience of schizophrenia
10:30–10:45	Coffee break and informal discussion
10:45–12:00	Treatment of schizophrenia
	The use of medication
	How it works
	Why it is needed
	Impact on outcome
	Side effects
	Other treatments
	Family psychoeducation and multifamily groups
	Social skills training
	Day treatment
	Vocational rehabilitation and supported employment
	Psychotherapies
	Megavitamin and other dietary treatments
	Management of the illness
	Health
	Diet
	Stress
12:00–1:00	Lunch and informal discussion
1:00–3:00	The family and schizophrenia
	The needs of the patient
	The needs of the family
	Family reactions to the illness
	Emotional reactions
	Common interactions
	Common problems that patients and families face
	What the family can do to help
	Family guidelines
	The problem-solving method
3:30–4:00	Questions regarding specific problems
	Description of the multifamily group process
	Having patience with the slow pace of improvement
	Keeping hope alive
	Wrap up and scheduling
	Informal interaction

Note. From Anderson et al.[108] (p. 76). Copyright 1986 by The Guilford Press. Adapted by permission.

sentation by a physician. It covers research findings related to various theories of etiology as well as the mechanisms that underlie psychiatric medication. Frequent breaks offer an opportunity to discuss each section and to respond to questions from families. The leaders continue clarifying relevant information that was covered in the videotape, such as statistics on incidence and prevalence, hereditary factors, neurological findings about brain physiology, and mechanisms of action for various psychotropic medications. After a morning break, the clinicians present information about leading treatment and rehabilitation methods, especially those being offered to the patients in the multifamily group.

The staff remain with the families during lunch, sharing in this more informal time. After lunch, clinicians take turns presenting illustrations of typical family members' reactions to the presence of schizophrenia in their lives. The leaders might start off with an example such as "Family members often report feeling perplexed and scared when their son became ill" or "I've heard family members describe how frustrated they became with some repetitious behavior that seems to make no sense." Family members may describe their own experiences of exasperation, fear, confusion, anxiety, guilt, anger, and sadness, if they wish. The leaders ask which methods family members have used to cope with the illness of their family member. Here, too, the clinicians normalize the answers by acknowledging that many other families have described these same responses and that they are natural responses to illness in general. Family members report such things as attempting to reason with the patient, ignoring the situation, centering all family life on the patient, and paying watchful attention to the patient's condition. Leaders can ask how these methods have been helpful and suggest that whereas they are natural and useful responses to some illnesses, they may not prove as successful with schizophrenia. Clinicians point out that they will be discussing alternative methods of coping with the illness using the Family Guidelines (to follow), which are based on the specific effects of schizophrenia on the patient and the families.

Family Guidelines

An afternoon break is followed by a discussion of the Family Guidelines (see Table 7.2). Each person present will have a copy of the Guidelines to which he or she can refer as the leaders go over them, one by one. Clinicians take turns reading a guideline, connecting it to the biological information discussed that morning and asking family members for their reactions, questions, and experiences. It is helpful to illustrate the Guidelines

TABLE 7.2. Family Guidelines

Here is a list of things everyone can do to help make things run more smoothly:

1. GO SLOW. Recovery takes time. Rest is important. Things will get better in their own time.
2. KEEP IT COOL. Enthusiasm is normal. Tone it down. Disagreement is normal. Tone it down, too.
3. GIVE EACH OTHER SPACE. Time out is important for everyone. It's OK to reach out. It's OK to say "no."
4. SET LIMITS. Everyone needs to know what the rules are. A few good rules keep things clear.
5. IGNORE WHAT YOU CAN'T CHANGE. Let some things slide. Don't ignore violence.
6. KEEP IT SIMPLE. Say what you have to say clearly, calmly, and positively.
7. FOLLOW THE DOCTOR'S ORDERS. Take medications as they are prescribed. Take only medications that are prescribed.
8. CARRY ON BUSINESS AS USUAL. Reestablish family routines as quickly as possible. Stay in touch with family and friends.
9. NO STREET DRUGS OR ALCOHOL. They make symptoms worse, can cause relapse, and prevent recovery.
10. PICK UP ON EARLY SIGNS. Note changes. Consult with your family clinician.
11. SOLVE PROBLEMS STEP-BY-STEP. Make changes gradually. Work on one thing at a time.
12. LOWER EXPECTATIONS, TEMPORARILY. Use a personal yardstick. Compare this month to last month rather than last year or next year.

with concrete examples based on the kinds of problems described by families during joining sessions. This is the first time family members have heard the Guidelines explained formally, as they relate to coping strategies. The clinicians should make every effort to be clear and to explain the underlying rationale for these suggestions (see Anderson et al.[108]). It is important to remember, and it may be helpful to remind participants that these approaches are in many instances counterintuitive and may require suspension of disbelief to be implemented. The leaders will need to stress explicitly that the Guidelines are based on a fair amount of experience, even though they may not seem helpful at first. Also, it is useful to acknowledge that some of them apply at different times and in different situations. For instance, setting limits may be necessary when the patient is losing control, whereas ignoring what one cannot change applies at times when symptoms may be present but also quite stable for a considerable period of time. A tone of hopefulness is used as the new ideas are introduced. Extra copies of the Family Guidelines are distributed at the workshop, with the suggestion that they be posted on the refrigerator or wherever they will be handy as a reference.

Concluding the Workshop

The clinicians close the workshop on a positive note, conveying their optimism about this approach. The format for the multifamily groups is outlined, emphasizing the problem-solving method and its usefulness for families and patients. The agenda for the first two meetings is presented. Leaders validate the advantages of having other families present to assist in devising and learning new coping strategies. Any questions or concerns about the ensuing work in the multifamily group or in single-family settings are addressed. Participants should be reminded about whatever mechanism has been established for contacting the clinicians in case of questions or crises between sessions. A brief discussion is held regarding the slow pace that clinical and, especially, functional improvement seem to require. Families are reminded that the slowness of the pace is a major issue that has faced other families in previous groups, even when later results have far surpassed anything that they might have hoped. The notion of "slow and steady wins the race" is used as the theme.

The leaders encourage family members to voice their reactions to the workshop, making sure to listen and validate every response. Some common reactions are relief at finally knowing some facts, anger at being kept in the dark too long, sadness, despair, hopefulness about this approach, and eagerness to get on with the work. Leaders make sure family members know the time and date of the first meeting of the multifamily group, usually 2 weeks after the workshop. Families are reminded that patients will be invited to all subsequent multifamily group meetings. It may be helpful to briefly discuss any misgivings family members may have about those with an illness being present. The clinicians thank all participants for coming to the workshop on a precious day off.

EDUCATION AND INFORMATION FOR PATIENTS

Providing education to patients has proved highly useful, but it must be informed by careful clinical assessment as to their capability for, and openness to, information about their illness and preferable methods for self-management. Because clinically unstable patients do not attend the psychoeducational workshop, they need to learn about the guidelines in a different setting. This can be done in a shorter workshop for patients only or in the whole group, as a repeat or an update, after the patients have achieved clinical stability. It is best to not force the issue of attendance or acceptance of the information with patients who are steadfastly committed to the idea that they are not ill. Clinicians explain guidelines to patients at the earliest possible time, depending upon their phase of recovery and ability to pay attention. Sometimes this happens during a joining session. Usually, the patient will better comprehend guidelines as they are applied to a specific situation, either in the go-round or problem-solving section of the group meeting. When the patient's psychiatrist is familiar with the Guidelines, he or she may also make use of them. It has become a general rule that if a patient joins the group 4 to 6 months after his or her last psychotic episode has resolved, he or she will profit from at least an abbreviated and clinically appropriate presentation of the psychobiological and family-management information, as well as the Family Guidelines. We have seen remarkable changes in some very paranoid and resistant patients following a sensitive and individualized educational presentation. Err on the side of inclusion if there is lack of clarity about the safety of inviting particular patients.

If the clinicians have the capability, newer cognitive and behavioral therapies for the individual patient may be beneficial, especially Hogarty and colleagues' approaches based on the same underlying clinical theory as family psychoeducation.[182]

Chapter 8

The Initial Sessions of a Psychoeducational Multifamily Group

Forming a Healing Network

WILLIAM R. MCFARLANE, SUSAN GINGERICH,
SUSAN M. DEAKINS, EDWARD DUNNE,
BONNIE T. HOREN, AND MARGARET NEWMARK

This multifamily group approach has a specific and somewhat unusual initial process. It begins with a planned process of social interaction that for the first two or three sessions avoids any emphasis on the clinical and rehabilitation goals and effort. Rather, considerable attention is paid to establishing a working alliance among all participants as quickly and as deliberately as possible. To a large extent, this is driven by the biosocial underpinnings of the entire model. We assume that empathic and yet knowledgeable social support is a key intervention in itself. The initial phase is intended to build group identity and a sense of mutual interest and concern prior to addressing any particular clinical issue. That has proved consistently to promote interfamily and interpersonal social support. As well, this approach is designed to avoid a number of potential processes that, although common in older multifamily therapy methods, risk excessive and negative emotional interactions that resemble expressed emotion on a group basis. They certainly appear to have the same negative effects. It is almost routine that more spontaneous, group-centered, initial techniques quickly degenerate into open intrafamily conflict, disagreement between families about the function of the group, anger, and even confrontation with the leaders. All too often, that causes the people with schizophrenia to become overwhelmed and leads to their hasty retreat from the group, often permanently, with the ensuing loss of several families from further participation. Given that outcomes depend on at least one member of each family continuing their participation for a lengthy period, dropout is viewed here as an extremely serious adverse incident. So although the overall approach is highly focused on the details of each patient's treatment and rehabilitation, that focus occurs after there has been a carefully orchestrated opportunity to develop trust, empathy, and a shared orientation and consensus about their predicament. Because the problem solving that follows depends on ideas being shared and, we hope, accepted across family boundaries, we have found it essential to proceed a bit more slowly toward that effort to ensure its success as the leaders create a healing network.

FIRST MEETING OF THE
PSYCHOEDUCATIONAL MULTIFAMILY GROUP:
"GETTING TO KNOW EACH OTHER"

After the joining sessions and the workshop, the psychoeducational multifamily group meets for the first time, now including patients, after they have had joining sessions and whether or not they have attended the educational workshop. The patients and families have been prepared to meet with five to eight other families for 1½-hour meetings every other week for at least 12 months, and monthly for at least another 12 months. Refreshments, including decaffeinated beverages, are provided by the clinicians to allow relaxed interactions before and during the group.

The goal of the first group is that clinicians and family members get to know each other in the best possible light. Everyone will be working together for at least 2 years, and it is important to begin to feel comfortable with one another. It is very helpful during this group meeting to think of it as any group of people who are meeting each other for the first time. In such a group, people tend to put their best foot forward. The clinician acts like a good host or hostess and guides the conversation to topics of general interest, such as how people travel to the group, where they live, where they were born and grew up, what kind of work they do both inside and outside the home, hobbies, how they like to spend their leisure time, and what plans they have for holidays or vacations. Serious topics may be discussed as well, so long as they have nothing to do with the illness.

The clinicians begin by introducing themselves. Then, they welcome the entire group and remind members of the format of future groups. For example, the clinician might begin in the following way:

> "This is our first meeting. We're going to be meeting every other week on Mondays from 7:00 to 8:30. We will be working together on solving problems to help prevent relapse and to design small steps toward greater social and job satisfaction."

The clinician continues by setting the agenda for this particular group. He or she might say:

> "Tonight we will be focusing on getting to know each other. Since we will be working together for a long time, we need to start to get to know each other. What we will do during this meeting is to go round the room and each of us will say something about ourselves. We will go one person at a time; everyone will have a turn. In case we run out of time, we can finish next week. It's normal under these circumstances to want to talk about the illness and the problems it presents. However, we want to ask you to hold that until the next group meeting. Tonight, we would like to talk more about the rest of life, about the good times and the things about you and your family of which you are proud. I would like to start by telling you about myself."

In telling something about her- or himself, the clinician needs to keep in mind that the families will closely follow the clinician's examples. It is therefore important that the clinician cover as many areas of life as possible, following the guidelines for the group. The aim is to present oneself as one wants to be known and hopes to be appreciated and respected. Sharing personal information may be a departure from the clinician's usual way of conducting groups. However, it is an essential part of this model, which relies on a collegial relationship between families and clinicians, and between members of the respective families. Clinicians often find it useful to rehearse with each other what they will say at this stage. (See also Chapter 6 on joining.)

For example, a clinician might say:

> "As I mentioned earlier, my name is Rosemary Hawkins. I am married and have two children. They are Danny, who is 3 years old, and Alice, who is 7. Alice is in second grade at Thompson Elementary. She really likes her teacher so far. My husband and I were worried about her reading at first, but now she's doing pretty well. Danny is in preschool three mornings a

week. I love to see the projects he brings home. Last week, it was a collage of colorful leaves to show what autumn looks like. He was very proud of it, and I must admit, so was I."

Or:

"I am a counselor and I work 20 hours a week, split between the hospital and the mental health clinic. When I'm not working—and when I have the time—I enjoy some of my hobbies. I like to cook, especially Italian recipes like lasagna and baked ziti. My husband and I both like to listen to music at home. We mostly like jazz, especially the Big Bands. We don't go to movies as much as we used to before the kids were born, but we do rent videos about once a week. The last video we saw was *Honey, I Shrunk the Kids!*, which made me laugh. We like to take the kids on short trips on the weekends to the zoo or that big new playground near town hall. There are two things I would like to do more of: reading and exercising. It seems like I never have time for those. But I'm signing up for an aerobics class next month down at the YMCA, so maybe that will help. The whole family is excited about Thanksgiving coming up. We always go to my parents' house; they live up in Longview. Everyone pitches in and helps with the cooking. I'll probably make the pies."

Then the clinician turns to the next person and continues around the circle, thanking each one after his or her contribution. The second clinician sits halfway round the circle and takes his or her turn in sequence, reinforcing the first clinician's modeling of sharing personal interests and life history.

Usually, group members follow the clinician's lead. However, the clinician needs to interrupt when: (1) a family member speaks for someone else, or (2) a family member follows the natural impulse to talk about the illness and its problems. The clinician can restate the purpose and format of this particular group. For example, the clinician might say:

"Right now I'd really like to hear about you."

Or:

"It's natural to want to talk about the illness and we'll be getting to that in the next group. For now, I'd like us to get to know each other. I think that in the long run, we'll all be more helpful to each other if we have a sense of each other's backgrounds and interests."

In situations in which a family member offers a minimal amount of information about him- or herself, the clinician asks questions to help the person give more details. The group will then get a fuller picture of each person's life. For example, the clinician may ask whether the person likes to watch TV (which shows?), read, follow the news, cook (what favorite recipes?), eat out (what restaurants?), listen to music, go to the movies (any recently that you liked?), follow sports (which teams?), do crafts, take walks (where?), belong to organizations (which one[s]?), go to church (where?), volunteer, or garden. If family members remain shy about speaking, the clinician can acknowledge the difficulty in talking in a group, while pointing out that with time and familiarity, talking usually gets easier. A patient or two may find saying anything at all overwhelming; the leaders simply acknowledge their presence in the group and invite them to join in later, or perhaps in a later group meeting. It is, indeed, an achievement for some people with schizophrenia simply to appear for a meeting, and that needs to be acknowledged, respected, and appreciated. Similarly, if some patients find it helpful to leave the meeting periodically, in order to regulate their experienced stress and symptoms, that is encouraged and facilitated. On the other hand, someone who leaves precipitously and unexpectedly should usually be followed, briefly assessed, and invited to return when they feel more comfortable, or, if that seems unlikely, to be allowed to return home and try again at the next session. Happily, these negative reactions to the first meetings are rare, but they can be disconcerting to novice group leaders. Participation by patients at any level is encouraged and welcomed, but failures to sustain full participation are accepted and not criticized. They are assumed to be caused by symptoms.

The group leaders should use a relatively low-key, matter-of-fact style in the first meeting. Given that this will be the patients' first experience of a multifamily group, it is important that the process be conducted in a benign, relatively warm and structured way. The aim is to avoid surprises and criticisms that might destabilize the patients and make families defensive. Thus, each person is heard equally and fully, except when that might interfere with another's comments. The pacing is relaxed and accepting, if a bit on the slow side, yet guided by an underlying agenda to include all participants on an equal basis. The principal techniques for shaping the process are validation and positive reinforcement. Occasionally, groups that have members with mood or substance abuse disorders will coalesce rapidly, with much conviviality and sharing in the first two sessions. We have found that this needs to be restrained somewhat, because it tends to provoke anxiety in other families and patients, and because sharing of some content will prove to be regretted later by its subject or other family members. These special situations only reinforce the need to structure the process in an orderly way and to emphasize not so much intimate details but, in the first session, strengths and accomplishments, and, in the second, personal reactions to the illness. If these kinds of overly intimate interactions can be anticipated, it is useful to mention that members need only share what they think others will view in a positive light. Untoward family historical information—criminal activity, addictions, incest, and so on—actually is of little help in problem solving and, if presently under control, is not especially pertinent.

The clinicians use opportunities to point out common interests in the group and to help the group members to see similarities among themselves. In particular, they emphasize themes that might begin to build cross-family relationships as means of building group cohesion and creating a positive, hopeful group milieu. There are also opportunities to highlight different approaches to things. These differences are defined as valuable and deserving of respect. In fact, they are one of the principal currencies of this approach: The diversity of ideas is the cornerstone of the success of problem solving in multifamily groups.

It is advisable to make explicit the rules of the group at the outset of the postworkshop phase. At a minimum, these include the following:

1. Attendance at each meeting is expected of all members of the family who have significant contact with the patient. The patient is expected to attend as much as possible but is not required to attend against his or her will, or when feeling vulnerable emotionally and/or symptomatically.
2. Families should attempt to share their difficulties openly when they see fit. There is no pressure on anyone to disclose anything that is thought to be inappropriate.
3. Material shared by any member of the group is to be treated as confidential by all other members of the group and its leaders.
4. Group members should feel free to interact with members of other families; this is encouraged and is the key to the effectiveness of the group. Comments or suggestions are to be taken as attempts to be helpful; no one is obliged to accept what is said.
5. No physical interaction will be allowed during the sessions. Participants should try to maintain emotional control. Interrupting others' comments is strongly discouraged.

6. Depending on the membership of the group, it may also be advisable to discourage attending the group while intoxicated.

These rules are described straightforwardly, with invitations for discussion, if desired.

This group meeting benefits from humor and a light touch. Since each clinician has joined with only half of the families present, he or she can use these individual presentations as an opportunity to get to know the rest of the families and patients in the group. The meeting ends with the clinicians' describing briefly the focus of the next meeting, explaining again why the groups will not focus on clinical problems for now, agreeing on a time and place, and thanking everyone for coming.

SECOND MEETING: "HOW SCHIZOPHRENIA HAS CHANGED OUR LIVES"

The clinicians have joined with patients and families, conducted a full-day educational workshop for the families, and have met with patients and families together in the first meeting of the multifamily group. The goal of the second meeting is to talk about how schizophrenia has affected everyone's lives. To continue the process of building a sense of trust and commitment among all group members, the second meeting has been designed to allow participants to share and explore the varieties of experiences that either having schizophrenia or having a relative with the disorder tends to exact. While the first meeting emphasizes the stronger qualities and people-as-people aspects of the participants, this meeting is intended to develop quickly a sense of a common experience that, although devastating and demoralizing, is nevertheless what is expected once this illness arises and begins to become chronic. This session is rarely uplifting in the usual sense, but to the extent that everyone comes to appreciate the source of their various miseries, there emerges a very strong group identity and sense of relief. This will be even stronger to the degree that family members have endured stigma and lingering guilt about imagined transgressions that may have caused the illness. This will be the first time that many family members will hear their ill relative share his or her inner experiences, past and present, and about the pain, humiliation, and terror that have accompanied symptoms and functional deterioration.

Both clinicians welcome members to the group as they arrive and direct them to the refreshments. To start the group, one clinician outlines the agenda for the meeting. He or she begins by saying:

> "I am happy to see everyone here tonight. Last week, we spent time beginning to get to know each other. Let's begin by chatting for about 15 minutes. That'll give us a way to catch up since the last meeting. Then, we'll talk about how the illness has affected each of our lives."

The clinician begins the socializing with a comment or question unrelated to the illness, such as the following:

> "I really enjoyed the Fall Festival this year. Did anyone else see the huge pumpkin exhibit?"

It is important to socialize for 15 minutes. The clinicians encourage participation by modeling, pointing out connections between people and topics, and asking questions. Talking on the side, interrupting, monopolizing the conversation, criticizing, complaining, and speaking for others are discouraged with positive, supporting, and redirecting remarks, such as these:

> "It's hard for me to hear when more than one person is talking."

Or:

> "That's interesting; I wonder if Mr. Smith has something to say about this."

Or:

> "Your wife says she thinks you're over the flu. How long were you sick?"

After socializing the clinicians move explicitly to the topic for this meeting. One of them might say:

> "As I mentioned earlier, we will talk tonight about how the illness has affected all of our lives. I'll start by telling you about my experience. Then, we'll invite each of you to tell us what your experience of this illness has been."

As in the first group, families and patients closely follow the clinicians' examples. It is helpful to share as much as possible about relevant professional and personal experiences. On the professional side, clinicians can describe how they became interested in the field, and how they have been affected by treating people with schizophrenia, including both frustrations and feelings of accomplishment. On the personal side, the clinicians may talk about any family members or friends who developed the illness or a patient with whom they were close. It is important to model talking about the feelings stirred up by these experiences, especially the feelings that family members commonly have but are reluctant to express. Examples of common feelings are anxiety, confusion, fear, guilt, embarrassment, frustration, anger, sadness, and mourning. It is also important to express some hope about new treatment approaches to schizophrenia, including family psychoeducation and multifamily groups. If clinicians feel uncomfortable talking about their own experience, it is useful to practice what they will say with a colleague. For example, a clinician might say:

> "My work is very much involved with the illness of schizophrenia. I have been a counselor at the hospital and the community mental health center for the past 5 years, and over half of my clients have this illness. I often work with them, trying to get the services they need, like medication, day programs or vocational programs, employment, and community residences. However, it can be frustrating, because there are not enough services available for the people who need them, and there is so much red tape involved. Before I worked here, I worked part-time in the emergency room at St. Joseph's Hospital. I think that's when I first became interested in helping people with schizophrenia. At first, I felt frightened of the symptoms I saw, but I soon learned that the patient was just as frightened and needed my help. I often felt guilty that I couldn't do more to really help. Since I started working with this approach, with families as well as the person with the illness, I have felt more optimistic.
>
> "From a more personal side, I have had the experience of a friend developing the illness. Gene and I were pretty good friends in high school. I remember feeling confused when he started being suspicious of everyone, including me. When his symptoms got much worse, he had to be hospitalized. I felt sad to see him so ill. I suppose this experience is one of the reasons that I started to work in the emergency room."

When the clinician finishes, she or he pauses, then turns to the person in the next chair. "How has it been for you? How has the illness affected your life?" The first clinician leads the process as people talk, going halfway round the circle. The second takes over leading the group, until everyone has had a chance to speak.

Some individuals may find it difficult to talk about their experiences. It can be helpful to ask persons questions about how things are different since the illness began, how the illness has affected their plans, and what they might be doing now if the illness had not developed. People can say as much or as little as they wish. After each account of an experience, the clinician thanks the group member for participating. He or she may point out that other group members have had similar experiences and responses. This group meeting may be the first time some families realize that they are not alone, and comments such as "I'm not the only one who went through this" may be voiced. The clinicians should support this theme by emphasizing how vital it is to share these devastating experiences with others who have had similar problems. Especially important is focusing on specific feelings that are nearly always expressed, including grief, confusion, guilt, stress, and concern about the fate of siblings and the ill member in the more distant future. At the same time, it is important to acknowledge feelings and experiences that are not shared but may equally be the result of the psychosis and disability that follow with schizophrenia. The theme can be explicitly developed as "Misery loves company" or some variation that fits the culture and apparent preferences of that group.

In comparison to the first group meeting, the tone of the second meeting is somber. The mood is usually one of sadness and mourning, with some anger and frustration expressed as well. Many patients and families take this opportunity to express dissatisfaction with the mental health system. If this happens, the clinicians validate the experiences that give rise to these feelings. It is important not to gloss over the reactions and to elicit concrete and specific details about group members' complaints. Of course, it is important to not let this discussion dominate the session. At the same time, it is common for family members to express sadness and even become tearful as they share these experiences. We have found that this process, though painful, deepens the involvement of the group members and tends to orient them to the value and function of the group. For patients, this experience is occasionally stressful, and their reactions may require delicate management and especially patience as they attempt to speak. On occasion, one or another member may fall silent, or even leave the room briefly.

Usually, that is all that is required, since even those with the most emotional reactions are also those who appreciate having the opportunity to share them with other, fellow sufferers. Again, it is valuable to have family members listen patiently and with interest to whatever their own ill member has to say about the illness, because it may be occurring in this clear and open way for the first time.

If group members begin to talk about specific problems that they want to solve immediately, the clinician helps them to return to the agenda of the meeting. The clinician might say:

"I can see that's a problem that's been bothering you a lot. We'll be working on solving specific problems starting in the next meeting, so I'd like you to keep that problem in mind. For now, though, let's talk more about how the illness has affected your life."

It is also appropriate to make a brief suggestion using a guideline or to offer to meet with someone after the meeting, or in the next day or so, perhaps with the psychiatrist, if it seems like a crisis.

It usually takes at least an hour for everyone to have an opportunity to speak. If time runs out, set aside a portion of the next group meeting to allow the rest of the members to tell about their experiences and feelings. At the end of the group meeting, the clinicians thank participants and acknowledge that everyone has had some very difficult experiences. If appropriate, they summarize the feelings and experiences shared by people in the group. It is important to acknowledge that expressing these feelings and describing such painful experiences can be unpleasant, but that it is also important for group members to put these experiences behind them as much as possible. It is helpful to emphasize that there is increasing hope with each passing year for treating and even preventing this illness, and that the members of the group will benefit from one of those developments, just by attending and participating in the group. The leaders also remind group members that during the next meeting, everyone will be working on solving problems similar to the ones raised in this meeting, and that previous groups have dealt with similar issues in surprising but successful ways, in just these types of sessions. However it is done, it is crucial to superimpose a sense of hope and a forward direction after these difficult conversations and send people home with a desire to continue or at least give the group a chance to help them.

Five to 10 minutes are set aside for socializing at the end of the group. The clinician might ask if people anticipate a difficult trip home or have special plans for the upcoming weekend, or if anyone is attending a local fair, performance, or special sports event.

GENERAL POINTS

Over time, experience has allowed us to see patterns of good and poor outcome arising from a number of lesser issues having to do with general techniques and approaches to conducting multifamily groups. We share here the most salient of those recommendations that apply to multifamily groups at any stage of development.

New Members

Entry into the group is a significant change for both new members and the group. Clinicians may find the following guidelines useful.

New members should have attended at least three joining meetings and an educational workshop before they join the group. Two or three new families enter the group at the same time whenever possible. The approach to the first session with new members is a condensed version of the first two sessions of the original group. When new members attend the group for the first time, the clinicians introduce themselves and ask others in the group briefly to do the same. In this meeting, members, new and old, are asked to share both general and illness-related aspects of their lives. The clinicians remind the group: "When we first met as a group, we all told a little about ourselves and our hobbies; the kinds of things we like to do, and what our interests are. It would also be helpful to hear how the illness [or hospitalization, crises, difficulties] has affected you." One clinician begins by telling something about him- or herself in a low-key and friendly manner. He or she then asks the new members to tell something about themselves briefly. The clinicians briefly review the format of the group (socializing, go-round, problem solving) and then start right in.

It is not unusual for persons with schizophrenia to require a lengthy period of recuperation before they begin to attend the multifamily group. For that reason, patients may join the group at any time, and they should be welcomed. Their first few sessions should be as comfortable and useful as possible. When a patient attends for the first time, the clinicians pay close attention to any cues suggesting discomfort or anxiety. Prompts should focus on areas that are known to be comfortable for the patient to discuss. The clinicians avoid making him or her the focus of attention, despite the temptation to lead off with clinical questions that may elicit defensiveness, such as the new member's medication compliance, substance abuse, or family disagreements. When it appears that a person is accommodating to the pace and tenor of the group, clinicians can ask him or her to join in problem solving and socializing in a more direct way. The go-round is a good place to inquire about how patients are feeling, what they are doing, and how they see the group and their own participation. Consistent with findings from expressed emotion research, the clinicians should use positive reinforcement and low-key validating comments in response to whatever the new patient is able to say.

Late-Arriving Members

When a group member consistently arrives late for a meeting, the clinicians acknowledge his or her arrival, state briefly the stage of the group, and turn their attention back to the group. The flow of the group is not interrupted. If the person arrives after the go-round, the clinicians check up on his or her concerns after the group meeting is over. It is usually a good idea to review the factors that keep patients from attending on time, if only to let them know that their tendency to arrive late disrupts the group and prevents everyone, them especially, from gaining maximum benefit from the multifamily group. Identifying legitimate barriers to attendance is also crucial, because, in many instances, the clinicians may be able to intercede and overcome these barriers. If they involve patients' employment resulting from the group's rehabilitative effort, procedures can be adjusted to accommodate a predictable late arrival.

Reminders about Attending

During the first 3 months of group meetings, it is a good idea to call all members ahead of time to remind them of the time and place for the meeting. In some settings, especially where families are facing poverty, discrimination, and community stress, reminders may need to be continued longer and, in some cases, indefinitely, simply because the members do not keep calendars and have many other crises impinging on their lives. We have seen many families that would never have attended without reminders, usually by telephone, the day of, or the day before, the meeting. Nevertheless, with such reminders, they attended regularly and made excellent progress. It has become clear that, in some instances, ensuring attendance is simply part of the leaders' responsibilities. The clinicians mention absent members in the transition from go-round to problem solving and share information that is appropriate, if the subject has not come up earlier. They follow up with absent members by calling them, telling them they were missed, and asking whether they need help to get to the next meeting. Clinicians also call absent members again, just before the next meeting, as a reminder. As the group becomes more cohesive and relationships begin to develop, much of the responsibility for following up, reminding, and even transporting members who have trouble attending can be assumed by the more capable and motivated members of the group. Clearly, this shift of responsibility must be arranged with some care, so as not to discourage those who extend themselves. However, we have been continually impressed with the generosity of participating families and the remarkable degree of camaraderie and solicitude that develops among multifamily group participants, which frequently translates into assistance and helpful advice at the interfamily level.

Crises and Emergencies

Threats of violence or suicide are dealt with immediately. The clinicians take charge and tell families what to do. In general, response to such emergencies is fully the responsibility of the clinicians and the available crisis services. However, as the group becomes more established and effective, its members can become increasingly useful as crisis intervenors, when the crises are less than life threatening. After the first 6 months or so, it is not uncommon for families to call each other to ask for advice. It is important to make sure that families are aware that they can also use the 24-hour access to group leaders as well, and that they are not calling other families' members because they cannot reach professional help or are reluctant to "bother" the family clinicians.

Communication and Interaction in the Group

A few general rules for communication within the group promote open and relaxed communication:

- The clinicians are careful not to speak for patients or family members.
- Whenever appropriate, families are encouraged to talk to other families as much as possible.

- The clinicians encourage the patients to participate, without pressing them to do so.
- The clinicians discourage all side conversations.
- Positive statements and requests for change in behavior are preferable to carping and criticizing.

SUMMARY

Before focusing more intensively on the clinical and rehabilitative issues facing persons with schizophrenia, it has proved nearly essential to conduct group sessions in which the emphasis is on the group members as people. In the first two or three sessions, the leaders use a structured social network engagement process that lays the foundation for later therapeutic work. The intent is that patients and their families will feel comfortable, supported, and attended to as people with strengths and potential for contributing to the effort to overcome mental illnesses in their own and each others' families. The risk in this approach is that some individuals at certain points may lose patience or fail to see the relevance of what is purposely a slow beginning. The leaders are launching a new social and community organization, which will provide support, ideas, opportunities, and a sense of belonging not only to those suffering from a dreaded mental illness but also to their families and, ultimately, to the clinicians themselves. We have found that care in developing the social and emotional ties among all the participants is crucial to eventual effectiveness and therefore highly relevant. The challenge for groups leaders is to develop sufficient confidence in the value of a social network, as a healing community, that this admittedly peripatetic method can be carried out with grace and efficacy. The ultimate goal is that patients and their families feel known and validated, hopeful that later meetings with these same people will indeed bring relief and a better life.

Chapter 9

Problem Solving in Multifamily Groups

A Psychoeducational Approach to Treatment and Rehabilitation

WILLIAM R. McFARLANE, SUSAN GINGERICH, SUSAN M. DEAKINS, EDWARD DUNNE, BONNIE T. HOREN, AND MARGARET NEWMARK

The structured, formalized problem-solving method presented here has been developed to capitalize on the biological and psychological knowledge about schizophrenia gained over recent years. It is built upon the unique supportive and creative capabilities of a group of families with various experiences of living with a major mental illness. By design, problem solving slows down the process of reaching a decision and planning for a new approach to a difficult dilemma, and is thereby better suited to deal with the sensitivity to pressure and the slower information-processing abilities of people with schizophrenia. Furthermore, these cognitive and psychophysiological vulnerabilities are sometimes shared by family members on a genetic basis. This method suits their tendencies and needs as well. The approach not only fosters input from each participant but also does not allow interruption. That combination facilitates the full development of a line of thought within a social setting, something that people with schizophrenia find particularly difficult. It is a social prosthesis, in that it achieves the following:

- It fosters concentration, by providing external cues and sequences.
- It reduces demands on short-term memory, by having all steps be explicit and written down.
- It provides an external framework for higher order executive cognition by delaying decision making until the possible options have been systematically evaluated.

It simplifies and makes sequential the problem-solving process, which for people with schizophrenia is usually slower and less effective because of prefrontal and limbic deficits, and their effects on higher order cognitive processes. After a few sessions, the process becomes a predictable ritual and is thereby reassuring and comforting to those participants for whom social interaction is anxiety-provoking. Because problems are broken down into their elements and each is considered with regard to its advantages and disadvantages, the process allows participants to forestall closure and to allow new options to develop. At the same time, it makes preferable cognitive methods explicit and overt, allowing patients to learn to internalize the technique and families to adopt the method for use outside the group.

Problem solving in multifamily groups prevents negative attitudes and previous experiences of failure from foreclosing other possible options. The diverse backgrounds and experiences of several families and their members greatly expand the available pool of ideas that can be brought to bear. Their ideas often are more adaptive than those of clinicians when the focus is on less clinical issues, because the group is drawing on the life experience of up to 20 people, many of them older and perhaps wiser than the patients or even many younger clinicians. The process capitalizes on the well-recognized ability to see counterproductive behavior and interaction in others, while not being able to see the same in oneself or one's family. The MFG encourages gentle and respectful observations about what might work better, without allowing them to be couched in directly critical comments. Rather, it fosters and encourages participants to make suggestions, rather than criticisms, and to direct these suggestions to the leaders, rather than to the involved family members, for inclusion in a list in which all suggestions are of equal value, at least at first presentation.

Problem solving in multifamily groups is a procedure that organizes participants' experience, valuing each person's possible contributions, and preventing premature closure before family members carefully plan a new approach. It stimulates brainstorming, while not allowing participants to criticize or dismiss anyone else's ideas. Then, it encourages the key participants to examine carefully and evaluate each option, and to make a considered judgment as to which idea or constellation of ideas and approaches they think might work for them. It allows any family member to veto an option that they find totally unacceptable but also encourages them to have an open mind and give at least one of these ideas a chance. That decision is then translated into an explicit, detailed plan, to be carried out over a short time period to assess its usefulness. It does so within the larger strategy of arranging an incremental and graduated approach to rehabilitation. Thus, ideas do not have to be brilliant, penetrating insights. Instead, they are good if they provide some alternative options for undertaking only the next step toward community integration, not necessarily the final and complete answer.

This approach is more specific and routinized than some therapies with which the reader may be familiar. By way of explanation, this approach was developed to achieve reliable results under a wide variety of circumstances, especially in clinics that serve severely ill people and are funded by public sources, therefore suffering shortages of staff, limited supervisory support, and inadequate physical facilities. Many alternative methods and techniques have been tried; this model has emerged from a process of trial and error. One implication of this process of development is that clinicians who set out to learn this model will find it advisable to use the approach as described, saving experiments with other methods for subsequent groups and later stages. In training and supervising even experienced clinicians, we have been impressed that major modifications of this approach have tended to be less successful, achieving poor outcomes or leading to higher dropout rates, or both. Thus, while we do not claim to have developed the most effective multifamily group model possible, this approach seems to be more effective than other methods that we and others have tested.

INTRODUCTION AND PREPARATION
FOR A GROUP SESSION

After the joining sessions, educational workshop, and first two meetings of the multifamily group, all remaining group meetings are centered around solving problems. The format of the 90-minute problem-solving group is the same each meeting, although the emphasis shifts from clinical issues and goals to social functioning and vocational rehabilitation as the group continues to meet. The format is as follows:

- Initial Socializing   (15 minutes)
- Go-round   (20 minutes)
- Selecting a Problem to Solve   (5 minutes)
- Solving the Problem   (45 minutes)
- Final Socializing   (5 minutes)

Each of these steps is discussed in detail in this chapter.

A meeting of the co-leaders 15 to 30 minutes before each group is advisable. They review several questions:

1. In what phase of recovery is each patient?
2. What problems and events are known or are likely to have occurred since the last group meeting?
3. What problem was used for problem-solving during the last group meeting, and what might be expected to have happened?
4. Which families have solved problems in the last several group meetings and which have not?
5. From present knowledge, on what problem would it be best to focus?
6. Are any absences expected?

In the beginning phase, it may be helpful for clinicians to plan a division of tasks, such as who will lead the socializing, the go-round, and the problem solving. These tasks are rotated, especially during the first 6 months of the group. The clinicians make sure that the room and equipment are prepared. They check the video equipment, if the session is being taped for supervision. Other equipment, such as chalkboard or conference pad, pencils and paper, copies of the Guidelines, and a worksheet with an outline of the problem-solving steps (see Appendix 9.1), is also useful. The clinicians round out the circle and bring chairs close enough so that people can communicate easily. Any extra chairs are removed. Clinicians sit across from each other during the meeting. Other recommendations include setting out refreshments, but caffeinated beverages should not be offered. Smoking is not allowed in the meeting room. Group members are told where smoking is allowed.

The clinicians make sure that the meeting will not be interrupted by such things as telephone calls or people walking through the room, except in emergencies. The session starts on time. Latecomers are greeted briefly by a clinician and told what has gone on up to that point; then, the group resumes the discussion from the point at which it was interrupted.

INITIAL SOCIALIZING

Every meeting starts with 15 minutes of social conversation, which underscores the collegial relationship among patients, family members, and clinicians. This random but upbeat and friendly socializing is intended to develop interpersonal relationships that will constitute a social network and expand the range of emotional and practical support available to each family and each patient. It helps people to relax with each other and to share the events that have taken place in the intervening period. That in turn helps families to continue to get know each other. It keeps the group and, we hope, its members from being totally problem-oriented. In addition, it allows group members to exercise social skills that may have atrophied as a consequence of the isolation that is so often a secondary effect of the illness. Clinicians can use this time to demonstrate their interest in the events of people's lives that have nothing to do with schizophrenia. This emphasis reinforces group members' sense of competence and mastery. The conversation can be light or serious, so long as there is a place for humor. For further discussion, please see Chapter 6.

At the beginning of each meeting during the first few months, one clinician reminds everyone of the agenda. Either clinician may begin the socializing section by saying something such as "Let's catch up on what's been going on in the last few weeks," and, if need be, takes the initiative in introducing a neutral but engaging topic of conversation. The content is kept light. The clinicians model the kind of small talk that they would like to hear from the group. Good openings include talk about holidays, weather, food, children, hobbies, movies, sports, TV, or local events. Complaints and criticisms about the patient are deflected, ignored, or reframed. The clinicians divert problem discussion by saying something like "We really want to hear about that, and we will get to it in the go-round stage in a few minutes. That's when we focus more on problem areas."

The clinicians attempt to balance participation among group members. It is ideal if everyone says something during socializing. Socializing works best when it is as natural as possible; that is, the clinicians do not ask members to go round in the circle, with each taking a turn. Members should be encouraged to participate but should not be pushed if they appear too uncomfortable. Also, one group member should not dominate this part of the session. Group members are encouraged to talk to each other directly and to respond in socially appropriate ways, without starting side conversations. The clinicians stop any side conversations and avoid being drawn into them. For example, the clinician may say, "Excuse me, I'd really like to hear what you're saying, but I can only hear one person at a time." The clinicians limit members' interrupting and speaking for others. For example, the clinician might say, "Can you hold that thought for just a minute?" or "Joe, your father says you think that's OK—does he read you correctly?"

The clinicians are careful to spend 15 minutes socializing and postpone talk about problem areas until the go-round stage. The socializing begins on time, regardless of late arrivals. The clinician is explicit when he or she is moving to the go-round section. The best transition from socialization to the go-round is to bring everyone up to date on members who are absent. Then, the clinician can say, "Now it is time to start the go-round section of the group. This is the time when we hear about problems and progress connected with the illness. That will allow us to focus on a problem or an opportunity for careful attention later."

THE GO-ROUND

This section of the group meeting has two goals: checking on the current concerns of each family about the illness, and selecting a single problem for the problem-solving section of the session. The families' concerns tend to fall into two areas:

1. Factors that might lead to relapse.
2. Issues that have to do with the next step in recovery.

The clinicians need to get enough information to determine the nature of each family's concern. Three to 4 minutes are allotted to each family, so that this section of the meeting takes no more than 20 to 25 minutes. Many clinicians learning this approach have found that to review each case effectively, but not exhaustively, in a few minutes is challenging. Eventually, it becomes manageable. The key is to stay focused on clinical assessment and evaluation of the family's immediate situation for indications of impending life events or unusual stresses.

The clinicians begin the go-round by turning to the family that solved a problem in the previous meeting. Family members are asked, "How did it go with the solution we settled on last time?" The clinicians briefly review the implementation steps and praise the family for its efforts. If the experimental solution or some other option tried by the family seems to have helped, the family is praised again. The clinicians thank all the group members for their participation in problem solving and point out any specific suggestions made by other families' members that contributed to a solution.

If the solution did not seem to help, the clinicians review the steps in greater detail, looking for factors they might have overlooked, such as reviewing life events or other demands on the family, taking on too much, or proceeding too quickly. When solutions don't work, family members tend to assume that it is their fault, that they have done something wrong. To counter this assumption, clinicians explicitly take responsibility for any failure of the solution. A possible statement might be "I'm sorry. I didn't realize that we were going too quickly for Sam" or "I forgot to take into account the employer's reaction when we were developing this solution." It is important to relieve the family of any burden associated with failure of a solution. Then, the clinicians may suggest an alternative solution to help the family to proceed in dealing with the situation. This suggestion may come from the list generated in the previous meeting, or it may arise from the review of the implementation steps. Occasionally, the problem can be addressed in the problem-solving phase of the group, so long as that does not preclude addressing a more critical issue in another family or passing over an individual family that has not had a problem addressed for several months.

After checking in with the first family, the clinicians move on to the next family. They inquire explicitly about specific areas of concern for that family, such as medication compliance, attendance at the day hospital, progress toward employment, and so on. Usually, there is a spokesperson for each family, but it is useful to check in briefly with all family members if time permits, especially the patient. As the group proceeds and patients improve, it is best to start the interview of each family with the patient. In the go-round, the clinician both looks for and inquires about evidence of prodromal signs, using the lists generated for each patient during the joining sessions. Clinicians also listen for any of the following changes or problems:

1. Safety in the home and community (e.g., smoking in bed, aggressive behaviors, suicidality).
2. Medication compliance.
3. Drug and alcohol abuse.
4. Life events (e.g., family celebrations, moving, deaths or other losses).
5. Outside agency events (e.g., changes in program, therapists, or financial aid).

6. Disagreement among family members.
7. Conflict with one of the Family Guidelines from the educational workshop (e.g., going too fast, expecting too much).

Frequently, families will spontaneously indicate the presence of an early warning sign without attaching significance to it. The clinicians must be sure to inquire further into the situation at this point, doing a brief clinical assessment and tracing the course of the sign or symptom. When a problem or change has been identified, the clinicians first acknowledge any feelings family members may have expressed, such as anxiety, satisfaction, discouragement, amusement, or frustration. Then, after all the families have had a chance to report, the clinicians briefly discuss each family's situation in turn. They have several options.

- Make a suggestion based on the appropriate biological information or Family Guidelines.
- Offer to intervene directly (e.g., change in medication, crisis intervention, rehabilitation services, residence, a single-family or individual session, etc.).
- Suggest that the family observe the situation and, if it continues, contact the clinician before the next meeting.
- Suggest that the situation might be used for problem solving at this meeting.

When clinicians decide not to work on a particular problem in the meeting, there are several options:

- Make a direct suggestion and ask the family to report on how that suggestion works at the next meeting.
- Offer to meet outside the group, if there is a crisis.
- Refer to any past solutions that may apply.
- Elicit, in more established groups, a previously successful solution from the other families.

If a patient is known to have difficulty with medication compliance or substance abuse, it is crucial that the clinicians ask him or her about it directly, if the information is not volunteered. Clinicians should not assume that all is well when the subject is not mentioned. The clinician might ask, for example, "John, how's the beer drinking been going the last 2 weeks?" and follow up with specific questions about when, where, with whom, how much, the effect (positive and negative), induced symptoms, medication taken that day, and so on.

In the following example of a go-round, the family who solved the problem in the previous group meeting has already taken its turn. Obviously, the dialogue is abbreviated.

CLINICIAN: How have things been with the routine in the past 2 weeks, Mr. Salinger?

MR. SALINGER: Well, it's the same old thing at our house. Norm is doing pretty well, except that he keeps sleeping late. He's in bed until 11:00 A.M. every morning. He seems to have no energy for anything . . . except the game shows on TV.

CLINICIAN: Is that right, Norm, you don't have much energy?

NORM SALINGER: Yeah. I just can't get out of bed any earlier than 11:00 A.M. I've really tried, but that's as good as I can do.

CLINICIAN: How long have you been home from the hospital?

NORM SALINGER: About 6 weeks now.

CLINICIAN: Well, that's pretty recent. It takes time to recover from an episode. It's a little like having a broken leg. Even after it's been set, you can't expect to go jogging right away. The brain is similar; it needs plenty of time to recuperate. It's a lot like recharging a battery—you can't rush the process without endangering a good outcome. Remember the guidelines "Go slow" and "Take one step at a time." It's common not to have much energy at this point. For now, do as much as is comfortable for you.

NORM SALINGER: Yeah, OK.

MR. SALINGER: I guess so.

CLINICIAN: I know it's frustrating at times. However, it's our experience that going slow pays off in the long run. Let's give it a try for a while longer. (pause) How are things with the job, Lisa?

LISA JACOBS: Pretty good, really. I feel like I'm ready for a new volunteer job. It gets pretty boring just stuffing envelopes.

CLINICIAN: How long have you been volunteering at that job?

LISA JACOBS: About 6 months. At first it was hard, but now it's too easy. I want something more interesting.

CLINICIAN: What does your supervisor tell you?

LISA JACOBS: I've been getting very good reports, right, Mom?

MRS. JACOBS: Yes, she's doing great. And she has been helping around the house. She seems to be doing much better.

CLINICIAN: That's nice to hear. So the question is, what is the next step? Lisa, if it's all right with you, I'll speak to the Volunteer Coordinator. I'll ask her about other possibilities for you right now. Would you like to meet with her and me?

LISA JACOBS: Yes, that sounds fine. I'd like that.

CLINICIAN: Good. . . . What's been happening at home the last 2 weeks, Mrs. Smith?

MRS. SMITH: We've been having a lot of trouble at our house. We're fighting almost every time we see each other or talk on the phone.

CLINICIAN: It sounds stressful for everyone. What are the arguments about?

MRS. SMITH: Mostly about our plans for the Christmas holiday. See, Bill doesn't want to come home from the community residence for the day. He says these family gatherings are boring. But getting together with relatives means so much to me.

CLINICIAN: How do you see it, Bill?

BILL SMITH: Well, it's not just that they're boring. These get-togethers make me very nervous. They ask me all kinds of questions that I just don't feel like answering.

MR. SMITH: When he was home these past two weekends, he was pacing in his room, too. I've been hearing him overhead.

BILL SMITH: So what?

CLINICIAN: Well, Bill, holidays are stressful for most people. If I remember correctly, pacing has been one of your early warning signs, one of the things that could signal another episode. It sounds like you're feeling a lot of stress and anxiety. This might be something to problem-solve tonight. Let's finish the go-round before we make that decision. OK?

MRS. SMITH: OK. We're so upset these days.

MR. SMITH: It can't hurt to talk about it, I guess.

CLINICIAN: And the Sullivan family. . . . Any changes since our last meeting?

DENNIS SULLIVAN: I don't like this medication the doctor has me on. It stinks.

CLINICIAN: What don't you like about the medication?

DENNIS SULLIVAN: My mouth is dry all the time. It feels like sandpaper. I'm thirsty, but I don't want to drink a lot of soda, because I'll gain weight.

CLINICIAN: That sounds unpleasant. Are you managing to take the medication regularly anyway?

DENNIS SULLIVAN: Yeah, but I feel like stopping.

MR. SULLIVAN: You'd better not. Remember what happened. I never want to go through that again.

CLINICIAN: Yes, the last hospitalization is upsetting to remember. Dennis, I'm glad that you're still taking the medication even though you're having some unpleasant side effects. Having a dry mouth is no fun. I think it would be helpful to talk with Dr. Anderson about your concerns. You and he may be able to work out a different combination of medications that will be more comfortable for you. In the meantime, I would suggest drinking lots of water, or those exercise drinks, and sucking on hard candies. They make some good sugar-free ones now that won't add pounds or harm your teeth. When do you think you could call Dr. Anderson?

DENNIS SULLIVAN: Maybe tomorrow afternoon.

CLINICIAN: Good. If you need any help getting through to his office, let me know.

DENNIS SULLIVAN: OK. I just want this dryness to go away.

CLINICIAN: I do, too. It often goes away with time. I'm sure that we're all glad to hear that you're staying on your medication even with the dry mouth problem.

SELECTING A PROBLEM TO SOLVE

The clinicians conclude the go-round by thanking everyone for letting them know how things have been going. They begin to discuss which problem needs to be worked on in this session. They confer openly in deciding which problem to solve. The selection of a problem usually takes just a few minutes. It is desirable to rotate the problem solving among the families, so that each family gets an opportunity to work on one of their own problems approximately every six meetings. All families benefit from the problem chosen, since they have struggled, or will struggle, with a similar problem themselves.

As mentioned in the preceding description of the go-round, the clinicians must be alert to two major areas of concern:

1. Factors leading to relapse.
2. Issues having to do with the next step of recovery.

The clinicians need to consider carefully any report of actual or potential exacerbation of symptoms. As mentioned earlier, areas of particular significance include the following:

1. Safety in the home.
2. Medication compliance.
3. Drugs and alcohol.
4. Life events.
5. Outside agency events.
6. Disagreement among family members.
7. Conflict with a Family Guideline.

The clinicians use their judgment when the group presents more than one problem that requires immediate attention. In order to decide which problem to work on, the clinicians ask detailed questions, such as how long the problem has existed, what has been tried so far, past consequences of similar situations, and time pressure for the problem to be solved. The scale of problems, at least in the first few months of the group, is also a factor in selecting the problem. Long-standing, complex, or previously intractable problems should be selected with caution and be addressed only if they can be broken down into more solvable subproblems (see "Solving Problems When There Is an Intractable Family Disagreement"). For instance, addiction to alcohol or drugs is rarely, if ever, addressed as a totality. Rather, first steps toward reducing consumption, easing burdens of the addiction on the family, or addressing one or another of the social or psychological drivers for the behavior can be selected. Here, the clear understanding is that a clinically satisfactory solution may take several steps, several different problem-solving sessions, and require considerable effort and patience to achieve. To build confidence and group cohesion, the leaders may strategically select somewhat simpler problems early in the group, so that the members learn the method, gain trust in each other and their collective capacity, and achieve a few successes. Clearly, problems that might alleviate the risk for relapse will have a high priority. As well, more critical and potentially dangerous situations will need to be addressed outside the group by the leaders and their clinical colleagues. That is preferable to tackling them in the group, failing, and leaving members feeling discouraged about their efforts. In the end, it is preferable that families and patients learn how to address problems using the problem-solving method rather than taking a chance on failing in an overly ambitious attempt.

There are other considerations to address at this phase of the group. First, when a patient or other family member attends the group for the first time, problem solving in the first session with that family is unadvisable. Second, the clinicians keep in mind the specific phase of recovery of each patient. As time goes by, they will notice a shift from problems related to symptom exacerbation to problems related to accomplishing the next step in the recovery process. Third, there may be a problem that a family does not wish to address in a particular meeting. They may be ready to do so at another meeting. This preference should be respected.

In the following example of how clinicians select a problem to solve in the group, the clinicians' names are Rosemary and Jack.

ROSEMARY: Let's review. Lisa, I'm going to call the Volunteer Coordinator and go over the possibilities with you next time we meet. Mr. Salinger, things are going pretty much as we would expect at this point in Norm's recovery. Hang in there. Going slow is one of the hardest things to do. Dennis, you're going to call Dr. Anderson tomorrow and let me know what he has to say. If I don't hear from you, I'll give you a call. In the meantime, try drinking lots of water and sucking on hard candy to help your dry mouth. And Mrs. Smith, we said we needed to spend more time talking about your Christmas plans. (*turning to the other clinician, Jack*) We need to decide which problem to work on tonight, Jack. What are your thoughts? I suggest we deal with the Smiths' situation.

JACK: Well, Lisa is getting ready to plan the next step at work, but that can be put off until we hear what the coordinator has to say. And Dennis is having a problem with side effects. His doctor may be able to help with that. Bill says he's nervous about Christmas, and Mr. Smith says he's worried about Bill's pacing. And pacing seems to be an early warning sign for you, Bill. This is especially important given that Christmas, with all its activity, is only 4 weeks away. So it seems reasonable to use this situation for problem solving today.

ROSEMARY: Is that all right with you, Bill, Mr. and Mrs. Smith? (*Bill and his parents nod.*) OK, everyone? These holidays are tough for all of us. To get started, we need a recorder. How about you, Mr. Salinger?

MR. SALINGER: OK.

ROSEMARY: Thanks.

SOLVING A PROBLEM

After the socializing, the go-round, and the selection of a problem or goal, the clinicians then lead the group in formal problem solving, using a six-step method based on organizational and business brainstorming methods and later adapted by Falloon and colleagues.[178] Forty-five minutes are allowed to complete this process in the group.

The goals and rationale of problem solving in a group will have been described to the family in the educational workshop and are reviewed at the third group meeting. The goal of formal problem solving in a multifamily group is to help families to use the biological information about schizophrenia and the guidelines that follow from this information. Using a structured approach follows directly from several Family Guidelines: go slow; keep things cool; set limits; keep it simple: and solve problems step-by-step. This model also draws on the experience of the other families, who contribute more ideas, options, and solutions than could one family and one clinician alone. An advantage of using this approach is that it breaks down problems into a manageable form, so that a solution can be implemented incrementally and, thereby, more successfully. Experiencing success in small steps gives families and patients a sense of momentum and hope that change is possible. Often, a small success will motivate families to continue applying the method to other aspects, eventually leading to a more wide-ranging and clinically significant effect. That is more likely to occur if everyone starts small and works up gradually and systematically to larger and more long-standing dilemmas.

To use formal problem solving, one clinician leads the group through the six steps. The other clinician ensures group participation, monitors the overall process, and suggests additional solutions. The clinicians choose someone to write down the six steps of the problem-solving process. This recorder can be a clinician, a family member, or a patient. The proceedings can be recorded on a chalkboard or a notepad, or both. The board has the advantage of being visible to all. The notepad of a preformatted worksheet, such as the one provided in Appendix 9.1, can be used to make copies as needed. In many clinical settings, the worksheet can itself serve as the medical record for that session and patient. Whichever method of recording is selected, both the clinicians and the family should have a copy to keep.

After a recorder is chosen, the clinicians carefully follow each step of formal problem solving:

- Step 1. Define the problem or goal. (Family and clinicians)
- Step 2. List all possible solutions. (All group members)
- Step 3. Discuss first advantages and then disadvantages of each in turn. (Family and clinicians, group members)
- Step 4. Choose the solution that best fits the situation. (Family)
- Step 5. Plan how to carry out this solution, in detail. (Family and clinicians)
- Step 6. Review implementation. (Clinicians)

Each step is important and will be covered here in detail. Both clinicians carefully track the process to make sure all the steps are completed and in the proper sequence.

Step 1. Define the Problem

The overall goal of this step is to narrow the definition of the problem or goal, so that it can lead to practical, concrete solutions. The clinicians return to the problem raised in the go-round. They gather information in order to reach a definition of the problem, usually in terms of the relevant biological information and the guidelines that apply. The clinicians question family members, gathering relevant recent historical, social–contextual, and clinical details. The clinicians ask additional questions about the situation from the perspective of how it relates to either relapse prevention or to the next step in the recovery process. When considering relapse prevention, it is important to review medication compliance, drug and alcohol use, life events, difficulties with agencies providing services, disagreement within the family and conflict, with a guideline. The definition of the problem must be one with which every family member present can agree. The more concrete and behavioral the definition, the more useful and focused will be the solution-generating and implementation-planning steps, and the more successful the overall outcome. It is very helpful to elicit each person's view of the problem and what he or she desires as an outcome, again, in behavioral and concrete terms.

The following questions, some of which may have been asked in the go-round, are often helpful:

- When did you first notice the problem?
- When does it occur?
- Is it related to biochemical factors, such as changes in medication or substance abuse?
- How often does it occur?
- Is it getting worse? At what rate?
- Does it occur with certain people or under certain conditions?
- Is it occurring more or less frequently than when it was first noted?
- Who is affected by the problem, and how?
- What has been tried to alleviate the problem in the past? What was helpful?
- With what activities does the problem interfere?

When considering the next step in the recovery process, the clinicians review the degree of symptoms, the present level of social or vocational activity, the patient's and family's goals, and characteristic reactions to higher levels of activity.

When a problem has been defined in a way that is acceptable to each member of the family, the clinician asks the recorder to write it down and read it back to the group. The following is an example of how a problem might be defined in a group meeting:

ROSEMARY: Mr. Smith, you said that you have been hearing Bill pacing in his room on his visits home. When did you first notice this pacing?

MR. SMITH: I think it was the weekend before last.

ROSEMARY: That would be about 10 days ago.

MR. SMITH: Yes. He comes home Saturday morning, and I first heard him pacing overhead two Saturdays ago.

ROSEMARY: How long did it last?

MR. SMITH: Oh, I'd say about 20 minutes, after dinner.

ROSEMARY: Did it happen again during that weekend?

MR. SMITH: Yes, on that Sunday, in the afternoon, I heard him, too. Then, the next weekend, it was about twice a day on Saturday and Sunday, and it lasted a little longer.

JACK: Is this how you remember it, Bill?

BILL SMITH: Yeah, I guess so.

MRS. SMITH: I noticed it, too.

JACK: Was anything else happening around the time of the pacing?

MRS. SMITH: I'll say. Every time we talked about Christmas, we ended up in an argument, and Bill went to his room mad.

MR. SMITH: Now that she says that, I remember it, too.

ROSEMARY: Bill, it sounds like you followed the guidelines and gave yourself some space. Good for you. Did any of you notice pacing at any other times?

MRS. SMITH: I think Bill paced once last Saturday, without an argument.

MR. SMITH: That's what I remember, too.

ROSEMARY: How about at your community residence? Do you pace there, Bill?

BILL SMITH: I don't pace there.

ROSEMARY: Before your last episode, pacing was one of the early warning signs. You also played loud music, didn't eat, and locked yourself in your room. Are any of these things happening now?

MR. SMITH: No, only the pacing.

JACK: Bill, what happens if someone asks you to stop pacing?

BILL SMITH: So far, no one has asked me to stop.

JACK: Are you having any experiences or thoughts that are unusual? In the past, for instance, you began to feel that people were against you.

BILL SMITH: Maybe a little.

ROSEMARY: Do these thoughts bother you?

BILL SMITH: Yeah, I guess so.

ROSEMARY: Can you give us an example?

BILL SMITH: (*pause*) Well, I think my parents might have some other reason for wanting me home for Christmas.

MR. SMITH: Oh, Bill. That's not so.

MRS. SMITH: How can you say that?

ROSEMARY: Hang on, folks. I just want to ask Bill a few more questions. Bill, have you been taking your medication and keeping your appointments?

BILL SMITH: (*hesitates*) Well, I missed my last appointment with Dr. Anderson.

ROSEMARY: When was it scheduled?

BILL SMITH: Last Wednesday.

ROSEMARY: How about medication?

BILL SMITH: Well, I forget sometimes lately, especially in the morning.

ROSEMARY: How many times have you missed a dose?

BILL SMITH: I don't know. A couple of times, I guess. Maybe four this week.

ROSEMARY: Thanks, Bill. This could be contributing to the situation. Jack, do you have any other questions?

JACK: No, I don't think so.

ROSEMARY: Then let's review the problem from what we know so far. Bill has been pacing in his room on weekend visits, starting about 10 days ago. At first, it was once a day for about 20 minutes, but more recently it's been twice a day. This pattern occurred before Bill's last relapse. This time, it seems to happen mostly after arguments and is not occurring at the community residence. He says he is bothered by thoughts about his family's intentions in wanting him at home for the holidays, which is itself a stressful time. Bill missed his last appointment with Dr. Anderson and about four doses of Prolixin. Have I skipped anything?

BILL SMITH: No.

MR. AND MRS. SMITH: I think that's it.

ROSEMARY: So we all agree that Bill is experiencing early warning signs now. Does that sound accurate to you, Jack?

JACK: Yes. There are two possible causes: Christmas and medication. I think we need to deal with the medication question first. Many times, stimulation like preparing for Christmas can be handled easily if medication is under control. I think the problem is how to help Bill reduce the early warning signs.

MR. SMITH: I guess that's what I'm most worried about now.

MRS. SMITH: Well, I can make sure he takes the medication.

BILL SMITH: I can take care of it myself.

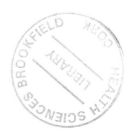

JACK: Good. Let's be sure those suggestions get on the list of possible solutions.

ROSEMARY: OK. Mr. Salinger, please write down the definition of the problem: "Helping Bill reduce early warning signs." Now, let's get the ideas of the family and the rest of the group about possible solutions to this problem.

Step 2. List All Possible Solutions

When the problem has been defined, the clinician asks the group members for suggestions. The object is to get ideas about how the problem might be solved, or how the goal might be achieved. The more possible solutions, the more likely there will be one that addresses the problem or goal well. This step is open to all members of the group, and it is desirable for each family to contribute a possible solution.

The clinicians might begin by saying

"Now that we have defined the problem or goal, let's hear from everyone in the group about possible solutions. This is a time for brainstorming. All ideas are taken seriously and recorded, even if a suggestion seems wild or a little silly; be as imaginative as possible. Then, we will discuss the advantages and disadvantages of each one."

At this time, the recorder is asked to write down each suggestion.

The following is a list of possible solutions that might be generated for the problem defined in Step 1, "Helping Bill to reduce early warning signs":

1. Call the doctor for an appointment.
2. Ignore the warning signs; they will go away by themselves.
3. Bill could stop going home on weekends.
4. Bill could take his medication as directed.
5. Everyone could stop urging him to be home for Christmas.
6. Bill should be told he's to come home for Christmas dinner, and that's final.
7. Mrs. Smith could supervise Bill's medication.

When group members are first learning this model, they may want to discuss the advantages and disadvantages as each suggestion is made. The clinicians need to delay this discussion until the list of solutions is complete. This is to forestall premature rejection of proposed solutions, which in itself inhibits the creativity of other group members. This process is most successful when all members of the group feel free to make any suggestions that come to mind, without censoring by themselves or any other group member. Furthermore, in more established groups, suggestions are more forthcoming and creative if they can be interspersed with humor and a even a degree of small talk, and if these comments are not critical or negating. It is especially important to remind more pessimistic family members to suspend judgment and see what the process yields, before they conclude that any particular suggestion is doomed or inadvisable. Studies have shown that the more participants are allowed to second-guess and criticize during this stage of the process, the fewer and less useful the suggestions. The clinician may say, "Thank you for your suggestion, and we will get to discussing the advantages and disadvantages in the next step. For now, we're focusing on gathering everyone's ideas."

The clinicians contribute their ideas without dominating this step. They should ensure that both sides of any disagreement are represented in the solutions list, so that all viewpoints on the situation will be discussed. The families themselves usually come up with the most creative solutions and the ones most likely to succeed. The families also benefit from helping each other in this step. When all the families have contributed suggestions—usually from 8 to 15 ideas—and when it seems that the most relevant solutions have been covered, the clinicians thank everyone for their contributions and move on to the next step.

Step 3. Discuss the Advantages and Disadvantages of Each Possible Solution

After the possible solutions have been listed, the clinicians move on to discuss first the advantages and then the disadvantages of each solution. The clinician asks the recorder to read each solution aloud, then asks the involved family and the group, "What are the main advantages of this solution?" After the advantages are recorded, the clinician then asks, "What are the disadvantages of this solution?" Advantages are always listed first, and there should be at least one advantage and at least one disadvantage for each solution.

For example, for the third solution ("Bill could stop going home on weekends") in Step 2, an advantage might be "There would be fewer chances for arguments" and a disadvantage might be "Bill would miss seeing his family." For the fifth solution, the advantage might be "Things would be calmer at home." Among the disadvantages, the clinician might add that disagreements are part of daily life, and it's too much to ask any family simply to stop disagreeing. We have learned that disagreements often subside when symptoms are under control. Also, notice that the clinician has redefined "arguing" as "disagreeing."

Sometimes group members want to stop the problem-solving process as soon as they discuss a solution that they feel has a strong advantage. The clinicians remind them that all suggestions will be discussed in turn before one is chosen, in case the best idea comes at the end of the list (which happens often). Sometimes group members may jump ahead to planning the implementation of a solution before it has been selected. The clinicians remind them that after a solution has been chosen, the group will focus in detail on how a solution can best be carried out.

Step 4. Choose the Best Solution

The clinician asks the recorder to read each solution aloud, including the principal advantages and disadvantages. Where the disadvantages strongly outweigh the advantages, the clinician consults the family and, if they agree, asks the recorder to cross off that solution. In addition, if any family member, especially the patient, is adamantly opposed to that particular item, he or she is allowed to exercise a categorical veto. After more discussion of the solutions, the family whose problem or goal is being worked on is asked which solution or combination of solutions suits family members best. Although the problem-solving process is done by the group, it is the family with the specific problem or goal that is most involved and will be carrying out the solution. For example, in the problem of helping Bill reduce early warning signs, the family felt most comfortable with a combination of solutions: "Call the doctor" and "Resume medication."

Step 5. Plan How to Carry Out a Solution

The clinicians help the group break down the solution into manageable, concrete, and specific steps. Once again, it is the family with the problem or goal that makes the final decisions. The family members are the ones who have the biggest investment in making the solution work, and they are usually the ones who take the most responsibility. However, group members can often be helpful in making reminder phone calls, giving rides, accompanying someone to an appointment, and providing names of helpful agencies or people.

The clinicians help the group to be as specific as possible in each step of implementation by asking questions such as "What needs to happen first?", "Who will be doing that step?", "When will that step happen?", "Where will people meet for that step?" The clinicians also help to troubleshoot things that might go wrong and formulate backup plans. When the steps of implementation have been specified as much as possible, the clinicians ask the recorder to read back the steps. The family and the clinicians both keep copies of the problem-solving worksheet. The clinicians thank everyone in the group for their hard work and help.

The following is an example of how the clinicians, Rosemary and Jack, might lead the group in planning to carry out the solution chosen for the Smith family's problem.

ROSEMARY: Mr. Salinger, you've been recording this process. Please read back the solutions that were chosen.

MR. SALINGER: It's a combination of solutions. One is for Bill to take medications as directed, and the other is to call the doctor for an appointment.

ROSEMARY: Thanks. Now, what needs to happen first to carry out the combination of solutions?

MR. SMITH: Bill needs to start taking his medication regularly again.

ROSEMARY: Yes, that's a good first step. Bill, do you think you could do that?

BILL SMITH: I don't know. I keep forgetting.

ROSEMARY: Would it help to have someone remind you?

BILL SMITH: Yeah. Maybe.

ROSEMARY: Who would you like to do that?

BILL SMITH: Well, my counselor, Anne, at the community residence is nice. I could ask her.

ROSEMARY: Good idea. When can you talk to her?

BILL SMITH: Tomorrow afternoon at the community meeting, I guess.

ROSEMARY: Good. How about on weekends?

BILL SMITH: My mom, I guess. But just don't nag me, Mom.

MRS. SMITH: I'll try. How about if I just mention it in the morning at breakfast?

BILL SMITH: Yeah. Quietly, just so I can hear.

MRS. SMITH: OK.

ROSEMARY: Sounds good. And I would like to call you, Bill, in a few days, to see if the reminders are helping you to remember. OK, Mr. Salinger, the first steps to write down are these:

1. Bill will ask Anne, tomorrow, to help him remember to take his medications at the residence.
2. Bill's mother will remind him quietly at breakfast on the weekends.
3. Rosemary will call Bill in 2–3 days to see how it's going with medications.

MR. SALINGER: OK. I'm writing those down.

JACK: What should happen next?

BILL SMITH: I suppose I should make an appointment with Dr. Anderson.

JACK: Sounds important. When can you do that?

BILL SMITH: Maybe tomorrow morning.

JACK: About what time?

BILL SMITH: Maybe after Men's Group at 10:00 A.M.

JACK: OK. Please add that step to the list, Mr. Salinger. What's next? (*silence*)

ROSEMARY: What happens if the situation gets worse before our next meeting?

BILL SMITH: What do you mean?

JACK: For instance, what if you start pacing more, Bill?

BILL SMITH: Well, maybe we should call someone.

ROSEMARY: I'd like you to call me. Remember, our treatment team is available 24 hours a day, 7 days a week. We want you to call.

BILL SMITH: OK.

JACK: Please write that down, Mr. Salinger, that Bill or Mr. Smith or Mrs. Smith will call Rosemary at any time if the situation gets worse. Can anyone think of any more steps that would be necessary? (*silence*)

ROSEMARY: OK. Thank you all for your participation. I think we've come up with a good plan. Mr. Salinger, would you read back the steps that were decided on and give a copy to the Smith family?

Step 6. Review Implementation.

In the go-round of the next group meeting, the clinicians ask how the implementation went. What steps did the family complete? What went well?

What did not go so well? The clinicians praise the family and any others involved for their efforts and point out any progress made. If relevant, the clinicians might suggest how to continue with the implementation, how to use a backup plan, or how to use an alternative solution. Sometimes the clinicians might suggest "taking a break" from working on the particular problem or goal. If it seems appropriate, it is important to ask the other families if the solution or any of the suggestions would be, or have been, useful and effective for them. If those types of indirect effects can be made explicit, it encourages all participants to see completed solutions as potentially applicable in similar situations in each family. Such generalizing will also alleviate any sense that a particular family is uniquely deficient because it is having that particular type of difficulty.

CLOSING WITH SOCIALIZING

After completing the problem-solving process, the group spends about 5 minutes socializing. The goal is to help people relax and think again about topics not related to the illness. The clinicians might say, "Everyone did a great job tonight. Now we'd like to spend the last 5 minutes just talking together. What are your plans for the weekend? Is anyone doing anything special after the group tonight?"

Time can pass very quickly in group meetings. It can be tempting to work on solving problems or achieving goals to the very last minute. It is extremely important, however, not to omit this socializing at the end. When group members end on a social note, they are more likely to return to the next meeting and want to work together again on problems.

GENERAL POINTS

Clinicians conducting these groups have found specific guidelines useful for leading MFGs over time.

Solving Problems When There Is an Intractable Family Disagreement

The behavioral approach to solving problems upon which this model is based depends on the family members coming to an agreement that (1) there is a problem, (2) they want help in looking for a solution, and

(3) they can, at least tentatively, agree on a definition as proposed by the group leaders. If these things do not happen and the family remains split, there is one alternative that has proved useful in allaying tensions and reducing the potential for stress to destabilize the family's ill member. This technique involves solving the secondary problems that follow from the existence of the disagreement itself. The underlying approach is to explore alternatives that might allow the family members at least to respectfully disagree, while not being manifestly and emotionally in constant conflict. At a deeper level, there are possibilities for paradoxical effects; that is, by discussing the things they might do to reduce tension, many families hear the conflict portrayed in stark and sometimes indefensible terms. This often becomes the view of other families' members, who will tend to empathize with the various positions being held but may also encourage the family to get past the conflict or let time work things out. As might be expected, the most common topics for such disagreements are those between the ill member and his or her parents regarding medication (non)compliance and substance abuse.

The procedure is not dramatically different. The leaders frame all positions as having credibility and validity given the vagaries of schizophrenia and its complex course and treatment. Age- and gender-related roles are validated as well. For instance, it is common for husbands and wives to disagree about the value of the patient, usually male, finding work as soon as possible. Each of the respective positions is related not only to common roles played by fathers and mothers throughout the society but also to the reality that this kind of disagreement is nearly universal in families in which a young adult member has a major mental disability. Empathy is expressed for the anxiety and pain that attends and drives each position. *The leaders should not make any attempt to adjudicate the conflict or to take sides.* Even members of other families are encouraged to not try to resolve the differences. Rather, the problem is defined as "How can the (disagreeing parties) deal with their disagreement such that feelings are not hurt and tensions do not provoke a relapse or deterioration?"

The rest of the procedure is similar to that in situations in which there is relative agreement. Ideas are encouraged, especially from individuals in the group who tend to be sympathetic to one or another of the positions. It is important to include suggestions, so that a balance is struck. For instance, around medication compliance, other patients may make suggestions sympathetic to the patient's struggles with side effects. The process needs to be carefully monitored and guided, so that there are not outbreaks of anger. What is being modeled here is the respectful and thoughtful approaches taken during conflict resolution and mediation: that all positions make sense within the cognitive framework and life experience of those holding particular positions and everyone is doing their best to help, but alternatives may simply work better. In the end, the underlying bias of this approach is that it is better to have a calm, stable, and, if possible, contented family than for one member to win out over the others.

The solutions proposed should address the consequences of the disagreement rather than the respective positions that generate the conflict. In many cases, this kind of definition promotes suggestions that have practical effects. For instance, ideas may include trying out variations on the respective positions, attempting a compromise, distancing interpersonally at times of marked stress (taking "time-outs"), or systematically noting, or even trying to alleviate, the consequences of the disagreement. Other families' suggestions can be remarkably helpful. Simple suggestions sometimes have alleviating effects on the degree of disagreement. These can include (1) talking about each position for no more than 5 minutes, (2) trying alternative approaches on different days or weeks, (3) having one member pretend to give in just to see the effect, and so on. Family Guidelines can be invoked, but only to the degree that they do not invalidate the position of any individual party in the disagreement. Judicious use of humor, especially from the other families' members, is often helpful in easing tension and making problem solving more productive.

It is important to allow the family members to comment on the suggestions in the "pros and cons" portion of the process. In the end, a plan should be developed that involves all family members, and an agreement reached that family members will try the plan in good faith until the next meeting. The results are often surprising. In many instances, by providing support and validation, one or another member has conceded, sometimes with positive clinical effects. For example, a patient agrees to try medication, provided it is a low dosage; or a father who agrees that his son is not quite ready to work supports a work trial period as his son's symptoms improve; or a young man agrees to drink no more than one beer per day, if his mother will not nag him about it.

Meetings with a Small Attendance

If at any one session the group is small, there will be time saved in the go-round. The extra time is spent on problem solving and, at the end of the group, socializing and planning for follow-up with absent families or members. In more mature groups, this can involve the families and their ill members contacting missing members and even paying a visit to those sidelined by illness.

Solving a Problem Shared by Most Families: "Generic Problem Solving"

In some groups it has proven useful to pose a problem shared by most or all families. This is more useful in the first month or two of the group's life, as practice in problem solving and as a means of developing group cohesion, confidence in the leaders, and experience with the methodology. It often generates interesting approaches to shared issues and also serves to avoid focusing on any one family or patient when group members or the leaders believe that they are not prepared for that intensity of focus. It needs to be said, however, that this is a far less effective method for addressing the real concerns of families and their ill members, simply because it does not lead to specific plans or means for testing them. Occasionally, more experienced and successful groups will use this method to develop strategies for improving the local mental health services. This can lead to a plan of action and advocacy that may even involve the patients. It is an effective technique; however, it may also occur when the members are avoiding seemingly intractable issues in one family or another.

Techniques for Longer Term Groups

After the group has been meeting for about 18 months, the clinicians usually arrange to meet on a monthly basis. By this time, the patients and families are usually prepared to deal with situations that emerge between meetings. The rate of change is slower at this point, an indication for less frequent meetings. As the group evolves over time, there is increasing value in spending more time on socializing as a rehabilitative analogue for competitive social situations in which the patients increasingly find themselves as they improve. In more recent work with individuals who enter the groups at the rehabilitation phase and achieve competitive employment, the groups have had meetings that are "purely" social outings, picnics and the like, specifically to help patients develop social skills that might transfer to the workplace. We have found that multifamily groups, composed as they are of people of two or three generations, different social classes and ethnic groups, cultures and background, are an excellent forum for developing and practicing free-form socializing. Because of the length of time that the groups persist, members develop an unusual degree of trust in their co-participants, which allows people with schizophrenia to extend themselves socially and interpersonally in ways that they find nearly impossible in a new and unfamiliar social context. Senior members of various families will nearly always take an interest in the ill members of another family, which helps the patients to feel sufficiently safe that they can begin to converse, tell jokes and stories, and generally interact in more normative and satisfying ways. In this process, a more challenging but relevant form of social skills training can take place.

Exits and Entrances of Group Leaders

Because these multifamily groups may continue meeting for unusually long periods of time, a leader may leave the group. Experience has shown that these departures tend to be emotionally difficult for some patients and family members. Often, the attachments that develop may be invisible and difficult to gauge, because so much emphasis is placed on problem solving and interfamily support. Nevertheless, group leaders should depart with preparation and careful attention to various members' emotional responses and even transferential reactions. Not to do so risks deterioration and even relapse in patients and dropout among family members.

Over time, a simple procedural approach has proven effective as a framework for ameliorating the effects of a clinician's departure. It requires identifying a replacement a few weeks in advance of the departure. Then, both the departing leader and his or her replacement are present for at least the last two, and if possible, three sessions before the departure. Across those sessions, the departing leader becomes less and less active, while the replacement leader begins to become more active. During the last session, the replacement leader is fully in charge, working with the co-leader, while the departing leader expresses appropriate sentiments and praise for the progress that members have made. It helps if he or she encourages everyone to continue participating. Often, group members will want to honor the departing staff person with a small celebration, and this should be encouraged. In essence, the goal is an emotional substitution of positive transferential feelings rather than a disruption and later necessity to rebuild new attachments. As simple as this approach may seem, it has largely alleviated untoward reactions to terminations by a clinician. Such problems do tend to occur when leaders' overlapping attendance proves impossible because of unforeseen circumstances.

SUMMARY

This chapter and Chapter 8 have described a method for conducting psychoeducational multifamily groups developed over the past two decades in clinical research studies, and now in widespread and routine application in the United States and overseas. The method proceeds through phases, addressing in turn the needs of persons with schizophrenia in the earliest days of an acute episode and in the later stages of reintegration into the ordinary life of the community and workplace. With appropriate modification across the course of that recovery, it serves as a remarkably cost-effective framework for carrying out treatment and rehabilitation, engaging several families and patients in not only supporting each other but also contributing materially to respective coping abilities. It is an individualized yet highly social method. In empirical studies, it appears to be effective across a broad cross-section of the affected population, although some patients fail to respond.

Although this approach may seem simplistic or overly rigid to many clinicians who have trained in the psychodynamic or family systems theoretical paradigms, in practice, it has proved to be flexible enough to meet the needs of most patients and their families, while not being so undefined as to risk being a clinical stressor in itself. In practice, the clinician should strive to strike an effective balance between stultifying rigidity and humorless adherence to a strict protocol and chaotic, unpredictable, anxiety-inducing formlessness and anarchy. Nearly every practitioner who has run a multifamily group has described the experience as enjoyable and deeply gratifying, especially as he or she has learned to find this balance in technique. As mentioned earlier, with experience and increasing comfort and confidence shown by group members, other technical modifications can be attempted. However, in the beginning stages of multifamily groups and for the novice practitioner, this predictable and intentionally practical method is surprisingly successful in achieving what most patients and families want: to become less symptomatic and be more capable of living life in the same manner as their peers.

APPENDIX 9.1. Worksheet for Solving Problems and Achieving Goals

STEP 1. WHAT IS THE PROBLEM/GOAL?

Talk about the problem/goal, listen carefully, ask questions, get everybody's opinion. Then, write down the exact problem/goal.

_____

_____

STEP 2. LIST ALL POSSIBLE SOLUTIONS.

Put down all ideas, even bad ones. Get everybody to come up with at least one possible solution. List the solutions without discussion at this stage.

1. _____
2. _____
3. _____
4. _____
5. _____
6. _____

STEP 3. DISCUSS EACH POSSIBLE SOLUTION.

Quickly go down the list of possible solutions and discuss the main advantages and disadvantages of each one.

STEP 4. CHOOSE THE "BEST" SOLUTION.

Choose the solution that can be carried out most easily to solve the problem.

_____

_____

STEP 5. PLAN HOW TO CARRY OUT THE BEST SOLUTION.

Determine the resources needed and major pitfalls to overcome. Practice difficult steps. Leave time for review.

Step 1. _____
Step 2. _____
Step 3. _____
Step 4. _____

STEP 6. REVIEW IMPLEMENTATION AND PRAISE ALL EFFORTS.

Focus on achievement first. Review the plan and revise as necessary.

From Falloon et al.[539] Copyright 1988 by The Guilford Press. Adapted by permission.

Part III

Applications in Other Disorders and Contexts

*Expanding the Range and Relevance
of Multifamily Group Treatment*

Chapter 10

Family-Aided Assertive Community Treatment

WILLIAM R. MCFARLANE AND SUSAN M. DEAKINS

RATIONALE AND BACKGROUND

In a comprehensive review and evaluation of the literature on treatment effects in schizophrenia, multifamily group, psychoeducational and behavioral family interventions, and assertive community treatment (ACT) were recently found to be the only psychosocial treatment models for which there is unequivocal evidence of efficacy.[109] This chapter describes how the two approaches have been integrated to yield Family-aided Assertive Community Treatment, or FACT.

ACT shares with the family intervention approaches its goal of improving community functioning and increasing community participation of persons with severe mental illness. Like family psychoeducation, it focuses on clinical goals and practical concerns, assuming that all but a very few individuals can live reasonably safe and satisfying lives outside institutions, but only with professional treatment, life skills training, and a full measure of social support from family and friends. Working in teams of 3 to 12, clinicians have on their caseloads a small number of patients (no more than 8–10) in the community, often after discharge from a hospital. The team helps them to learn community living skills by acquiring, relearning, and practicing those skills through actual experiences and placements in the community. Key elements of the model include outreach; in-home coach-

175

ing; tightly organized teamwork; proactive, highly individualized treatment and rehabilitation planning; on-the-job training; frequent contact and site-specific job preparation; and development.[324]

There have been several replications of the model, in rural settings,[325] in an inner city,[326] in mental health centers,[330] and as a statewide policy.[328] More recently, Test and her colleagues have been investigating effects of a refined version of this approach (Program of Assertive Community Treatment [PACT])[329] on young patients to determine if the early course of the illness might be altered. It has been remarkably successful in at least 11 published trials.[330, 331] The effects on rates of rehospitalization, daily functioning, and work adjustment were all significant when compared to traditional hospitalization. The rehabilitation effort in ACT has been shown to yield better job placement rates.[332] Increasing numbers of states have incorporated the approach into the range of services routinely provided. At the present time, it is far more widely disseminated than the family intervention approaches, in spite of dramatically higher costs and cost to benefit ratios.

Given their greater effectiveness, combining psychoeducational multi-family groups and ACT seems a promising, empirically supported approach. The combination extends the strategy inherent in both approaches of fostering maximum possible coordination between all of the key people and social forces that influence a given person with a major mental illness, which means assisting them to actualize their rehabilitative, educational, vocational, and social goals, while improving clinical and functional outcomes. The merger of these two treatment methodologies formally integrates the family as a partner in the ongoing treatment and rehabilitation work being conducted by the ACT clinicians. It combines the unique efficacies of each approach, potentially enhancing outcomes additively or perhaps synergistically.

In spite of the effectiveness of these treatment strategies in reducing relapse and enhancing community functioning, each contains a crucial limitation: ACT has not adequately addressed family participation in treatment, while the family approaches do not adequately deal with the needs of those with especially severe mental illness and additional personal factors that complicate treatment or even impede it altogether. Like the prevailing clinical methods of the time, the original ACT project (then termed Training in Community Living) emphasized "constructive separation" from the family in times of crisis.[333-335] This approach was based on the assumption that the family's interaction with its ill member may hinder crisis resolution and that continued family contact represents excessive dependence. In general, families were involved only on an ad hoc basis, when intervention was deemed necessary by the team. The clinicians promoted the almost-mandatory separation of the patient from his or her family following crisis episodes. Furthermore, patients were encouraged to live away from the family home and restrict their contact with family members, who usually were not included in the treatment effort. Early papers by Marx and colleagues, which set the stage for the ACT approach, refer extensively to the family literature of the 1950s, which emphasizes pathogenic characteristics of the family bond in schizophrenia.[333, 334] It is not surprising that the early ACT clinicians avoided engaging the family in treatment unless absolutely necessary. Patients who lived with their families were seen as suffering from pathological dependence, simply perpetuating the behavior that they had manifested toward the hospital.

Subsequent variations have been more pragmatic, supportive, and individualized.[331] Some replications have demonstrated that including families does not exacerbate patient symptoms and, in fact, may reduce family burden.[302, 336, 337] Some have provided crisis intervention, education and, in a few instances, guidance, occasional family therapy, and constructive separation intervention. More recently, Test's Wisconsin Group has made more of an effort to include family members. However, neither PACT nor any of the ACT replications currently include family interventions as part of their routine treatment approach. This is an important deficiency given the youthful age of typical community-based patients, the high probability of their living with family members, and the demonstrated beneficial effects of family psychoeducational intervention.

The argument for a weakness in the family approaches is based largely on our clinical research experience and is consistent with experience reported to us by other family clinical researchers. These methods rely heavily on alterations in family affect, behavior, and attitudes. When outcome is determined more by negative *patient* factors, family interaction, even if ideal, is less likely to affect the course of treatment positively. This is particularly evident regarding co-occurring substance abuse, personality disorders, poor prior employment achievement, or severely debilitating negative symptoms and cognitive deficits. Also, because the family models conform to an outpatient therapy profile, they rely on conventional substance abuse treatment programs, vocational rehabilitation services, and other ancillary services. If these are unavailable, ineffective, or refused by the patient, recovery and rehabilitation are much less likely to occur. Treatment noncompliance by the affected individual often prompts families to decline or leave family intervention, including multifamily groups. In addition, our work has shown that approximately 15% of those treated in multi-family groups suffer from repeated relapses and rehospitalizations that are likely to be preventable with assertive, proactive outreach intervention, as is routine in ACT. Additional positive effects on substance abuse and independent living through ACT-like interventions can be expected. Adding intensive case management capacity to multifamily groups should further reduce family burden through instrumental relief and create a broader, more heterogenous social network.

Given these considerations, we came to the conclusion that combining ACT and psychoeducational multifamily groups would lead to enhanced outcome compared to ACT or psychoeducation alone, because each compensates for crucial deficiencies in the other model. It seemed likely that these differences would be most evident when addressing such challenging issues as co-occurring substance abuse, noncompliance, or finding and retaining competitive employment. Furthermore, neither ACT nor single-family psychoeducation significantly expand the patient's or the family's social network, whereas a multifamily group, by definition, does exactly that, thereby adding an additional increment of efficacy.

Ultimately, the primary justification for FACT is that it fosters maximum possible coordination between all the important people and social forces that influence a given patient. It is all too easy for conflicts, contradictory treatment interventions, simple confusion, poor communication, and uncertainty to dominate the functioning of the patient's social network. Although both of the source treatment models in FACT espouse and create continuity of care, each has been somewhat deficient in bringing all the components of the patient's treatment under one coordinated system. FACT makes possible a broader array of interventions and supports, and can reduce the likelihood of contradictions and disagreements among those who are invested in the treatment and rehabilitation effort.

At the practical level, family members become collaborators by assisting providers in early crisis intervention, relapse prevention, and stepwise functional progression. The family is encouraged to expand its social network within the multifamily group by cross-family problem solving and emotional support, as well as out-of-group socializing. The overarching framework is that the patient's social support system (including families and ACT providers) becomes something of a task force, in which experts from various sectors of the patient's total network share knowledge, prior experiences, information, planning, and the creation of new ideas and options. The professional team's job is then to attempt to realize these possibilities. In this manner, all aspects of a patient's network are brought to bear in a coordinated fashion on the effort toward rehabilitation. Expanding that network through the connections established in the multifamily group can gain each patient access to a greatly expanded pool of potential opportunities and a larger set of resources with which to realize them. It is important that the integration into such services does not add to a family's level of burden. So while family members and friends are encouraged to gather information on job possibilities, all the actual work of job development, preparation, planning, coaching, and ongoing employment support is carried out in the field by members of the team.

This more intensive intervention is necessary when the individual has especially severe deficits in attention, concentration, higher order sequencing skills, planning capacities, social skills, arousal dyscontrol, or sensory gating. The same holds true in the presence of major substance abuse, personality disorder, persistent clinical deterioration, and resistance to involvement with the family and/or clinical treatment. The extra effort is also required when the goal becomes successful, long-term competitive employment. All these factors demand that a professional stay in close contact and teach skills in the context in which they need to be used. This means spending much more time with each patient than the psychoeducational approach provides. Because the family approaches all intend to reduce family burden, there is a limit to what can be asked of family members. So FACT expands the professional time and effort available, and puts those members of the team in the community to work closely with the affected individual. As can be expected from the broad range of deficits that require ACT, the needed kinds of community-based intervention vary widely, including training in living skills such as shopping, using public transportation, doing laundry, and cooking on one extreme, and, on the other, résumé writing, socializing on the job, and preparing tax forms. Throughout the process, daily delivery and supervised administration of medication is usually necessary.

In the presence of these complicating factors, it is more likely that family members will develop exasperation that can contribute to higher expressed emotion and negativity in their interaction with the patient. For that reason, intervention with *both* patient and family may be necessary and ethical as the means of reducing the tension level in the home. In these extreme situations, FACT is necessary above and beyond the effects of multifamily groups on family stability and well-being. Studies of expressed emotion have documented the negative effect of patient hostility and provocative behavior on family members' expressed emotion ratings.[248, 338] This self-perpetuating cycle is one of the indications for referral to a FACT program. Thus, intervention that improves the functioning of the patient will be expected over time to lower or prevent family members' anxiety, exasperation, and hostility, if present. That, in turn, will enhance patient clinical stability, and social and vocational functioning.

The enlarged social network is especially therapeutic when the family member is a socially isolated single parent who is attempting to support and protect a young, substance-abusing man with a psychotic disorder. Also, as will be seen in the later sections of this chapter, a larger network appears to be more effective when the goal is to enter the demanding arena of competitive employment. In addition, the larger social milieu is especially useful when the issues—high-risk behavior and entrance into the mainstream workforce—intersect more directly with stigma and the social barriers that still exist for patients and families. There is probably no group in which shame is more pervasive than in families of patients in whom substance abuse and mental illness co-occur. Similarly, entering the world of work often puts individuals face-to-face with the most glaring and rejecting forms of stigma. These young people and their families need the extra support of the multifamily group and the ACT team to feel empowered enough to stay the long course of treatment that is usually required. As we saw in Chapter 4, in FACT, patients with severe schizophrenic illnesses and at least one major complicating factor and their families experienced reduced isolation, less conflict, better coping, less perceived burden, and better work outcome over the course of treatment.

ASSERTIVE COMMUNITY TREATMENT: A BRIEF SYNOPSIS

Because the reader may be unfamiliar with specific features of ACT, we describe them here, dividing the model into its constituent elements for heuristic purposes and into aspects that, unique to FACT, deal with the specific features and applications of psychoeducational multifamily groups when led by members of a FACT team.

As it has been applied in most instances, ACT is a comprehensive, biopsychosocial intervention designed to improve the community functioning of those with severe mental illness, thereby diminishing their reliance on inpatient care, while improving quality of life. ACT, essentially a training program for living in the community, assumes that the vast majority of affected individuals can live satisfactorily outside institutions. The strategies are derived from PACT in Madison, Wisconsin. Because ACT has been well-studied and described over the last two decades, we provide only a brief synopsis here.[329, 339]

Integration of the Patient's Life into the Community

This approach, conceived as an alternative to hospitalization, provides the patient with a viable support system in the community. This calls for an assertive approach with considerable outreach and proactive monitoring, in which ACT staff function as direct providers of individualized therapeutic and rehabilitation services rather than as service brokers.

In Vivo Teaching of Coping and Problem-Solving Skills

In order to meet the demands of community life, patients must not only have adequate access to all material resources but also learn how to use them effectively. In addition, problems of daily living and vocational adjustment arise frequently and require an array of problem-solving skills. As much as possible, teaching these skills takes place *in vivo*, that is, side by side in the patients' natural settings.

Prevention of Relapse and Crisis Intervention.

Monitoring social stressors such as life events or transitions and responding immediately and assertively are essential for the prevention of relapse. This requires a proactive stance and an awareness of prodromal signs on the part of the treatment team. Medication management and monitoring are integral features of this approach and require close collaboration with the prescribing psychiatrist, who is usually a member of the ACT team. The team is available on a 24-hour basis to respond to client emergencies and is reachable by all concerned parties.

Graduated Increase in Patient Responsibilities

The ACT approach maintains a continuous rehabilitative stance in looking for opportunities to help the patient move in the direction of his or her established goals and independence. An assertive but graduated approach is maintained to support patients in their striving toward higher functional levels. However, we also recognize that precipitous and premature advances can contribute to the resurgence of prodromal symptoms and ultimately lead to a relapse. Therefore, an increase in support, advanced guidance for family and friends, careful preparation, and symptom monitoring accompany any significant increase in functional demands.

Support and Education of Community Members

Community members, especially the patient's family and employers, frequently react to patients' behavior in ways not supportive of community tenure. The goal of the FACT team is to aid these key community members by providing them with ongoing support and guidance.

Team Approach

FACT is provided by an interdisciplinary team whose members are known to all the team's clients and serve relatively interchangeable functions. It functions within a tightly organized, pragmatic and hierarchical structure, with an emphasis on goal-oriented treatment planning. Daily schedules and staff assignments are based on client needs and staff availability. The team reviews every case daily and does in-depth treatment planning once or twice weekly, focusing on individual cases.

WHEN ASSERTIVE COMMUNITY TREATMENT AND MULTIFAMILY GROUPS ARE COMBINED

The original intention in combining psychoeducational multifamily groups and ACT was to enhance outcomes by adding the clinical effects of each modality to those of the other. As we learned, in very high-risk, treatment-resistant populations, there appears to be a limit to the reduction in clinical morbidity that is possible with these methods and pharmacotherapy. However, there are additive effects for the family intervention in the functional domain, especially in employment, relief of family burdens, and improvement in family members' emotional well-being. What can account for these effects? The following section describes processes that occur, perhaps uniquely, in FACT when multifamily groups are conducted by a team that is also working intensively with the ill member of the family.

The most obvious effect is that all efforts, whether by professionals, family members, friends, or others in the community, can be coordinated. The multifamily group then functions as a clearinghouse for all the various actions taken by and on behalf of the person receiving services. It is crucial to ensure that contradictory directions are not being suggested to the patient by family, clinicians, and rehabilitation professionals. Especially for people with schizophrenia, contradictory instructions are destabilizing at best, and debilitating at worst. This coordination is especially valuable with individuals who have multiple diagnoses and personality disorders. Family members are commonly faced with wrenching dilemmas and need to act confidently in tense situations precipitated by patients' drug abuse, minor criminal activity, and lack of compliance with all forms of treatment. The multifamily group serves as a place to plan out what the family will do in these situations, and what the team will do as well. Even if an agreement is not reached, at least all parties are aware of what the others will tend to do. Just having clarity eliminates many of the effects of conflicting actions that are usually carried out without awareness of the others' actions, leaving the person with the illness to try to sort out what is happening. Given the cognitive and social skills deficits that are so common in schizophrenia, sorting it out is an overwhelming challenge for many patients. The alternative, which involves the team's routine and regular sharing of immediate and longer term next steps with the family, allows discussion and melds intentions and actions into a coherent plan.

At the more general level, the regular meetings of the group promote sharing of appropriate information of all types, in all directions—among patients, family members, and clinicians, across families, and even between groups. Over the three decades that multifamily groups have been in use, it has been noted repeatedly that patients speak more openly, honestly, and coherently that in individual therapy or single-family settings. Family members find that the presence of other families is conducive to more open communication. Multifamily group leaders often observe that they learn more from families about the life events that might trigger decompensation during friendly socializing than during more focused interviewing. Members of different families regularly share information about resources and opportunities in their communities, some of which may be unknown to clinicians or rehabilitators. This sharing of information is routine within natural networks and is one of the group's most valuable functions. Therapy modalities have rarely been defined as having this function. However, in situations with complicating factors, or when patients attempt to find and keep mainstream employment, the challenges are great enough that all available resources need to be known, exploited, and coordinated. This happens readily in a multifamily group but occurs with difficulty or not at all in other treatment or rehabilitation formats.

Information sharing and coordination make possible comprehensive treatment, which means that multiple interventions can occur simultaneously. For instance, while encouraging compliance with a substance abuse treatment program carried out by the FACT team, the family can bolster compliance, reduce availability of substances in the home, attend Al-Anon support groups, problem-solve in the group the practical aspects of treatment that threaten to derail the combined effort, and derive emotional support from other families in the group. Meanwhile, other ex-substance abusers in the group can reinforce the dangers of abuse and share the benefits of reducing their intake. While any of these interventions might fail when applied alone, the combination is often irresistible. Though the total effort expended is greater than would be applied in any of these interventions alone, no individual has to do any more than he or she would do in the single-intervention mode. Later, we discuss examples of the same comprehensive result when this approach is applied to vocational rehabilitation.

Especially for high-risk individuals, crisis intervention tends to be more successful, as a result of better reporting of prodromal symptoms. It is rare that a psychotic or substance-abuse relapse occurs completely by surprise in FACT. The team is in contact with each person at least twice a week. Families usually learn to alert the team to upcoming major life events in advance, so everyone is prepared. Stresses engendered by treatment and rehabilitation are anticipated by the team, the family is alerted to their effects and what to do to compensate, and the individual is educated about what his or her initial response may be to new challenges. Contact with family and friends can be increased as stresses loom or events impinge. Self-induced events, such as the resumption of substance abuse, romantic disappointments, minor criminal behavior, and episodes of violence, will need rapid responses. Because team members have ongoing and usually mutually supportive relationships, involving the family in crisis intervention starts at a different and more efficient level. All participants know and trust each other rather well, and know the basic guidelines for managing relapse. When families know that this kind of response will occur, they tend to stay much more calm, which in itself tends to reduce the risk of relapse. It is quite common for family members to reach out for assistance and support to other members of the multifamily group, which also tends to reduce the ambient anxiety surrounding the patient. With regard to the team, family members have repeatedly expressed gratitude that various team members respond as needed, with speed being the highest priority, rather than waiting until the primary clinician is available. For the family, the professional network is visible, present, and anything but an abstraction.

Compared to multifamily groups operating in a more conventional clinic or mental health center context, the FACT multifamily groups are free to be more purely supportive of family members. Of course, this fits with the severity of stresses that they generally face if the team is specializing in high-risk cases. Because many of the case management and treatment planning functions are carried out by team members in the course of their daily work, problem solving is more focused on generation of new ideas and incorporation of new information coming from the lay members of the group, rather than carrying out the proposed solutions. Implementation is a task usually assumed by the team. Although there is greater likelihood that families of high-risk cases will be disorganized or manifest more deeply rooted interactional problems, the supportive function of the group tends slowly to replace those interactional patterns with more functional transactions. This is almost impossible to carry out in ACT alone, unless the team clinicians are unusually well-trained and sensitive family therapists and can devote a considerable portion of their time to the effort. The groups especially help families that are isolated and/or enmeshed, by giving family members an opportunity to develop cross-family relationships gradually. These new relationships, though not necessarily deep friendships, tend to reduce anxiety and exasperation.

The FACT team, through its familiarity with the ill individual, can carry information back that tends to validate the person in the eyes of his or her family. The same occurs in interactions with the other families in the group. These validating interactions are particularly important in the two domains to which FACT has been applied to date: high-risk cases and vocational rehabilitation. In both these challenging situations, reinforcement of more functional behavior needs to occur in as many domains of life as possible. However, family members are often not in a position to see, or may be biased against seeing improvements. The team's and other families' reporting of improvements that do occur is a crucial factor in furthering functional improvements. An extension of this process is particularly therapeutic for individuals who attend the group regularly. The multifamily group experience is often a laboratory for relating to people who, though not members of the family, are concerned and empathic, and are not being paid to be so. That sense of validation and acceptance by nonprofessional, nonfamilial citizens often provides a person with the first experience of positive attention and regard since he or she became ill. It is invaluable in breaking the cycle of misbehavior and failure, and the resultant diminished self-esteem and loss of personal control.

Once these cross-family relationships have developed, there is a practical side. These relationships provide social contacts that can accelerate and facilitate the person's engagement in the community, but not with people that might offer drugs, criminal activity, and other complicating factors as the price for social acceptance. Rather, other family members and other patients in the groups can constitute a quasi-natural social network, with real activities outside the group contributing to rehabilitation and normalization. The normal sequence is reversed—emotional engagement precedes social engagement and out-of-group activities—but the outcome is similar—improved social skills and a sense of acceptance and belonging, as well as shared interests and entertainment. The team has a pool of contacts and relationships that can be used judiciously to foster social skills development and social rehabilitation. These contacts can have considerable value in providing links to social settings, jobs leads, or entertainment that are needed at critical times in the process of treatment and rehabilitation. Occasionally, they lead to community resources that are unknown, but should be known, to the team.

Problem solving in which families and team members combine their ideas often leads to more sophisticated solutions for the team to implement. Given that most teams are assigned difficult cases that have failed in previous treatment, the usual clinical approaches used by the team are highly likely to have been tried before and proven unacceptable or ineffective. The brainstorming that occurs in multifamily groups can generate options and new ideas that might not always occur to professional therapists. Sometimes these ideas can break a therapeutic impasse. The very process of attempting to find new approaches can signal to individual patients that there is still hope, and that they should have open minds and give the new options a reasonable try. Often, the fact that ill individuals can exert veto power shifts their motivation and breaks them out of oppositional or defiant behavior.

The psychoeducational approach takes the middle path between indefinite protection from demands and immediate, intense immersion in rehabilitation. The ACT approach more aggressively places people as rapidly as possible in natural settings and full-time community participation, and sometimes separates individuals from family or other objects of dependence. For reasons rooted in the psychobiology of schizophrenia, the FACT approach favors a more gradual pace, but with no less ambitious eventual goals. It is assumed that the treatment and rehabilitation process is capable of presenting stresses at least as formidable as those in life in the community. It is also assumed that the specific deficits in schizophrenia do allow patients to develop new skills and more demanding adaptations, if taken at a pace that permits mastery before new demands are made. This stepwise approach is well described in Anderson's writings and has been advanced as the preferable and natural course of community adaptation by Strauss[343] and by Sullivan and colleagues.[19] The method is no different than that described earlier, but it alters the strategies used by an ACT team in the rehabilitation phase. On the one hand, it uses a more psychobiological framework for deciding on the pacing of treatment and rehabilitation. On the other hand, the FACT model assumes that family and friends can speed rehabilitation, and make it more likely to succeed, when they work directly with involved professionals.

TREATMENT OF HIGH-RISK PATIENTS

FACT was developed specifically to address the poor outcomes observed in a small minority of individuals in the New York Family Psychoeducation in Schizophrenia Study, described in Chapter 4. The selected population included patients with schizophrenia and one of several additional complications, including noncompliance with drug treatment, frequent hospitalizations, substance abuse, criminal activity, unwanted pregnancies, and homelessness. We compared outcomes in ACT and only minimal family crisis intervention with FACT, in which multifamily groups and ACT were made available to all participants assigned to that cohort. Although improved clinical outcomes were expected and achieved, the principal result was a marked superiority in employment rates (see Chapter 4).

The family intervention component in high-risk cases need not be modified extensively when it is done by a full-scale, faithfully replicated ACT team. The groups should be smaller, averaging five rather than six cases. Two members of the team lead the groups, with families assigned on the basis of which team members have primary responsibility for the patient members. The format for the groups is as described in previous chapters.

The problems presented for solution are often formidable. In the study referenced, they included the following:

- How to keep the patient from stealing the family's material possessions to buy crack cocaine.
- How to prepare the ill member of the family to return home from a prison term.
- How to avoid contracting HIV in the course of intravenous drug use and promiscuous sexual activity.

On average, families were more disorganized and conflicted, and tended to miss sessions more frequently. Therefore, one of the differences between

FACT and ACT is that the team will need to expend more effort in reminding and even transporting some families to the multifamily groups. For
some families, the team clinicians will need to make frequent home visits,
both to reengage continually with members and to handle crises. Although
there were about the same number of engagement sessions, it became apparent that more single-family contact is required in the beginning and
throughout the treatment to involve key family members successfully.

The groups often focus on substance abuse. For that reason, problem
solving includes dealing more often with the consequences of a disagreement than in lower morbidity contexts. Usually, the family and the clinicians inherently agree about the need to reduce or eliminate drug and alcohol consumption, while the patient is usually uninterested, unconcerned,
and annoyed that the issue is even being discussed. The same holds for
most of the high-risk issues that make a case eligible for FACT. The usual
strategy is to work simultaneously on finding solutions in the multifamily
groups that reduce the conflict and tension about the issue, while focusing
the team's efforts on the primary behavior that stimulates the conflict. Family members can agree to make their strong desire for reducing intake
known in a nonprovocative manner, the group can explore ways in which
to avoid overt conflict, other group members can express concern, and former abusers can be encouraged to share their experiences and encourage
abstinence. Meanwhile, the team intervenes with the individual, using cognitive-behavioral, motivational, and/or self-help interventions on an individual basis outside the group and in the field. The other key parameter is
time. This method is effective but not immediately. It is not unusual in a
given case for the group to focus on substance abuse for over a year before
change occurs. On the other hand, we have found in case after case that
persistence brings the desired reward. In the large New York study, 36% of
the sample met DSM-III-R criteria for substance abuse disorder. After 2
years of intervention, there were no patients using clinically significant
quantities of drugs or alcohol in single- or multifamily cohorts, with the exception of those regularly using crack. Interestingly, change often occurs in
other family members with substance abuse diagnoses, even though their
use is not directly addressed or even openly acknowledged.

Family-Aided Assertive Community Treatment in Action:
A Case Example

The case of a 23-year-old man is presented to illustrate the interaction between psychoeducational multifamily group and ACT interventions. Mark,
as he is called for this purpose, was in the midst of his first episode when he

joined the FACT project. He had become assaultive toward his mother and sister, was disruptive by shouting in public, and had refused medication. Members of his family, while also opposed to medication, were at their wits' end when they applied for treatment. Less than a month following his intake into the study, Mark had threatened to kill his mother with a knife he had been concealing, convinced that he was part of a white supremacist group aiming to rid the country of communists. This led to his first and only hospitalization, for 2½ months, during which he was first given antipsychotic medication. He became less agitated and his psychosis remitted to the point that the family tolerated his return home. This acceptance was in part related to the family's beginning multifamily group meetings while Mark was still an inpatient. As stipulated by his mother, and reinforced by the FACT team and the multifamily group, a contract was negotiated for Mark's release that included monitoring his medication and his refraint from reading and ordering incendiary and weapons-oriented literature. When a mercenary magazine arrived in the mail 3 months later, Mark's mother reported this to the multifamily group and the ensuing problem solving enabled her to confront Mark about it for the first time and with positive results. During this time, FACT staff visited the client at home to assist with daily life skills and medication monitoring. Upon recommendation of the team, Mark began to attend a day treatment program and was shortly thereafter evaluated for a vocational rehabilitation program at a sheltered workshop. An initial placement in a shoe factory was not successful, and FACT staff assisted Mark in securing a part-time job with the sanitation department. The staff made regular visits to him at the job, later, when he returned to the sheltered workshop, and throughout a third work-trial with the Parks Department. By that time, Mark was assigned responsibility over his medication intake. His intermittent compliance raised his mother's concerns and prompted another problem-solving multifamily group session. A number of life events ensued, including a move and the death of an aunt, throughout which Mark and his mother received extra support from the multifamily group and the FACT team.

For the next year, Mark remained actively involved in vocational rehabilitation. Repeated family events required attention in the group, while Mark began to expand his social circle to include a number of substance abusers. He started to experiment with his prescribed medication and became overtly psychotic, requiring active psychiatric intervention. In spite of these setbacks, FACT staff continued to help him with job applications and two work-trials, one a state-run betting parlor, and the other a picture framing workshop. He worked on his résumé and prepared to enter longer term employment, which he eventually obtained.

FAMILY-AIDED ASSERTIVE COMMUNITY TREATMENT AS VOCATIONAL REHABILITATION

Prior Outcome Studies

We have seen in preceding chapters that family intervention promotes functional adaptation. Kopeikin and Goldstein,[170] Falloon,[341] Hogarty, Anderson, and colleagues,[342] and our research team[171, 186, 343] have reported high rates of community participation—in work rehabilitation, competitive work, or school—during or after family intervention, with trends favoring multifamily groups.[186] The absolute levels of employment outcomes have been modest—30–50% compared to the 90–95% rates for the general population—but they have been dramatically higher than these samples' previous levels, and clearly higher than expected rates.[229, 300] A stark contrast emerges when one examines what a person with a major psychotic disorder could expect from previous methods of vocational rehabilitation. Until recently no single study had reported a significant effect for competitive employment,[344] which remains the stated goal for most members of the affected population and their families.[345] Only about 10% have been successfully employed in mainstream jobs and occupations.[229, 344]

Newer approaches, including ACT[169, 329] and individual support and placement,[346] attempt to provide jobs in competitive, integrated settings, doing whatever is necessary to help a client to find and retain normative employment. These methods provide skills training in job interviews, assurances of reliable work activity to employers, on-site job coaching, and special positions suited to those with mental illness. Integration and close coordination of clinical treatment, support, and rehabilitation services are inherent and routine. These methods are individualized and do not involve congregating or segregating participants. Recent studies support their efficacy.[332, 341, 342, 347–349] On the negative side, these community-integration approaches, because of their greater costs, can only achieve cost-effectiveness by reducing service utilization and raising the ultimate earning power of the individuals served.

A Practical Application of Family-Aided Assertive Community Treatment: Toward Real Jobs and Career Development

The goal is straightforward: holding a meaningful job in the regular economy for an extended period. Most people who have been stabilized clinically desire to rejoin the workforce. The same hopes for their affected member persist in family members. While income is somewhat attractive as the end point for a job, for most, the depth of the desire to work can only be attributed to the social role played by work in contemporary postindustrial societies. Working defines a large part of the identity of most people who are free of mental disorder. The same is true for those who are afflicted. In surveys of consumers and families, assistance in getting a job is one of the highest priorities.[350, 351] The following describes how FACT is modified to achieve this often ambitious and highly prized aspiration, a decent job in the mainstream job market.

The groups are led by a clinician, usually a psychiatric social worker, psychiatric nurse, occupational therapist or psychologist, and an employment specialist, usually a rehabilitation counselor. The more experienced the clinician and the rehabilitation counselor, the better will be the outcome. It is assumed that a psychiatrist is closely affiliated with the group leaders, preferably as the team psychiatrist and the single physician, with medical/psychiatric responsibility for all of the patients in the group. The psychosocial treatment responsibility rests with the clinician/group leader and most, if not all, the vocational effort is provided by the employment specialist. Groups meet biweekly, then monthly after 12 to 18 months, for 1½ hours. Both clinical and vocational rehabilitation supervision should be available to the leaders.

The employment specialists have several specific tasks when the goal of most members of the group is finding work:

- Lead the Vocational Pathways sessions and groups, using a format developed by Balser and Harvey,[352] that establishes individualized vocational goals and plans for all participants.
- Work with each individual to identify potential employers and develop a plan to contact them.
- Develop jobs for the entire multifamily group cohort.
- Find cooperative potential employers.
- Coach participants on and off the job site in the initial month or two of employment, or longer if necessary.
- Provide technical assistance as clinical teammates assume the job-coaching function.
- Assess work-readiness, assist participants to prepare resumes and practice interviewing skills.

The groups are larger, usually starting with seven or eight cases, in order to enlarge the pool of ideas and resources that might produce both job leads and social support after jobs have been found and taken. The groups are also larger because there is more focus on everyday experience during problem solving; that is, the more people that are involved, the greater the chance for diversity of experience, the broader the cross-section of the community represented in the group, and the greater the chance for success in finding jobs. Clearly, groups are assembled on the basis of persons' having some interest in working. Those who emphatically do not want to work tend to retard the progress in the groups and may eventually drop out as more people become employed.

The specific modifications include special adaptations of engagement, family education, early sessions, and the ongoing group format. Work with the family begins with a minimum of three joining sessions, in which the patient's primary clinician or rehabilitation counselor meets with the family. One session is held with family members alone, one with the patient, and all others are left to clinical judgment, usually determined on the basis of the degree of symptom recovery and family harmony. There is at least one separate meeting with the patient to assess and begin to address vocational preferences, key clinical issues, and any vocational issues that can be dealt with before starting the treatment.

The responsible employment specialist also begins a goal-setting and evaluation process with the person with the illness. In carrying out rehabilitation, the essential starting point is goal setting, with the patient as the central focus. For both philosophical and practical reasons, patients' perceived desire for their vocational and social lives is the nucleus of work done by both the FACT team and the families in the multifamily group. Thus, the first, crucial step is getting a sense of the patient's previous work history and his or her interests in starting employment, continuing a career already started, or changing career directions.

Simultaneous with the engagement sessions, the cohort of patients due to join the multifamily group meets together for nine sessions, beginning in tandem with the engagement sessions for families. In these class-like meetings, the team teaches the patients how to set a goal, decide on the steps necessary for its achievement, and deal with barriers that might impede success. When all of the families have completed the joining process, the FACT team conducts the educational workshop, usually with invited patients attending. In this presentation, we also closely follow Anderson's format except that there are additional guidelines and other components specifically geared to the vocational rehabilitation phase. In particular, the employment specialists present the general outline for finding and keeping jobs, discuss job development and coaching, and describe the stresses that may be encountered, as well as the methods commonly used to overcome them.

Following the educational workshop, the first meeting of the ongoing psychoeducational multifamily group has a special format. Patients are strongly encouraged to attend and actively participate. The first session's structure is similar to that described in Chapter 8. However, the topic is "What work have I done and what work would I like to do in the future?" All group members comment on the topic in whatever way they see fit. The second session addresses the barriers that people have experienced in achieving their hopes in the world of work. In particular, patients and family members are invited to comment on the role that mental illness has played in frustrating those desires. The intent is that the theme of work is set as the dominant focus from the very beginning. Discussing hopes, achievements, and impediments imposed by the illness is designed to emphasize the commonality of these issues across all families and between well and ill members within families. The leaders should share their own personal and professional experiences as workers to facilitate the discussion and set the stage for equal participation in the problem-solving process to follow.

In the meetings following the introductory sessions, the multifamily group has as its goal to help ill members secure and keep jobs that they want and find meaningful. The group achieves employment for its members largely by using the group-based problem-solving method described in Chapter 9. Families are taught to use this method as a group function and are encouraged to use it outside the group in a single-family format, without a professional leader. It is the core of the approach, one that has been especially effective when the issues faced by the individuals seeking employment are less clinical and more similar to those faced by all citizens, both employed and unemployed.

The first phase concentrates on problems experienced by the future employee as he or she begins to reenter the world outside the protection of inpatient or partial hospitalization. A central goal during this phase is prevention of relapse, achieved by limiting functional expectations and demands, and reducing the level of stimulation and stress in the social environment. The rehabilitation phase in FACT should be initiated only by patients who have achieved clinical stability by successfully completing the community reentry phase. However, if patients have been clinically stable for over 6 months prior to entering the multifamily group, the reentry phase is accelerated in proportion to the time the person has been stable and the degree to which both positive and negative symptoms are in remission. In determining readiness, positive symptoms are clearly indicative of heightened vulnerability to stress, but in their absence, negative symptoms are used as a measure of degree of recovery from past episodes. If negative symptoms are not only severe but also very persistent over 12 months or more, rehabilitation can be undertaken as soon as the relationships with staff and other families in the group have been comfortably established. However, the steps taken into the workforce will need to be smaller and slower than those for individuals without such high levels of negative symptoms.

In the employment-directed version of FACT, a major goal of psycho-educational multifamily groups is to lower stress in the home and other social settings. An optimal home environment permits patients to tolerate greater stresses in their employment environment without relapse or job loss. Families need to compensate for those stresses by creating an unusually calm and protective milieu at home. Most family members can understand and implement this concept; they contribute to the effort enthusiastically. Because many families are highly motivated to see their ill relative work, they are more likely to adopt the specific stress-reduction strategies advised by the group leaders. It is also common for families to encourage the group leaders, who are also the job developers and job coaches, to pursue work goals in behalf of the ill family member.

As stability increases, the psychoeducational multifamily group in FACT functions in a role unique among psychosocial rehabilitation models: It operates as an auxiliary to the *in vivo* vocational rehabilitation effort being conducted by the clinical team. In an informal way, it becomes an employment agency. The central emphasis during this phase is the involvement of the family and the group in helping each patient gradually, step-by-step to resume responsibility and socializing. The clinicians continue to use the group-based, problem-solving/brainstorming approach to identify and develop jobs, and to help individual patients obtain job placement and enrich their social lives.

This process often involves some reduction or postponement of previously held vocational goals. Those goals are often held as strongly by family members as by the patients themselves. Therefore, the outcomes of the goal-setting classes are reported to the multifamily group. This occurs systematically during the early phase, when the Vocational Pathways component is nearing completion. This allows each family to express doubts, reservations, and opinions, as well as support, so that the final result of goal setting has been discussed and ratified by the patient's own family in the public arena of the multifamily group. Reconciliation of goals and disagreements about work among family members is crucial to alleviating the ambivalence held by many of those who have been out of the workforce for long periods. Furthermore, the other families in the group are aware of each patient's intentions, making vocational success the project of the entire group. Once success occurs, it helps to define a positive group identity. Reciprocally, the family's or other families' ideas, opinions, and information can be taken back to the goal-setting process or to individual sessions with the employment specialist and be incorporated into the rehabilitation plan.

After the group completes the goal-setting phase, a group meeting is devoted to developing a list of possible job opportunities derived from the members of the group, their extended kin, and friends and associates. Potential jobs may be located in the homes or businesses of group members, in those of relatives and friends outside the group, or in those of their kin or friends. In this way, potential jobs may be with members of other families in the multifamily group and/or within their extended networks. Jobs may also be identified that are known to group members by simple informal connections, through chance encounters (e.g., seeing "Help Wanted" signs), or through deliberate inquiry and community advocacy. Ultimately, families, in collaboration with the team and local family advocacy associations (such as chapters of the National Alliance for the Mentally Ill), may create jobs for the patients through community action. In general, jobs developing out of the multifamily group are potentially less stressful, because they are embedded within the social network of the group and involve social connections that are inherently more familiar to the patients. To a large degree, we modeled this approach after the usual methods—involving networks and personal connections—that are normally used to get a job or to ferret out job leads.[132, 146, 266, 353, 354] Family members may be asked to gather additional information on these possibilities between meetings, but final implementation (i.e., actual job development and placement) is usually carried out by the team clinicians.

This general process is continued in another form, and with another focus, after job opportunities have been identified. The vocational or social rehabilitation process for each patient is broken into steps that are attempted sequentially. The achievement of the next step toward employment is raised as a focus in the problem-solving portion of the group, focusing now on specific individuals. Other common problems or topics include specific barriers to employment, social anxieties and/or rejection on the job, and reasonable accommodations that might improve work performance. The members of the group and their extended kin are polled as a source of ideas to overcome barriers to employment and to obtain, if needed, alternative jobs leads, with specific reference to one particular patient in the group. In this brainstorming process, various ideas are generated by participants in the multifamily group. These suggestions are then reviewed by the patient and his or her family, after which a final plan is developed. This nearly always involves aspects of job preparation, job development, coaching, planning, and problem solving, all carried out in the field by the FACT team. The results of these efforts are then reported back during the team's rounds and/or treatment planning, *and* during the initial reporting-in portion of the next multifamily group. If necessary, the process is repeated if initial results were disappointing.

Case Example of Family-Aided Assertive Community Treatment as Vocational Rehabilitation

A recent case illustrates the interaction between an employment specialist working directly with the person and the multifamily group. Joan is a middle-class woman in her 30s with schizophrenia and a severe anxiety disorder. As she entered the work world, she wanted a job oriented toward helping others but did not want to work within the mental health system. She thought that she would do better working with the elderly. The employment specialist and Joan worked on the application to a nursing home for a part-time receptionist position that involved working weekends and as backup for the other staff at the home. The initial difficulty Joan encountered was a somewhat complex, seven-line telephone system, which she operated while she greeted visitors, sorted mail, photocopied, and completed a number of incidental office tasks. The employment specialist and Joan developed a log sheet and a simple system that allowed her to manage the telephone calls.

Once on the job, however, Joan encountered a more serious problem. She tended to develop extreme anxiety whenever she became bored. Even worse, she would sweat profusely and, by the end of the day, often appear rather unkempt. The occupational therapist visited Joan at her home to organize her clothing. Also, Joan's mother made several jumpers for her that were easy to care for and looked more professional. However, Joan's tendency to become panicky when she became bored persisted. This situation was brought to the multifamily group for problem-solving. In the group, the problem was framed as "How can Joan control her anxiety on the job, especially when she becomes bored?" In the group, the other members helped Joan to develop a list of "Anxiety Busters" that she could use to control her anxiety: "This too shall pass," "Do one thing at a time," and so on.

As she continued to apply these simple solutions, Joan gained confidence on the job. She was able to keep it long enough to allow her to explore carefully other job possibilities with more regular hours. Although Joan initially received one-on-one job coaching, presently she uses only the multifamily group and occasional visits with the employment specialist as supports needed to maintain her job and pursue other career options.

SUMMARY

In an effort to capitalize on the specific advantages and efficacies of ACT, multifamily groups, and family psychoeducation, and to eliminate their most salient deficiencies, we have combined them in a more comprehensive treatment system, Family-aided Assertive Community Treatment (FACT). Throughout the treatment, the aim is that the psychoeducational multifamily group become a clinical–rehabilitative task force, in which professionals, patients, family, and friends share experiences, information, planning, and the creation of new ideas and options, especially in the difficult area of vocational rehabilitation. The professional team's job is then to take these possibilities and make them real. The assumptions are that all aspects of the patient's network should be brought to bear on the effort toward community adaptation and employment, and that expanding that network through the quasi-natural connections in a multifamily group can gain for each patient access to a greatly expanded pool of emotional and social support, potential jobs, and social opportunities. This total process is the major factor contributing to the higher employment rates achieved in our experimental outcome trials of the FACT approach.

Chapter 11

Training Staff of Supportive Housing Programs in Principles and Practices of Psychoeducation

Creating a Family-Like Social Environment

BONNIE T. HOREN AND JULES M. RANZ

In the aftermath of the early phases of deinstitutionalization, those adults with schizophrenia who cannot live alone or with their families begin living in a variety of supportive housing situations. In these arrangements, staff provide support, either on a 24-hour basis, in which case the term "supervised residence" is often used, or as regular (once or more per week) visitors to the client's home, usually called "supported housing." As this type of housing unfolds, the relationship between staff expectations and client outcome come under scrutiny. In an article that set the early tone of that debate, Lamb and Goertzel[355] compared a low-expectations boarding home to a rehabilitation-oriented halfway house. The residents of the high-expectations halfway house achieved higher instrumental performance levels. They spent more time out of the hospital, although they did suffer a higher hospitalization rate. The authors concluded that the low-expectations environment provided insufficient stimulation and a resultant poor quality of life for its residents. In 1978, Carpenter[356] reviewed the literature on supervised residences and reported a growing concern that low-expectations environments were creating back wards in the community.

In the 1980s, however, studies on environmental factors in supportive housing programs[357-359] began reporting that too much stimulation can increase the danger of relapse. Cournos[360] reviewed these studies in 1987, and concluded that a delicate balance must be struck in residential settings between placing too many and too few demands on adults with severe mental illness. She commented that highly confrontational and controlling environments are counterproductive to the slow and steady rehabilitation needed by these adults with severe mental illness. Segal and Holschuh[361] reported that residences that provide supportive approaches foster the development of social networks more effectively than those that utilize high-expectation approaches. These articles suggest that the development of more carefully paced, supportive approaches for housing staff are needed. In this chapter, the term "supportive housing" refers to both supervised residences and supported housing.

The psychoeducational model, developed specifically for adults with schizophrenia and their families, is an approach well suited to meet this need. As developed by Anderson and colleagues,[108] the model is derived from two bodies of research: expressed emotion (EE) studies and attention-arousal studies. The latter studies have suggested that schizophrenia is an illness characterized by arousal dyscontrol (i.e., limited tolerance for intensity, negativity, complexity, and relationship disruption), while the EE studies indicate that there are optimal social environments for schizophrenia. These include social interactions that are calm, benign, flexible, and relatively simple, with known social structure and behavioral limits. Rules and guidelines for behavior need to be appropriate to the severity and phase of illness, with major emphasis on the gradual redevelopment and day-to-day use of social and vocational skills. In addition, carefully controlled performance expectations and a high degree of predictability are important parameters. Weinberger has emphasized the need for social interventions that accommodate underlying brain dysfunctions.[60] Finally, introduction of current research and clinical knowledge about psychiatric medication and ongoing medication monitoring is an integral feature of the psychoeducational approach.[108]

Previous clinical trials of psychoeducation have been predominantly carried out with adults with schizophrenia and their families. McFarlane and Dunne[362] reviewed the results of numerous studies, noting an impressive average reduction in yearly relapse rate across studies, from 47.5% for individual supportive therapy to 11.5% for family intervention. Our group has replicated these results in two studies, one of which had 172 chronic state hospital subjects. Even though schizophrenia is by far the most common diagnosis of adults in supervised residences, Cournos[360] noted that very little attention has been paid to the use of psychoeducational techniques in such settings. She suggested modifying the principles used for family intervention in schizophrenia to train residential staff to provide social structure and a low-key supportive environment. In an article published in the late 1980s, Drake and Osher[363] reported several anecdotal examples of success with a psychoeducational approach for individuals without families. In a review of supportive housing, Lehman and Newman[364] suggested that psychoeducational approaches offer the best opportunity for clients and staff to come to an increased understanding of the illness, as well as pointing the way toward resolving problematic situations as they arise. They commented, in this regard, that the approach we describe[365] is promising.

The treatment model underlying the supportive housing psychoeducation program was developed by McFarlane and his staff, adapting the psychoeducational principles of Anderson and colleagues,[108] with additional elements of a behavioral approach (primarily problem-solving and communication skills) developed by Falloon and colleagues.[178] McFarlane[179] adapted these single-family models to a multifamily group approach, creating a social and instrumental support network and enlarging the pool of ideas for problem solving. Ranz and colleagues[365] adapted this model for supportive housing settings.

There are obvious differences between supportive housing and family settings. Supportive housing staff are paid employees whose commitment to the patient is circumscribed by staff members' continued employment and the patient's stay in the housing situation. Nonetheless, the same behaviors that are problematic for families cause trouble in supportive housing: Clients sometimes neglect to take medication, do their chores, or go to programs. Just as families are likely to react to such behavior with frustration and criticism, staff members tend to become controlling and subtly punitive. The resulting arguments are destructive to patients and debilitating to both families and supportive housing staff.

Severely mentally ill patients encounter incessant difficulties in daily living. Staff working with these patients in supportive housing facilities inevitably focus on what is not working, either offering concrete suggestions or solving the problems themselves. These are common reactions to negative symptoms (apathy, amotivation, anhedonia, etc.) that are particularly disabling to this population. Supportive housing staff need help in the following areas: managing problem residents, prioritizing corrective statements for maximum impact, allaying fear of unpredictable behavior, and increasing the ratio of positive (praising accomplishments) to negative (attending to problems) feedback.

Derived from research findings, psychoeducation is based on the premise that recovery from an acute episode of severe mental illness is a lengthy and gradual process. Traditionally trained staff require reorientation to the concept that progress occurs in microsteps and that the solutions devised are necessarily temporary. Psychoeducational guidelines have been developed to give staff and clients simple, practical concepts they can use while learning to implement a psychoeducational program. A list of staff psychoeducational guidelines, the same as those developed for families (see Chapter 7), is presented in Table 11.1. The guidelines are designed as the framework for creating an optimal social environment for recovery and rehabilitation in a broad range of psychotic disorders.

OVERVIEW OF THE MODEL

The approach is informed by the recognition that recovery from an acute episode of schizophrenia can take at least 2 years. Thus, for people recover-

TABLE 11.1. Staff Psychoeducational Guidelines

Here is a list of things everyone can do to help make things run more smoothly:

1. GO SLOW. Recovery takes time. Rest is important. Things will get better in their own time.

2. KEEP IT COOL. Enthusiasm is normal. Tone it down. Disagreement is normal. Tone it down, too.

3. GIVE EACH OTHER SPACE. Time-out is important for everyone. It's OK to reach out. It's OK to say "no."

4. SET LIMITS. Everyone needs to know what the rules are. A few good rules keep things clear.

5. IGNORE WHAT YOU CAN'T CHANGE. Let some things slide. Don't ignore violence.

6. KEEP IT SIMPLE. Say what you have to say clearly, calmly, and positively.

7. FOLLOW DOCTOR'S ORDERS. Take medications as they are prescribed. Take only medications that are prescribed.

8. CARRY ON BUSINESS AS USUAL. Reestablish family routines as quickly as possible. Stay in touch with family and friends.

9. NO STREET DRUGS OR ALCOHOL. They make symptoms worse.

10. PICK UP ON EARLY SIGNS. Note changes. Consult with the physician.

11. SOLVE PROBLEMS STEP-BY-STEP. Make changes gradually. Work on one thing at a time.

12. LOWER EXPECTATIONS, TEMPORARILY. Use a personal yardstick. Compare this month to last month rather than to last year or next year.

ing from an acute episode, a 2-year plan is followed. The first year is devoted to the creation of a calm, warm, low-key environment in the home, with high-intensity activity and critical or confrontational interventions kept to an absolute minimum. A clear set of minimum expectations for responsible behavior is maintained, with careful attention to the goal of symptom stabilization. The second year, the goal is gradually and progressively to raise functional expectations, and vocational and social performance, being careful to stay within the limits of residents' susceptibility to increasing symptomatology. This follows the strategy that guides family intervention in the psychoeducational multifamily group model. The approach requires minimum staff time, so that a small, largely paraprofessional staff in an ordinary supportive housing context is able to implement it.

The goal is a feasible and effective treatment model. Thus, the environment is tailored to the known biological and behavioral characteristics of patients with severe mental illness, especially schizophrenia. The model recognizes and accommodates the common limitations of publicly funded housing for this population, especially the usually minimal training and clinical supervision provided to the paraprofessional staff. In the following section, we review the principles underpinning the treatment model, briefly review their theoretical rationale, and describe their translation into five treatment components: (1) staff training, (2) staff supervision, (3) problem solving, (4) psychoeducational resident groups, and (5) general interventions. It is important to note that in most supportive housing settings, the clients are in various stages of recovery. The model is sufficiently flexible to tailor the approach to individual clients.

KEY CONCEPTS THAT INFORM THE
PSYCHOEDUCATIONAL APPROACH

Avoidance of Criticism

A rapidly expanding literature on expressed emotion has found that criticism of the patient by a key relative on interview is one of the most powerful and reliable predictors for early relapse in schizophrenia.[143, 232] Similar findings have emerged for bipolar affective disorder and depressive episodes.[366] Brown and his colleagues[229] originally noted high rates of relapse in parental homes and in larger board-and-care homes. They assumed that the factors precipitating episodes would be similar in the two contexts but chose the family environment, probably because it was easier to gather a large sample of families. Subsequent studies[367, 368] showed that the excessive arousal usually noted in adults with schizophrenia could be dramatically lowered by the presence of an accepting, supportive person well-known to the patient. This finding reflects characteristics of the illness itself and its effects on interaction with anyone in close, regular contact with the ill person.

The principal psychoeducational strategies designed to minimize criticism are (1) education about severe mental illness and schizophrenia and (2) training in preferable styles of interaction. Through staff education, we attempt to convert annoyance with residents' deficits into a more accepting stance. Staff are trained to recognize that negative symptoms are nearly universal sequelae to acute episodes, to more disabling subtypes of schizophrenia, and to poorly recompensated affective episodes. This change in attitude toward negative symptoms happens rapidly and consistently after educational programs are presented to families. We have seen essentially the same response by paraprofessional and professional staff to the scientific information and guidelines for illness management that constitute a major portion of the initial training sessions in our approach. Some of these guidelines, notably "Keep it simple" and "Lower expectations, temporarily," are direct expressions of this first psychoeducational principle: avoidance of criticism.

Most staff are enthusiastic about attempting to apply the model. Others have more difficulty because they do not see how the model can be helpful. Staff become more comfortable with the model and the use of guidelines as they apply them successfully to specific situations with specific people. Finding that this supportive approach works to manage difficult problems is reassuring to staff and encourages them to keep at it. Families work in conjunction with psychoeducational multifamily group leaders over a period of time in order to become comfortable applying the model. Similarly, ongoing consultations with a supervisor help housing staff keep to the model, using psychoeducational guidelines to develop management strategies.

Positive Reinforcement

The usefulness of positive reinforcement as an alternative to criticism has been established by family behavioral treatment research as a more effective method of altering problematic behavior in adults with schizophrenia.[369] In this model, positive reinforcement is the major interactional style for staff to use with mentally ill residents. In the training and supervision, we present various methods for staff to notice and comment on small examples of residents' improvement in daily functioning. Any change in participation in group meetings and new (even if minor) accomplishments are highlighted. We have found that this entire process acts as a positive reinforcer by placing emphasis on desirable and gratifying experiences rather than failures and deficiencies. In the group supervision process in our first experience with the process, each staff member found that he or she could shift focus to the positive. In doing so, the atmosphere in the home improved.[365]

The family psychoeducational model emphasizes the importance of building on existing strengths. The goal is for clients to learn to identify positive experiences, even if seemingly trivial, and to ignore or downplay their negative counterparts. These groups model for residents how to interact positively, warmly, and supportively with one another, and to focus on pleasant and/or gratifying aspects of their own and fellow residents' lives. A detailed description of these positive socialization groups follows.

Adjustments of Intensity of Stimulation

Based on numerous studies linking stimulation, hyperarousal, and attentional dysfunction in schizophrenia, the psychoeducational approach has emphasized the importance of reducing the intensity and frequency of interaction with these clients.[43, 49, 370] The findings have formed the basis for the psychoeducational approach's emphasis on establishing a calm social environment, presenting fewer and less complex stimuli and reducing the total amount of information that adults with schizophrenia must process in a given time interval. These techniques have proved remarkably effective in reducing symptomatology and relapse rates in family intervention studies. Similarly, these are effective techniques in any environment in which patients with severe mental illness live.

Many studies,[49, 108, 269, 360, 371] and the psychoeducational model itself, suggest that there is therapeutic value in a style of interaction that is accepting, somewhat emotionally neutral yet warm, and empathic and sensitive to cues that the patient is becoming overwhelmed. This is summarized in the psychoeducational guidelines, "Keep it cool" and "Give people space." Previous research also suggests that staff use a simple, uncomplicated, slower conversational style and learn to detect when a resident is being overstimulated by too much incoming information. Therefore, another of the psychoeducational guidelines, "Keep it simple," refers to spoken interaction with residents. In training and supervising, we emphasize this skill, teaching staff to use simple, short declarative sentences, checking periodically to see if they have been understood. Staff learn to keep their tones calm, relatively warm, and matter-of-fact. They can help each other use this approach during tense interactions in the residence. During supervision sessions, these transactions are reviewed in a search for alternative techniques via problem solving.

Client Choice

Supportive housing philosophy places a high priority on client preferences as a guide to housing selection.[372] However, at times, staff pay insufficient attention to individual preferences toward housing, vocational goals, or social cooperation.[373] In a supportive housing context, attention must be paid to what the resident wants and whether he or she perceives that a given housing or job opportunity is feasible and likely to be rewarding.[374] For example, a client may ask to move into more independent housing, although staff believe the client is not ready for this move. Instead of engaging in confrontation, use of the psychoeducational model's problem-solving technique (see below) allows for planning a step-by-step process to reach that goal.

Graduated Performance Expectations

Resumption of role functioning is a major goal of any rehabilitation program. Adults with severe mental illness tend to be readily overwhelmed by abrupt changes in expectations and/or actual performance. There is considerable evidence that adults with schizophrenia have increases in symptoms and relapse following stressful life events.[315] Often, as in family deaths or transitions to college or the military, these events also involve major changes in social context and physical setting.[316, 317] A new job is an especially stressful life event for adults with severe mental illness. It requires that he or she enter a new physical setting, learn new, often cognitively difficult skills, and interact socially in a preexisting network. The evidence demonstrates that for adults with schizophrenia, information processing is hampered by increased arousal levels, such as those that accompany major life events. Such a transition, if entered suddenly, can be overwhelming and lead to relapse.

Consistent with its emphasis on fostering a slow, gradual recovery from psychosis, the psychoeducational approach emphasizes a gradual, stepwise resumption of social and vocational functioning. During the first year of implementation of the approach, major emphasis is on symptom stabilization. Vocational rehabilitation becomes the major focus in the second year, since improved functioning depends upon symptom stabilization. This approach may appear to prolong rehabilitation, but it is a more reliable method that eventually yields higher levels of functioning. The design of the problem-solving groups encourages a consistent but gradual increase in responsibilities and level of vocational functioning. A detailed description of problem-solving groups appears below.

Flexible Social Milieu

Residents often complain that they feel oppressed by staff's seeming preoccupation with rules and regulations.[373] They are usually unaware of the ways in which their disabilities tend to frustrate staff. Moos[375] reports that residents invariably prefer and generally do better when such control is exerted in moderation. As Lehman and Newman[364] report, supportive housing staff complain most about negative symptoms and behaviors that accompany severe mental illness, such as difficulties with personal hygiene, lack of consideration for privacy of others, issues involving safety of clients and staff, and substance use and abuse. In our model, we encourage staff to deal with these issues in a calm, matter-of-fact way, setting priorities according to the severity of the situation. Two psychoeducational guidelines form the core of the approach to many of the more minor issues that commonly crop up in these settings: "Ignore what you can't change" and "Keep it cool." The former encourages dealing with only the most serious of residents' symptomatic behavior. The family intervention models suggest that talking about symptoms, trying to correct delusions, and trying to understand the underlying meanings of thought-disordered conversation are all counterproductive. "Keep it cool" refers to the desirability of dealing with potential confrontations in a calm, patient manner. Discussions about symptoms tend to become intense and frustrating interchanges accompanied by critical or angry remarks. This, in turn, may exacerbate these same symptoms. Thus, staff, like family members, are urged to attend only to appropriate behavior and comprehensible conversation. Obviously, threats of violence or suicide, or severely bizarre and disruptive behavior, are not to be ignored but should be dealt with promptly and definitively.

Nevertheless, rules and regulations are necessary in a supportive housing setting. The psychoeducational and family behavioral approaches have advanced the technical aspects of handling limit setting. Whenever possible, limit setting is couched in terms of the general social welfare of the house rather than with reference to external rules. The simplest approach is to ask a resident to do something because a reasonable person wants, and would explicitly appreciate, his or her help and compliance.[376] Sometimes it is helpful to problem-solve such issues in a group, because group participants may help by suggesting ways to avoid confrontations. In this approach, the staff prioritize limit setting, reserving hierarchical interactions for truly serious situations.

In summary, this psychoeducational approach educates staff about modern concepts of mental illness and brain function, specifically alters staff–resident interaction and the social climate of the residence, enhances symptom control, and fosters a gradual improvement in role functioning. Taken together, success in achieving these intermediate goals leads to longer community tenure.

THE PSYCHOEDUCATION APPROACH FOR SUPPORTIVE HOUSING PROGRAMS

This approach consists of the following components: (1) staff training, (2) staff supervision, (3) problem solving, (4) psychoeducational groups, and (5) general interventions.

Staff Training: Joining and Education

The initial training session is attended by staff working in the residence. Joining with staff is basic to the success of this approach and precedes educational meetings. The first step when using the psychoeducational approach is the creation of a working alliance between supervisors and staff, toward the ultimate goal of helping staff engage with residents. A series of meetings is held to gather information about the concerns of staff, problems they see in the operation of the housing program, and specific questions about specific clients. During this process, the supervisor can offer information about the nature of the illnesses, introducing the psychoeducational guidelines as a framework for translating concepts into action and validating staff concerns. This offer of information and support fosters the development of a working collaboration between supervisors and staff.

The curriculum for training includes introduction to psychoeducational theory, current concepts of etiology and symptomatology of schizophrenia, phases of treatment in the psychoeducational model, elicitation of concerns and issues of the residential staff, and special applications of the model in the supportive housing setting. Sessions include didactic presentations, audiovisual material, and role playing. These training sessions typically last one full day, with half-day refresher courses scheduled annually.

Staff Supervision

Residential staff needs ongoing support to implement this model, in the same fashion as recommended for mental health center and outpatient clinic staff working in the multifamily group setting. The clinical supervisor runs regular weekly or biweekly supervision sessions for all staff working in the psychoeducational approach. Supervisory sessions should continue throughout the entire intervention, because, as simple as the concepts appear, implementation is more complex. The psychoeducation model suggests that staff behave in a manner that may appear counterintuitive. In the face of low functioning, it is a natural reaction either to be critical or to offer enthusiastic encouragement for increased activity. The staff psychoeducational guidelines recommend other approaches, such as "Go slow" or "Give them space" or "One step at a time."

Each time a new problem arises, staff must figure out how to apply the psychoeducational principles. In our experience, it takes a long time for staff to apply this model independently. Psychoeducational guidelines are not logical and do not follow common sense. Instead, they are counterintuitive, requiring reflection on the nature of the biological disorder and on the particulars of the individual's course of illness. It would be natural to remind a client regularly to take a shower every day, but the guidelines call for a plan that is feasible for that particular person. Most people learn to use the guidelines by practicing them many times, and in many different situations

Supervisory meetings should begin with an explicitly identified socialization period, during which the supervisor and all staff members share everyday personal experiences, as in the multifamily group model. This models and provides practice for socialization with residents. Following socialization, there is a discussion of staff success in implementing psychoeducational guidelines, carrying out solutions, and maintaining a "cool and calm" demeanor. Each staff member is invited to give feedback about his or her experience and any suggestions for improvements in the approach. Progress by staff in reaching objectives, no matter how minor, is validated. Positive reactions and praise are elicited from other staff. The supervisor positively reinforces successful use of psychoeducational guidelines (e.g., "Ignore what you can't change," "Keep it simple") that reduce potential confrontations and thereby contribute to lower stress levels. During this period, called the "go-round," complaints, descriptions of failed interventions, and anger will occur. Common complaints include frustration with repetitious, negative resident behavior, distaste for some resident language, annoyance at efforts by residents to gain special favors, and so on. These feelings positively denote productive ventilation, which helps prevent displacement onto residents. Staff are encouraged to evaluate the behavior in terms of psychoeducational principles and knowledge of the illness, in order to prioritize their concerns.

Problems identified in the go-round may be specific to a given resident. Discussion of the problem in psychoeducational terms tends to generalize the issue in a way that relates to the entire residence. These issues are then prioritized using the psychoeducational guidelines in order to decide which one(s) to problem-solve. At times, suggestions for new house rules may be the desired outcome. Occasionally, it is necessary to proceed with a specific resident's problem.

Problem Solving

Once the problem has been defined, a structured procedure is followed to elicit ideas and suggestions, one-by-one, from each staff member and supervisor. To encourage everyone to participate, each person is asked to contribute just one idea. During this step, the ideas are not evaluated. After all suggestions have been gathered, each item on the list is discussed and evaluated separately. Continuing an emphasis on positive connotations, the supervisor elicits the advantages of each idea before any discussion of disadvantages. To encourage full participation, each staff member's suggestion is received positively. As the discussion proceeds, it usually becomes clear which suggestion(s) applies most to the situation at hand. The supervisor guides this process, promoting suggestions that are consistent with the psychoeducational guidelines. A detailed plan is devised to implement the preferred solutions during the following week. At this point, role playing, using this structured psychoeducational problem-solving method, may be appropriate. Each supervisory meeting closes with another brief period of socialization. This may include talk about plans for the weekend, upcoming life events, or vacations.

The supervisor inquires about the task in the go-round discussion at the next supervision meeting. Any difficulties that have been encountered are framed as the responsibility of the supervisor (e.g., the task was inappropriate for the phase of the problem). Acceptance of responsibility by the leader for unsuccessful tasks models a similar process that should take place in resident groups.

One goal of supervision is to encourage staff to use psychoeducational guidelines and underlying concepts in their interactions with clients, formally and informally, whether in individual or group contexts. These interactions create an optimal environment for recovery, one that is calm, with relatively low, but not absent, performance pressure. Rehabilitation progress is conceived as gradual. Positive interactions are maximized. The goal is an environment that enables residents to develop greater resistance to stress. Learning to solve problems in an orderly fashion, along with carefully planned preparation for each next step, contributes to stress reduction, with maximum likelihood for avoiding symptomatic relapse and achieving functional progress.

Psychoeducational Groups

It is feasible to implement psychoeducational concepts within the context of informal staff–resident interactions, or within existing groups (e.g., psychotherapy or skills training groups). However, the ideal approach is the creation of discrete groups specifically designed to maximize the impact of the psychoeducational intervention. Three possible formats are described as follows:

Positive Socialization Groups

A group organized to focus entirely on structured socialization derives from the concept that a supportive environment reduces interfering arousal for severely mentally ill residents. These groups provide built-in opportunities for maximal positive feedback. The approach helps to expand a protective buffer zone between the residents and stressors in their environment. Also, it counteracts demoralization and negative thoughts by reinforcing positive experiences, thoughts, and interaction.

In such a format, each group member, including leaders, spends 5 minutes talking about positive experiences, which may include observations and/or thoughts since the last meeting, current or past events, a favorite movie or television show, new friends, favorite food, or good job-related experiences. Residents often participate in this process spontaneously. Staff can encourage more retiring residents to present their own experiences. Residents who are reluctant to offer anything are thanked for their attendance and encouraged to join in whenever they are ready. Staff can lead the residents in responding positively to each member's report, for example, "I like that food, too" or "I'd like to see that movie." Any negative or critical reaction is interrupted by the leader, who might remind the resident that this is a time for good news and help him or her to make a positive response.

Medication Groups

Medication groups are best run jointly by a trained medication educator (e.g., a nurse or physician) and a case worker, with the goal of improving knowledge about medication and increasing medication compliance. The purpose of medication group meetings is to develop patient–staff collaboration concerning psychiatric medication as an integral part of the psychoeducation program.

The appropriate use of medication takes into account both general principles of pharmacotherapy and specific, individual patient characteristics. The risk-to-benefit balance for a medication decision may change according to the specific patient's clinical condition and the setting in which the medication is used. The more often a patient is able to decide the risk-to-benefit balance, the more likely it is that he or she will be able to participate in a collaborative alliance with the treatment staff. The goal is to improve adherence to an appropriate medication regimen. The term "adherence" is used in preference to "compliance," in order to clarify that active participation in medication decisions facilitates patients' commitment to continuing appropriate medication.

Each group meeting starts with a discussion of residents' current medication experience, which then serves as the springboard for a formal discussion. Some of the topics covered in these discussions include current pharmacological categories, the benefits and risks of medications for severe mental illness, positive and negative symptoms, and common side effects. The leaders explain the importance of distinguishing symptoms from side effects. Symptoms such as agitation, depression, and irritability can easily be confused with side effects.

Problem-Solving Groups

A structured procedure for identifying and solving problems is an effective path to rehabilitation. The staff attempt to generate solutions that are based on the psychoeducational guidelines. In this approach, staff learn these principles and procedures, and practice problem solving in supervisory groups. They can then apply the model with residents in similarly conducted, small groups.

Problem-solving groups meet for 1 hour and focus on helping individual residents problem-solve, plan, and carry out the next step in their rehabilitation. Group-based problem solving is fostered as the primary means of addressing difficulties that represent threats to symptom stability. The concept of group problem solving is well known, but we describe its specific implementation as a psychoeducational strategy in a residential context.

Each group starts with a socialization period, during which residents are encouraged (but not required) to participate. Staff are expected to contribute their own comments to this process. This format follows the model used in the supervisory groups and normally takes 5–10 minutes.

The go-round occurs next, consisting of a structured process for eliciting residents' reports and complaints. With the support of the leaders, each resident gives a capsule summary of his or her progress since the last group meeting. The following areas are explored: (1) medication adherence; (2) drug and alcohol use; (3) life events; (4) conflicts within the home; and (5) conflicts with outside activities and programs. Staff observations that validate these reports may be discussed at this time.

By the end of the go-round, the leaders identify one or two residents whose situations should be explored further during that meeting. The selection by staff of residents for discussion in the group is a primary means of individualizing the rate of rehabilitation. The extended discussion is structured as a formal, step-by-step, problem-solving sequence. The leaders conduct a group-oriented brainstorming period focused on one resident's issue. Each group member assists by presenting ideas and strategies. The leaders encourage residents to participate and offer suggestions, one by one, by validating and recognizing residents' ideas and perceptions. Reaction to the suggestions by other group members is postponed until all ideas have been collected. The leaders keep the process light and relaxed, while eliciting group interest and support. They try to operate in the midrange between residents' hopelessness and denial.

Once all the ideas are collected, each in turn is discussed. The advantages of each idea are discussed before considering its disadvantages. Every attempt is made to frame disadvantages in terms of impracticality rather than inappropriateness. This procedure quickly eliminates unproductive suggestions, while highlighting the solution that yields a workable strategy. Everyone participates in choosing alternative functional possibilities and methods of implementation. A plan is then created with specific steps for implementation, including assignment of who does what, when, where, and how often. Whenever possible, the task is devised to include another resident as a partner. In this regard, we are striving to make the group serve as a stable social network that provides a supportive base for the resident making a transition to a new work or social setting.

Each group meeting ends with a 5-minute socialization period, which may include mention of plans for social activities or upcoming special events. At the following problem-solving meeting, progress with the tasks is evaluated by leaders and residents during the go-round segment. As modeled in supervision, any difficulties that may have been encountered are framed as the responsibility of the leaders.

General Interventions

In addition to psychoeducational resident groups, psychoeducational principles can be introduced into ongoing resident–staff interactions and community meetings. Increasing staff familiarity with the biosocial information underlying severe mental illness and increasing use of psychoeducational guidelines allow the staff to weave these ideas into the daily life of the residence.

The following example is drawn from experience in our pilot study[365] in a transitional residence in a suburban setting (described below in "Adaptations of the Staff-Psychoeducational Model"). A resident demanded second and third helpings at mealtimes to the detriment of his health. Although this request was generally not met, at times there ensued an upsetting interaction between staff and the resident. Staff normally attempted to reason with the resident, using logic and health information to persuade him. This produced a negative response of anger, frustration, and increased arousal for the resident, who then started to exhibit symptoms. Discussion of the problem with other staff using psychoeducational principles helped develop a strategy for staff to use to help the client at mealtimes. Speaking in a calm, low-key manner, staff would remind the client that this meal consists of one helping and that there will be a snack and another meal, followed by another snack. If the client still felt hungry at the end of the day, he was encouraged to tell his case manager the next day, in order to arrange an extra snack, if necessary. All staff present in the dining room were alerted to this plan. The requests from the client for more food tapered off as he experienced a validating, positive response to his perceived hunger

In family behavioral approaches, there is strong emphasis on family members making frequent statements about what behavior they want and expressing praise and appreciation when it occurs. When negative statements are made, they are framed as preferences of the family member as opposed to criticisms of the patient. In the residential setting, staff remind the resident of the appropriate rules in a brief statement of fact, and in a calm manner. They then end the interaction by moving on to the next activity. This avoids heightening arousal that may lead to symptoms. A calm resolution to the situation encourages staff to handle this problem similarly the next time the request occurs. If the resident is unable to accept the rules and continues to become agitated, staff can refer to the appropriate guidelines of "Keep it cool" and "Give people space," in order to plan a response. For example, the resident may be asked to take a brief time-out by going to another room before the discussion continues.

ADAPTATIONS OF THE STAFF-PSYCHOEDUCATIONAL MODEL

In midtown Manhattan, the staff of a newly organized, supervised long-term residence serving homeless people with severe mental illness requested a psychoeducational consultation to help develop a conceptual framework with which to provide services. Over the course of several years, residential aides, social workers, maintenance staff, nurses, and administrators met with the consultant monthly. It was decided that this would be the most practical and efficient route to disseminating psychoeducational ideas. After initial sessions introducing the principles and concepts, a format evolved that mirrored the psychoeducational model. Staff psychoeducation meetings always began with chat about everyday events, then moved on to a go-round, in which all staff had a chance to raise any questions, whether about a specific client, a specific group, a floor issue, or an organizational issue. One of these issues was selected for closer scrutiny using the problem-solving format. Suggestions were elicited, each discussed in turn—advantages first—and finally a plan was generated with a specific description of what was to happen. Staff found the psychoeducational principles useful in providing a framework for thinking about difficult problems, while discussing these questions in a calm, humorous, and thoughtful manner, and producing a concrete result (a plan that could be implemented).

For example, one problem concerned a resident with a very severe activities of daily living (ADL) impairment. She neglected to brush her teeth, launder her clothing, or wash her hair. Most disturbing to staff was the fact that she did not shower regularly enough. Many staff members had tried to help but all met with frustration and some anger. There was talk of asking the resident to leave, since she was unable to comply with the house ADL expectations. The staff members threw up their hands in helplessness. Clearly, the stress level of the staff had risen in response to the situation. The guidelines specifically recommend keeping stress at a minimum by such means as setting limits, keeping interactions calm and low key, and communicating in a brief, concise, and simple manner. Using the psycho-educational problem-solving format allowed for the expression and validation of staff reactions, while brainstorming alternative options that would follow the guidelines and lead to new solutions and a specific plan. In the end, a staff member who was comfortable working with the resident volunteered to implement the plan, which called for adding one shower every 2 weeks, with staff assistance, to allow the resident to experience some success before trying to take on more responsibility. In the next staff psychoeducation meeting, the staff member reported only partial success; as the resident had taken only one shower that past month. In line with the key concept of implementing progressive performance expectations, the task was reviewed and evaluated as to relevance to the particular client. It appeared that two showers a month was too ambitious given the resident's level of functioning, and the group decided to set the goal at one shower a month for the next month and, if that proved successful, to proceed to two showers a month. Stepping down the rate of expectation in this way proved effective. The client showered twice the following month. The staff could then move on to consider increasing the frequency to three times a month, following the psychoeducational guideline "One step at a time." This slow-paced strategy of gradual increases in responsibility was successful.

A group of young men had developed a pattern of harassing female residents in the smoking lounge in the early evenings. The women residents were distressed by this and somewhat afraid the situation might get out of hand. When questioned by staff, the young men complained that they had no way to release sexual tension, and that this was what they considered a relatively harmless alternative for them. At the monthly staff psychoeducation meeting, the problem was raised for brainstorming. Some staff members were very concerned for the safety of the women, while others were wondering, only partly tongue-in-cheek, how to help the young men, perhaps by renting "hot" videos or by paying for a visit to a prostitute. The staff members were divided as to how to proceed with such a highly charged issue. Meanwhile, stress levels for residents were increasing in the lounge. A plan was needed. Brainstorming allowed staff to discuss each suggestion in a calm and humorous way, looking at all the advantages and disadvantages. Even the most controversial ideas were treated in a respectful manner. Rather than being rejected out of hand, these ideas were dropped when more productive skills-building solutions emerged. The solution chosen was that two staff members would volunteer to run a short-term group with the young men, focusing on management of difficult impulses, with the goal of helping the men become less stressed and more considerate of other residents. They planned 10 sessions to help resolve the issue. Shortly after the group started to meet, the horseplay dwindled away, and residents could all mingle freely again. Both the staff and the consultant felt that the solution worked because the highly charged issue of sex was treated in a matter-of-fact and organized manner, and that through the resident group meetings, the men were able to develop better coping skills to manage their impulses.

A new resident had been homeless for so long that he was no longer comfortable sleeping in a bed. He preferred sleeping on a couch in the lounge or on the floor. Using the psychoeducational model and problem-solving the issue led to a gradually paced strategy of encouraging the resident first to try the floor in his own room, while becoming acclimated to the residence. The move to the residence represented a major life event, with accompanying higher levels of stress that could lead to symptom exacerbation. Asking him to make a small adjustment at first allowed the resident time and space to stabilize before facing the next challenging level, a real bed.

A more extensive adaptation of the model was implemented in a 24-bed, supervised residence newly opened on the grounds of a New York State psychiatric center in a New York City suburb. The residents had spent some time as inpatients at the psychiatric center but were not yet prepared for independent community living. Being on the grounds of the hospital allowed them to adjust to more independence in familiar surroundings. The manager of the residence was enthusiastic about adopting the psychoeducational model. He was supportive, providing incentives (food) to the staff to participate and attend supervision meetings. It was clear that inviting family members to attend a regular meeting was logistically very difficult in this setting, due to distances and inadequate public transportation. However, staff training, supervision, and the development of resident groups were well received. Increased understanding of the nature of severe psychiatric illnesses enabled staff to better comprehend residents' behavior as symptoms of their illness, which helped decrease staff frustration and blaming of the residents.

Positive socialization groups were organized to meet weekly, providing staff and clients an opportunity to share a time of everyday give and take about ordinary topics such as sports, movies, television, magazines, the weather, and so on. These group meetings were difficult at first for both residents and staff but soon became relaxed and effortless. Residents looked forward to the meetings as a time to share experiences in a nonjudgmental, positive context. After this group format was well established, two other formats were created to alternate with the original socialization groups on a 3-week cycle. Problem-solving groups focused on social and vocational rehabilitation issues, paying attention to one or two individuals at each meeting. Medication education groups included didactic lectures on specific topics suggested by the residents, followed by specific discussions of related medication problems that members were experiencing.

An example of a problem-solving group issue was how a resident could increase the hours of a part-time job in order to earn more money. Since change is stressful for these clients, staff were taught that it is helpful to plan how to make that change in a step-by-step manner to minimize the impact of the increased stress for that resident. This client was already working 8 hours per week and wished to increase the workload to 12 hours over the same days. Any larger increase in hours would be too demanding, and changing days of work would mean changing two things at once. The staff supported a gradual effort by monitoring the client for any sign that increased stress was destabilizing. In that event, a new discussion would have led to a new plan to incorporate the new information. In the end, the client decided to try gradually increasing work hours in 2-hour increments. His employer agreed to a schedule that increased from 8 to 10 hours for 3 weeks. The client had little difficulty with the first increase, so he added another 2 hours the following week, reaching his goal of 12 hours per week and earning more money. The client remained stable during the increase of work time. The use of these three group formats produced a calmer, more low-key atmosphere in the residence and helped clients with steps they wished to take in their rehabilitation efforts.

GENERAL ISSUES

Residential staff are, by and large, nonprofessionals. Previous psychoeducational efforts have focused on professional staff on the one hand, or family members on the other. Each of these groups present special challenges because they have prior experiences that hamper their acceptance of the psychoeducational approach. Professional training often runs counter to the psychoeducational model. Instead of a therapeutic contract, this model necessitates a contract for management of the illness. Thus, the psychoeducational approach focuses on the behavior that springs from the biological disorder rather than insight and feelings. Families with severely mentally ill members have a history of being criticized by mental health professionals. Practitioners have to be careful that suggestions for changes in family members' behavior are not experienced as further criticism. Despite these factors, psychoeducation has proven to be highly effective for professionals working with family members. In our experience, nonprofessional residential staff are no more or less amenable to these ideas than professional staff or family members. Residential staff are alternately mystified and frustrated by the behaviors exhibited by adults with severe mental illness. The staff psychoeducational format offers staff members the conceptual basis necessary to understand how to work with these adults, as well as practical, ongoing supervision to support their efforts.

It is worth noting that, when feasible, a multifamily group is a worthwhile addition to the residence program, because it provides an opportunity for residents, family members, and staff to collaborate on troubling issues in the management of severe mental illness. However, adults in supportive residences often say that they have lost contact with their families. Reasons for this are that many family members may have gotten older and are possibly unable to travel to visit relatives, or there may have been a history of unhappy interactions with both the relative and the mental health system. Nonetheless, we have learned that even when residents say they are not in touch with their families, closer examination reveals that there is usually at least infrequent contact around holidays and birthdays. This level of contact would not be sufficient to allow the organization of regular multifamily groups. However, residential staff can engage family members on a case-by-case basis as participants in the psychoeducational approach to the management of their relative's illness. For example, if a resident has phone contact with a family member once a month, staff can suggest that she ask her family at that time if it would be all right for a staff member to call. Usually, families are very interested in speaking with professionals involved with their relative and would appreciate the opportunity. A follow-up letter sent by a staff member can maintain contact with family while sharing relevant information. Planning for monthly family open-house meetings held in the evening allows family members to stay in contact at their convenience and keeps them informed about their relative.

CONCLUSION

Our experience is that psychoeducational training and supervision of supportive housing staff produces the desired low-stress atmosphere, while providing a technique for staff to help residents pursue their own social and vocational rehabilitation goals in a gradual yet persistent manner. This approach draws its strength from the fact that it is derived from up-to-date biological information about schizophrenia and other severe mental illnesses. It is, moreover, appealing in its conceptual simplicity and down-to-earth pragmatism. Supportive housing staff who learn about this model generally respond with enthusiastic recognition that the model fits their own work experience.

We wish, however, to emphasize a point made previously. As simple as these ideas are, staff find that putting the ideas into practice is far from easy. Everyone knows how hard it is to remain calm and positive in the face of difficult behavior on the part of residents. Successful implementation of psychoeducational guidelines requires training and is best done in ongoing consultation with an experienced supervisor.

The approach is relatively low cost, because staff are not being asked to do more than they were otherwise doing. Moreover, the cost of supervision is low, because, after the initial training, ongoing supervision can take place as infrequently as once a month. As indicated earlier, the approach is flexible enough to be implemented in a variety of formats, so that it can be tailored to the needs of a particular agency. Administrative and clinical staff of agencies providing supportive housing might well consider this approach when developing their programs.

Chapter 12

Multifamily Groups
for Bipolar Illness

DAVID A. MOLTZ AND MARGARET NEWMARK

As the power and effectiveness of the psychoeducational approaches to the treatment of schizophrenia became clear, interest developed in extending these models to other conditions as well. Psychoeducational approaches did more than provide information; they were supportive to families in a number of important ways (see Table 12.1; see also Anderson and colleagues,[108] Steinglass,[377] and Chapter 16) and made a real difference in the course of the illness. Bipolar disorder, which shares important characteristics with schizophrenia and can be equally challenging to families, seemed especially appropriate for a psychoeducational multifamily group approach, such as the model developed by McFarlane and associates. However, bipolar disorder also differs from schizophrenia; clinical characteristics, course, and effects on the family are all different in important ways, requiring significant modifications to the model.

In this chapter, we describe an adaptation of the multifamily group approach that we have used for families with bipolar disorder. This model was developed and first implemented at a municipal mental health center in the South Bronx of New York City, and later at a community mental health center in coastal Maine. The model has been effective when applied in these very different settings.

TABLE 12.1. What Psychoeducational Approaches Do

1. Provide a safe environment
   - Nonblaming
   - Collaborative
   - Affectively modulated and controlled

2. Provide information
   - Relieve anxiety
   - Correct misconceptions
   - Avoid mystification
   - Alleviate blame and stigma
   - Lessen isolation
   - Help organize experience
   - Encourage treatment compliance

3. Facilitate discussion
   - Correct distortions and misperceptions
   - Encourage safe discussion of difficult subjects

4. Develop strategies to prevent, modify, or manage future episodes
   - Identify precipitants
   - Define specific prodromal syndrome
   - Develop specific strategies and coping skills

5. Develop supportive network
   - Therapists and treatment team as allies and supports
   - Encourage development of natural support system
   - Multifamily groups as support system

SIMILARITIES BETWEEN BIPOLAR DISORDER AND SCHIZOPHRENIA

Biopsychosocial

Like schizophrenia, bipolar disorder is a biologically based illness whose course and manifestations interact with the psychosocial context.[378–381] This suggests that a psychoeducational approach that both acknowledges the biological basis of the illness and focuses on modifying its impact on the family, as well as the individual, could be as useful in bipolar disorder as it has been in schizophrenia.

Course

Although bipolar illness is by definition episodic, like schizophrenia it has a chronic course, and future episodes are likely to occur.[378] In addition, recovery from episodes is not always complete,[382] and a significant proportion of affected individuals continue to experience symptoms and/or a decrease in level of functioning.[383, 384] Therefore, an approach to treatment that addresses the long-term and variable course of the illness is necessary.

Burden

Bipolar illness is generally considered to be a less ominous diagnosis than schizophrenia. However, its consequences, both to the individual and to the family, can be equally devastating. Because symptoms are affective, they elicit strong affective responses. The interpersonal environment tends to be highly charged, and conflict with or about the affected person is common. This interferes with problem solving and can lead to volatile interactions that are difficult to modulate or control. In addition, since individuals with bipolar disorder marry more often than those with schizophrenia, they are more often a spouse or a parent, and this multiplies the effects of the illness on the family. The affected individual may be the family's main source of income or the primary parent. When these roles are compromised by an episode of illness, the repercussions on the family are profound. Finally, as a result of poor judgment during an episode, especially of mania, the individual may engage in behaviors that are dangerous, criminal, or socially shameful and damaging to the family. Because of the relative preservation of personality and the manic individual's ability to debate, argue, and intimidate,[385] family members may have great difficulty intervening in or modifying this behavior. This can lead to mutual frustration, blame, and recrimination concerning the individual's behavior and the family's response to it. Thus, the family burden in bipolar disorder, while experienced differently, can be at least as great as that in schizophrenia. The information sharing and mutual support inherent in a multifamily group have been helpful in alleviating this burden and providing much-needed social support.

Stigma

The social stigma associated with bipolar illness can also be devastating. Episode-associated behaviors such as hypersexuality, substance abuse, or social inappropriateness can be highly shaming to the family, as well as to the individual who has recovered from the episode. Symptoms such as irritability, argumentativeness, or arrogant, self-centered disregard for the needs of others can have severe interpersonal and social consequences. Stigma is intensified because depressive or manic behavior is often not clearly distinguished from "normal" behavior or personality.[386] Because, to the outside observer, the individual may not appear to be "sick," he or she is often held morally responsible for his or her behavior and its consequences. Similarly, family members are often criticized either for not controlling the individual or for being too controlling. A multifamily group, which combines information and problem solving with a supportive social network, is helpful in alleviating the isolating effects of stigma.

ISSUES SPECIFIC TO BIPOLAR DISORDER

One strength of the psychoeducational model is its recognition that, over time, illness shapes the family.[386, 387] It follows that different illnesses present different challenges to the family and will have different effects on family functioning. The multifamily group model developed for schizophrenia by McFarlane and associates is based on psychoeducational principles that are generalizable to other psychiatric illnesses. These principles emphasize the importance of allying with the family, sharing information, designing specific and concrete solutions to illness-related problems, focusing on aspects of the individual and family that are not compromised by the illness, and combating isolation and stigma. These principles are expressed in elements of the structure of the model that are essential to its effectiveness and should not be changed. However, other elements are responses to specific characteristics of schizophrenia, and because bipolar illness differs from schizophrenia, modifications in the content and structure of the approach are necessary. (For more detailed discussion of these issues, see Moltz.[386])

Episodic Course

Bipolar illness is, by definition, episodic. Although residual symptoms and impairment of functioning are more prevalent than previously believed,[383, 384, 388] there is characteristically a pattern of remission and relapse. This is different from the typical course of schizophrenia, which, while characterized by acute exacerbations, tends to be unremitting and does not generally include periods that approximate the level of functioning the individual experienced prior to the onset of illness.

The on-again, off-again pattern presents specific challenges to the family. During an episode, roles shift for everyone in the family, especially when it is a spouse/parent who is affected. Parenting functions and other responsibilities often must be redistributed. Decision making and access to financial resources may be changed. The affected individual may require close and continuous monitoring for his or her protection, as well as the safety of others. Social institutions such as police, hospitals, or child protection agencies may become involved. Every aspect of family functioning may be altered. Then, when the episode has subsided, all these functions must shift again, often with little time for transition, as the affected individual resumes his or her previous roles and functions. This process can be tremendously confusing and stressful, especially when in some episodes the individual is manic and in others depressed, or when rapid cycling allows little or no recovery time.

Another important consequence of the episodic nature of the illness is the preoccupation for family members, and often for the individual as well, with the possibility of relapse. The effort to identify and head off episodes can lead to a characteristic hypervigilance, in which the affective state of the individual becomes the major focus of family life.

Affect

The hallmark of bipolar episodes is that they involve changes in affect, and affect tends to be "contagious."[389, 390] Living with someone who is depressed can be a depressing experience, and family members are at risk for becoming depressed themselves.[391] In the case of mania, it is the irritability and intensity that tend to be contagious. Family members in close contact with an individual who is manic or depressed may react strongly themselves, or they may withdraw from any interaction as a way of controlling this reactivity.

Another consequence of the affective nature of bipolar episodes is the widespread confusion between symptoms and normal moods. This can be expressed in several ways. Family members, acquaintances, and even the affected individual may minimize the seriousness of affective symptoms and recommend that he or she "just get a hold of yourself." The failure to do so can lead to anger and accusations, and to a profound sense of failure and isolation on the part of the individual. This misunderstanding can also result in an underestimation of the need for treatment.

At the other extreme, the similarity between affective symptoms and normal mood variations can lead to the pathologizing of ordinary manifestations of mood. Because affective changes are associated with the onset of serious episodes, family members may respond with concern to any expression of emotion. When the individual expresses appropriate sadness, anger, or even happiness, a family member may ask, "Have you taken your medicine?" This is a common source of conflict in families living with bipolar illness.

Influence on Personality

The effects of bipolar illness on personality are complex. Compared to schizophrenia, personality and social functioning are relatively preserved. Affected individuals may be highly competent and successful both professionally and socially, and recovery between episodes may be essentially complete. Even during an episode, the individual may be able to function appropriately, at least for short periods of time. Affect can be controlled, logical explanations offered, and a facade of rationality, self-control, and responsibility maintained. Paradoxically, this may increase the difficulty and burden for family members. A person whose judgment is impaired may be able to maintain a semblance of competence, effectively disarming family members who are attempting to set limits or to temporarily take over decision making. An individual who is manic, threatened with police intervention or hospitalization, may be able to "pull himself together" and act appropriately long enough to forestall immediate action.

Although personality is relatively preserved, bipolar episodes are characterized by such dramatic changes in affective tone that it may seem that the individual has taken on a new personality. A spouse who is warm and loving may become selfish, arrogant, and aggressive. A parent who is strong and supportive may become clingy, needy, and frightened. Family members may be left confused and uncertain, wondering whether the personal qualities they previously appreciated and respected are genuine, or whether the characteristics displayed during the episode define "the real person."

Practical Effects

Any chronic psychiatric illness can be devastating to a family. However, bipolar illness may be unique in its potential for real-world consequences. As discussed earlier, the affected individual may be a parent and spouse who occupies a central role in the family, and the consequences of disruption of that role may be extreme. The family's financial security may be threatened by loss of a job, unwise investments and business deals, spending sprees, or poor judgment. Staggering debt, eviction, divorce, damage to extended family relationships, automobile accidents, promiscuity, sexually transmitted disease—all may be consequences of bipolar episodes.

The manifestations of bipolar illness, as described earlier, can be confusing and mystifying both to the family and to others. The "on–off" cycling, the resemblance of symptoms to normal moods, and the complex effects on personality are all subject to misinterpretation and misunderstanding by friends, acquaintances, colleagues, police, court officials, and even therapists and inpatient staff. Families often feel blamed and misunderstood, and this contributes to a deep sense of isolation. These issues are specific to bipolar affective disorder and differentiate its effects from those of schizophrenia and other illnesses. Each of them must be addressed in designing a psychoeducational multifamily group model for bipolar disorder.

A MODEL FOR BIPOLAR DISORDER

Although psychoeducational approaches have been used in treating affective disorder,[392-398] only one other group has published a report of a psychoeducational multifamily group approach.[387, 399] Anderson and associates[399] compared a "family process" multifamily group to a psychoeducational multifamily group for treating inpatients with affective disorders. Although the groups each met only once for 4 hours, several significant differences were found in pre- and postgroup testing for both formats; however, there were few differences in outcome *between* groups. It appears that meeting in a multifamily group was more important than the distinction between process and psychoeducational models, and that even a single multifamily group session was useful to individuals and families dealing with affective disorders. One of the few significant differences between the groups was that those attending the psychoeducational group reported greater satisfaction than those attending the process group. Thus, whether or not the psychoeducational format had measurable clinical advantages, it was more valued by family members. (See Holder and Anderson[387] for a description of their model, which includes a one-time, multifamily educational workshop.)

Based on the specific characteristics of bipolar illness, as outlined earlier, we set out to adapt McFarlane's model of psychoeducational multifamily group treatment. This involved modifying each phase of the model.

Joining

Structure

As in the model for schizophrenia, initial joining sessions are held separately for the affected individual and for the family, respectively (see Table 12.2). However, the rationale for this separation comes from the nature of bipolar illness. The individual with schizophrenia is seen separately to protect him or her from the stimulation of prolonged, complex social interaction (see Chapter 6). In bipolar disorder, the goal is to avoid the intense and escalating family conflicts that frequently occur when illness-related issues are approached. These conflicts, related to the affective nature of the illness, can best be managed when the clinicians have established solid working relationships with both the family and the individual, and the separate meetings facilitate this process. As with schizophrenia, both the family and the individual benefit from the opportunity to discuss their experiences and perspectives in a more modulated and controlled environment.

Another difference is the format of the joining sessions. In the schizophrenia model, sessions with the individual are usually shorter, to accommodate his or her difficulties in focusing attention and maintaining concentration. These sessions serve primarily to introduce the therapist as a supportive ally in the achievement of the individual's goals rather than to gather or offer information.[400] However, in bipolar illness, cognitive capacities and social functioning are often relatively intact; the individual is more able to participate fully and often insists on the opportunity to do so. Therefore, in the bipolar model, the individual and family meetings have similar structure: The individual's perspectives on the illness and its effects are elicited, and the same topics are explored as in the family sessions.

Content

The content of the joining sessions is also modified to reflect the specific impact of bipolar illness on the family. While there is extensive discussion of the history of symptoms and course of illness, with particular attention to identifying precipitants and prodromal signs, there is also an emphasis on attitudes and attributions. Individual family members, and the affected individual, may entertain widely different explanations of the illness. For example, a family member may believe that prodromal signs such as lack of sleep or excitement are the cause of an episode, while the individual may dismiss their importance and accuse the family of overreacting to normal behavior. Conversely, the family member may believe that the individual "could stop it if he really wanted to," while the individual insists that the behaviors in question are out of his control. Such differences seem to be characteristic of bipolar illness and are related to such issues as its effects on personality and the ambiguous boundary between affective symptoms and normal mood variations. Because these differences in attribution may lead to ongoing conflict or to difficulty discussing the illness at all, it is important to air them early on.

In addition to a discussion of functioning during episodes, the family and the individual are asked about life when it is *not* dominated by an epi-

TABLE 12.2. Bipolar Multifamily Group Outline of Joining Sessions

I. Structure of sessions
   A. Minimum three sessions; more are usually necessary
      1. Initial sessions with family members alone and individual alone
      2. Later session(s) together
      3. One or both therapists for initial sessions, both for later session(s)
   B. Begin and end with "chatting."

II. Therapists' tasks
   A. Create and maintain a safe, controlled environment.
   B. Be responsible for modulating and moderating interactions and affect.
   C. Hear from everyone.
      1. Accept all "I-statements" as valid.
      2. Normalize experiences: "This is common in depression"; "Family members often report similar concerns."
      3. Be actively engaged and helpful in concrete ways.

III. Sessions with family (and individual) alone
   A. Begin and end each session with 5 minutes of "chatting."
   B. Same topics for family and individual
   C. Survey of present state
      1. Mood, symptoms
      2. Level of functioning, for individual and family members
      3. Attitudes toward the individual (family)
      4. Attitudes toward the illness
      5. Attitudes toward treatment
   D. Episodes
      1. Onset
      2. Symptoms
      3. Precipitants (life events, seasonality, drugs/alcohol, sleep deprivation)
      4. Who does what; what helps, what does not help
      5. Role changes
      6. Emotional reactions
      7. Experiences with treatment
      8. Resolution: what worked
      9. Attribution/explanation of the illness
   E. Life when not dominated by episode
      1. For the individual; for family members
      2. Roles; relationships
      3. Attitudes: toward individual, family, illness
      4. "Mutual influence": In what ways has the illness dominated your lives? In what ways have you been able to escape its influence?
      5. Other issues, not illness-related

IV. Conjoint sessions
   A. Initial "chatting"
   B. Summarize previous meetings, highlighting themes in common (e.g., mutual concern; mutual wish for improvement; previous successes).
   C. Review of each person's experience of illness, episodes, course
      1. "Keep it safe."

(continued)

2. Hear first from the individual, then from each family member in turn, the story of the influence and impact of the illness on their lives.
3. Guide the recital to highlight common themes.
4. Ensure calm by blocking critical, angry comments and all interruptions. Response should be supportive and respectful ("You'll have your turn.")

D. Preparation for the workshop
E. Preparation for the multifamily group
F. End with "chatting"

---

sode. How do roles, relationships, attitudes, and interactions change when the individual is well? Because of fear of recurrence, the periods between episodes can themselves be sources of stress for families struggling with bipolar illness. After repeated episodes, family members may lose some of their flexibility and continue operating as if the individual were acutely ill, even after the episode has resolved. A discussion of interepisode functioning can highlight and begin to address this problem. The discussion also helps remind the family, the individual, and the therapist that the illness is not the whole story, that there are aspects of life, for both the family and the individual, that are free from domination by the illness. This is the beginning of the important process of "externalizing" the illness[401] and "putting the illness in its place" (see also Chapter 16).

Conjoint Sessions

After several sessions with the family and the individual meeting separately, they are seen together for one or more conjoint sessions facilitated by the two therapists together (Table 12.2). For families dealing with bipolar disorder, useful discussions are often stymied by the widely differing perspectives of the individual and of family members, and by the rapid escalation of affect that may result when these differences are approached. The conjoint sessions are closely managed to provide a safe, modulated context in which to highlight areas of agreement and common purpose, while allowing discussion of the differences that have been identified in the earlier, separate sessions. The therapists use the connections they have developed with the individual and the family, a tight structure, and the technique of active listening to create and maintain a safe, calm environment for this discussion. To the extent that this is successful, the family and the individual will develop a sense of possibility and hope for future progress.

The importance of the joining sessions cannot be overstated. For many family members, these sessions are the first time that their experiences have been recognized as important and valid by mental health professionals. It is the first indication that this treatment model will be different from those that they have previously experienced, as illustrated in the following vignette:

> Mary came to the first session tense and angry, prepared to talk about her daughter's illness and how previous treatments had failed them. When the therapist said that she wanted to hear about *her* experience, and not her daughter's, Mary first looked surprised, and then sat back in her chair and said, "You mean you want to know about me?" The rest of the meeting was spent talking about her life and how it had been affected by her daughter's illness. This attention to her perspective was a new experience for her, one that she found positive and validating.

It is interesting that several families participated in the joining sessions but did not go on to the workshop and group meetings. While some families were reluctant to participate further, others appeared to have benefited from the joining sessions alone and did not feel it was necessary to continue.

> John, a man with frequent episodes of mania, came to the joining sessions with his wife and three children, ages 7 to 15. The couple had serious conflicts that prevented them from joining the group; however, in the joining sessions, the children were active participants in the discussions about the nature of bipolar illness and its effects on them and their family, and John reported that the meetings were helpful in improving his relationship with them. Two years later, the couple had separated, but John maintained close relations with his children.

> In another family, the parents had allowed their concern for their severely depressed 20-year-old son to dominate their family life, to the extent that their daughter, who was still in high school, had moved away from home and was staying with the family of a friend. In the first joining meeting, with the parents alone, it was clear that they felt powerless in relation to their son and had difficulty setting any limits because of their concern for him. The therapist treated this as an emergency situation and helped the couple to structure their time and attention to include their daughter, suggesting, for example, that they take her shopping for clothes and leave their son at home. The importance of caring for the rest of the family (one of the family guidelines) was a new and powerful concept for the couple. They came to the next

session with their daughter and discussed with her what would have to be different for her to be willing to return home. They also decided to explore alternative living situations for their son. The son, who refused to participate in the sessions, was never seen. The couple felt they had gotten what they needed from the two sessions and decided not to continue in the program. On follow-up, 1 year later, their daughter had returned home and successfully completed high school, and their son was living in a staffed residence.

Educational Workshop

The structure and format of the bipolar workshop are similar to the schizophrenia workshop except that the affected individual is included. In the schizophrenia model, the individual is given information a little at a time, to accommodate the need to limit stimulation. However, the individual with bipolar disorder is often able to participate fully and can attend with other family members. This can be an important step in helping family members to talk calmly together about the illness.[387]

In our experience, affected individuals are able to tolerate the workshop quite well, especially if they are not experiencing an acute episode. Even the inclusion of symptomatic individuals has not been as disruptive as anticipated. The structure of the workshop helps to focus attention and modulate behavior, and if the individual cannot tolerate long periods of concentration, she or he can leave or take a break. On occasions when an individual has been hypomanic or even manic, other workshop participants have been surprisingly tolerant; the other families are familiar with similar behavior and do not appear to be unduly upset by it. This acceptance by others may be a new and encouraging experience for the individual's family. If a particular individual is unable to participate or is too disruptive, the workshop leaders should be prepared to help him or her to leave, as part of their responsibility for maintaining a safe environment. In this case, the leaders should arrange for the individual to have access to the workshop information at another time.

The content of the workshop is determined by the characteristics of the illness (see Table 12.3). Symptoms of affective episodes, both manic and depressed, are described, with an emphasis on their differences from "normal highs and lows." The issue of "willpower" is addressed, as is the question of the "real personality." In addition to discussion of acute episodes, issues concerning the long-term course of the illness are emphasized. Topics include patterns of frequency and type of episode; presence or

TABLE l2.3. **Bipolar Multifamily Group Outline of Workshop**

I. Description of the illness
  A. Definition: A recurrent, episodic disorder, characterized by changes in mood, as well as in other areas.
  B. Episodes: Mania, depression, and mixed states
    1. Different from normal highs and lows: you can't pull yourself out of it.
    2. Symptoms (may vary in opposite directions for mania and depression)
      a. Mood
      b. Energy level and interest
      c. Activity level (thought, speech, physical)
      d. Physiological changes
      e. Thinking (concentration, decision making)
      f. Irritability
      g. Self-esteem
      h. Judgment
      i. Suicide and self-destructive behavior
      j. Hallucinations and delusions
    3. The question of "willpower"
  C. Course: The pattern of episodes over time
    1. Much variation between individuals, but fairly regular for a given individual
    2. Type of episode
      a. Mania or depression
      b. Pattern of onset
      c. Severity
    3. Frequency
      a. May increase over time, then plateau
      b. May be seasonal
    4. Precipitants
      a. May be present, absent, or ambiguous
      b. Problem of cause versus effect
      c. Life events, positive or negative, major or minor
      d. Drugs/alcohol/medication
      e. Sleep loss as final common pathway
    5. Functioning *between* episodes
      a. May be dramatic, "on–off" difference
      b. May be residual symptoms or decreased function

II. Effects on the family
  A. From the episode
    1. Role changes
      a. May be dramatic changes, for everyone
      b. Then shift back again, when it's over
    2. Dealing with symptoms (mania and depression)
      a. Demanding, intrusive, but unresponsive; nothing helps, but you can't leave.
      b. Poor judgment, so others have to take over
        • Financial, child care
        • Dangerous situations
        • Self-harm and suicide
      c. Appearance of responsibility and control makes this difficult.

  3. Dealing with practical consequences
     a. Financial
     b. Legal
     c. Social: shame and embarrassment
 B. Long-term effects
   1. Depends on type, frequency, and disruptiveness of episodes and on degree
      of recovery
      a. Residual symptoms
      b. Residual consequences
      c. Damage to relationships
   2. Fear of recurrence
      a. Ongoing sense of instability and unpredictability
      b. Fear of precipitating an episode, by confrontation
   3. Consequences of this fear
      a. Hypervigilance
      b. Mistrust of emotional expression
      c. Difficulty talking about stressful topics, especially the illness
      d. Worries about others in the family becoming ill

III. Causes of the illness
 A. It *is* an illness.
   1. Familial: higher incidence of unipolar and bipolar illness in relatives of
      bipolar individuals.
   2. Genetic patterns
      a. Identical twins have higher concordance than fraternal twins.
      b. Adoption studies
   3. Prominence of physiological symptoms: sleep, appetite, diurnal variation
   4. Patterns of recurrence even in absence of precipitants
   5. Specific response to medication (mood stabilizers)
 B. Biological theories
   1. Neurotransmitters
   2. Biological rhythm dysregulation
 C. The biopsychosocial model
   1. Less than 100% concordance for identical twins, so it's not simply genetic.
   2. Biological vulnerability *and* psychological state *and* social stressors, in
      varying proportions in different cases and across time
   3. Important implications
      a. The family didn't cause the illness and can't fix it.
      b. The individual didn't cause it and can't fix it.
      c. The family and the individual *can* affect the illness in important ways.

IV. Treatment
 A. Two distinct goals
   1. To stop an episode
   2. To prevent or minimize recurrence
 B. Medication
   1. *None* of them cure it.
   2. Mood stabilizers (lithium, carbamazepine, valproate, lamotrigine,
      topiramate)
      a. Only lithium and valproate are FDA-approved as mood stabilizers.
      b. Primarily for maintenance and prophylaxis

(*continued on next page*)

TABLE 12.3. (*continued*)

      c. Generally work better for mania than depression

      d. Benefits and risks of each

   3. Antidepressants

      a. Treatment and prophylaxis of depression

      b. Risk of precipitating mania, or rapid cycling

      c. Major classes, with benefits and risks of each

   4. Neuroleptics

      a. Acute treatment of mania

      b. Newer "atypicals" may be useful for maintenance as well, and have less risk of tardive dyskinesia.

      c. Major classes and benefits and risks of each

  C. Electroconvulsive therapy

   1. Useful for both depression and mania

      a. Urgent situations

      b. When medical condition precludes medication

      c. When medication is ineffective

      d. Maintenance treatment

      e. Risks

  D. Hospitalization

   1. To prevent imminent danger.

      a. Suicide

      b. Violence

      c. Severely impaired judgment

   2. For medication and stabilization when not possible in the community

   3. When family/caretakers are exhausted and cannot provide needed support.

   4. Problems

      a. Decisions about care are out of the family's hands

      b. Solutions don't address context, and problems may recur on discharge.

  E. Psychosocial treatments

   1. Individual, group, family, multifamily group, community support, housing, Assertive Community Treatment, self-help

   2. Provide information, support, problem solving

   3. Useful during episode, but especially over time

      a. Help with recovery from episode and with consequences.

      b. Help prevent recurrence.

         • Ongoing monitoring of affective state

         • Support for medication: information, discussion, monitoring

         • Address family issues

         • Ongoing stability and continuity

V. What families can do

  A. "Normal" reactions

   1. Depression: despairing, hopeless, not functioning, not helping self

      a. Response: encourage, energize, convince, argue, berate; try to get him or her to change

      b. Result: no change

      c. You both feel more helpless, more misunderstood, more of a failure

   2. Mania: euphoric, overconfident, unrealistic, argumentative, irresponsible

      a. Response: reason, cajole, debate, argue

      b. Result: escalation, intensity, anger, frustration

   3. End result: helpless, angry, guilty, demoralized

B. What to do instead
  1. Assure safety
    a. To prevent suicide, violence, catastrophe from poor judgment
    b. Use family and social network, hospital, police, as necessary
  2. Set limits
    a. Only when necessary (pick your battles)
    b. Medication and treatment
    c. Violence or harmfulness to others
    d. Any abusive behavior
    e. According to *your* needs
    f. *Don't* argue, scold, debate, convince, threaten.
    g. *Do* keep it simple, clear, specific, firm.
  3. Allow space, once safety and limits have been established
    a. Be available, but low key
    b. Avoid unnecessary demands or criticism
    c. Encourage only if it helps
    d. Accept her or his experience; don't join it, but don't deny it
  4. Care for yourself and the rest of the family
    a. Continue with your life
    b. Important, for you, for family, *and* for her or him
    c. Difficult; get support from family, friends, therapist
    d. Groups such as the National Alliance for the Mentally Ill (NAMI) and the National Depressive and Manic–Depressive Association (NDMDA) can be very helpful
C. Between episodes
  1. Talk about previous episode
    a. What happened, and how you each experienced it
    b. What helped, and what didn't
    c. Can be helpful in correcting misunderstandings and misconceptions
    d. This won't be helpful *during* the episode
  2. Talk about the likelihood of recurrence
    a. May be difficult to consider, but can be very important
    b. Identify early warning signs
    c. Differentiate these signs from normal mood changes
    d. Agree on a plan of action
  3. These discussions may be difficult, and it may be helpful to have outside assistance
  4. Maintain treatment
    a. For monitoring and maintenance
    b. For addressing issues
    c. For continuity and planning

---

absence of precipitants, including the significance of reduced sleep in precipitating mania[402]; seasonal variation; effects of drugs and alcohol; level of functioning between episodes; and the importance of identifying prodromal signs. This focus on course as distinct from episodes is often very helpful to family members, who may not have made the distinction before.

The discussion of the effects of the illness on the family continues the theme of distinguishing between acute episodes and the impact of the illness over time. Acute effects include the dramatic role changes that are required of family members; the frustration of dealing with symptoms that are intrusive, demanding, and unabating; the need to assume responsibility for important functions that the individual may not willingly relinquish; and the need to deal with the practical consequences of the individual's behavior and poor judgment. Long-term effects on the family result from the fear of recurrence; ongoing confusion between symptoms and moods; and the difficulty discussing illness-related issues with the individual in a calm and productive way.

Theories of etiology of the illness are addressed in the workshop, with emphasis on the biopsychosocial model, and with a clear statement that the family did not cause the illness but can have a major role in modifying its course in a positive way.

Treatment is also divided into short- and long-term strategies. Benefits and risks of mood stabilizers, antidepressants, antipsychotic medications, and electroconvulsive therapy are discussed. An integrated psychopharmacological/psychosocial treatment model is presented. The importance of long-term treatment and the benefits of a long-term relationship with a treatment team, for both the individual and the family, are emphasized.

The discussion of management guidelines, or "What Families Can Do," again addresses both short- and long-term issues (see Table 12.4). We begin with a description of typical "helpful" responses to an individual who is experiencing depression or mania. Like Anderson and colleagues,[399] we have found that the low-stimulation environment emphasized in the schizophrenia workshop is less important than interrupting the negative interactional sequences that are common in mania as well as depression. Rather than emphasize "going slow," we emphasize how to respond (and not respond) to affective intensity. For depression, we recommend being available, "but at a friendly distance"; for mania, setting clear limits and assuring safety, but otherwise avoiding arguments and debates, and "allowing space." For the long-term, we emphasize the importance of talking to-

TABLE 12.4. Bipolar Multifamily Group Family Guidelines for Bipolar Illness

1. Assure safety (for everyone).
2. Set limits as needed.
3. Be clear, simple, and direct.
4. Allow space.
5. Support medication and treatment.
6. Care for the rest of the family, too.
7. Between episodes, talk together and plan.

gether: sharing experiences of past episodes, identifying characteristic precipitants and prodromal patterns, and planning for future episodes. Finally, we emphasize the importance of long-term treatment and of an ongoing relationship with a treatment team that will be available when needed.

The workshop has been well received by all participants. New information is helpful, but recognition and validation of their own experiences, in the descriptions of episodes and course, and especially the effects of the illness on the family, have been equally important. As in the schizophrenia workshops, a classroom setting provides a comfortable way to meet other families. The encouragement of questions and discussion, along with frequent refreshment breaks, allows each person to titrate her or his level of participation and socialization. As expected, some affected individuals may decide not to attend the workshop or may leave early, but, as a rule, most have participated fully. Family members and individuals can often be seen exchanging glances and smiles of recognition as particular aspects of the illness and its effects are presented, and the workshop seems to have something to offer to all participants.

A recent innovation in some workshops has been the addition of a panel of community providers. This group, which may include crisis intervention workers, police, hospital emergency room and inpatient staff, and others, discusses how to access community services. This has been very helpful to family members and also provides useful feedback to the providers.

Ongoing Group Meetings

The structure of the multifamily group meetings is essentially unchanged from that of the schizophrenia model (see Part II). The first meeting focuses on the participants' lives apart from the illness, in order to emphasize that the illness is only one part of their lives. The second session starts with 10 minutes of "chatting" and then concentrates on how bipolar illness has affected each member's life. The group leaders contribute their own experiences in both sessions, underscoring the nonhierarchical relationships established in the joining sessions. Each subsequent meeting starts with a period of non-illness-related "chatting"; the meeting then moves into a structured "go-round," during which there is discussion of illness-related experiences since the last meeting. From this discussion, a problem is selected and defined, and group members engage in a structured problem-solving process. Finally, the group ends with another period of "chatting."

Throughout the meeting, the concepts initially presented in the workshop are highlighted, with an ongoing focus on distinguishing between the person and the illness. Problems and potential solutions are discussed in terms of these concepts and the management guidelines derived from them.

Although the format of the groups is the same as that for schizophrenia, the groups themselves tend to be very different. The emotional tone of the groups is heightened; the meetings are often livelier and more energetic, with active participation by affected individuals as well as family members. In fact, it would be difficult at times for a naive observer to know who is the affected individual and who is the family member. This tone can be expressed in joking and spontaneous conversation, as well as in arguments, confrontation, and crisis.

The formal structure of the group sessions is extremely important in containing and directing this energy. Bipolar illness is characterized by frequent crises, emotional reactivity, and a strong sense of urgency. The insistence on initial chatting before discussing the illness or crises gives a clear message about the importance, and the possibility, of "keeping the illness in its place." The structure of the problem-solving process, with its well-defined sequence of steps, also conveys the message that no problem is too urgent for an organized, thoughtful approach to its solution. The explicit nature of the structure provides a way to convey these messages without criticism or confrontation.

> In the joining sessions, Harold was quite focused, in a critical way, on the behavior of his wife Gladys, who was seriously depressed. In the first group meeting, where the task was defined as introducing oneself, separate from the illness, he began, "I'm Gladys's husband. She has manic–depression, and that's a real problem, because . . . " Rather than challenge him directly, the therapist interrupted with, "That part of the discussion will be next time. Today, we're introducing ourselves separate from the illness." Harold started over again, introducing himself as a retired typesetter, and went on to discuss his current hobbies and interests.

Over time, characteristic themes emerge. The problems and solutions raised in the problem-solving segment of the meetings tend to be different from those in groups for schizophrenia, with less emphasis on maintaining a low-stress, "one step at a time" environment, and more emphasis on issues of control versus autonomy. This is predictable given the nature of bipolar illness.

The theme of hypervigilance, initially presented in the joining sessions and workshop, is central to the experience of both family members and affected individuals, and comes up repeatedly in the course of the groups. It is one of the main areas where questions of autonomy versus control are played out. Family members, wanting to intervene as early as possible to prevent recurrence of an episode, often become concerned at any change in mood or sign of affective intensity. Since prodromal signs in bipolar illness may consist of positive changes, such as increased sense of well-being, energy, or ambition, or may be indistinguishable from appropriate anger or discontent, the family's concern may clash with the individual's view of the validity of these feelings. It is often difficult in the groups to distinguish between hypervigilance on the one hand, and useful and appropriate concern on the other. In a given situation, the therapists and the other group members, using the problem-solving structure, may help the family and the individual think this question through, using past experiences, prodromal patterns, and current observations to make the distinction.

A related theme is the differentiation between the person and the illness. This is sometimes expressed as "Is this the individual speaking, or is it the illness?" This question can be useful therapeutically, as part of externalizing the illness, but it is also a real issue that often confronts individuals and families living with bipolar illness. With the frequent and sometimes drastic changes in personality accompanying episodes, family members often become confused about whether a particular manifestation is the "real" personality, a symptom of the illness, or even an effect of medication. As one man with rapid-cycling illness put it, "Sometimes I'm a jerk with bipolar illness, and sometimes I'm just a jerk." This frequent topic of discussion in the groups is often not easily resolved.

Since individuals with bipolar illness are frequently employed, stigma is often experienced in the workplace. The members of one group in particular became quite knowledgeable about state equal rights statutes, and several members successfully challenged workplace discrimination.

Sylvia, a 45-year-old woman with bipolar disorder, attended the group with her husband and young adult daughter. She had worked for many years in a bank without incident, but following a hospitalization for mania, her colleagues learned of her diagnosis, and her supervisor told her she was unsuitable for her job and threatened to fire her. With the help of a plan developed in the group problem-solving process, Sylvia filed a complaint with the State Human Rights Commission and following an investigation, the company assured her of continued employment.

CHALLENGES TO GROUP
FORMATION AND MAINTENANCE

In the course of these groups, a number of issues related to specific characteristics of bipolar illness have presented challenges to group formation and process.

Diagnostic Ambiguity

Although bipolar disorder is a clearly defined syndrome, in practice, there is significant overlap of key, defining symptoms with a number of other conditions, including schizophrenia, substance abuse, and personality disorder. Therefore diagnostic ambiguity is inherent in the clinical picture and not simply a question of the evaluator's acumen.[403] Especially when the individual is already taking maintenance medication at the time of referral, the diagnosis of bipolar disorder may be provisional at best, even with a careful history and review of past evaluations. This can have significant implications for treatment.

> Michael is a 40-year-old, married man with a long history of abusing drugs and alcohol, and several psychiatric hospitalizations for problems with mood. His last hospitalization, 3 months prior to referral, resulted in the diagnosis of bipolar disorder, treatment with a mood stabilizer, and referral to a multifamily group. Initial evaluation, including history from Michael and his wife and review of hospital records, suggested, but did not clearly confirm, the diagnosis of bipolar disorder. The couple attended the multifamily group regularly but with no benefit. In the course of the group, Michael never described himself as being upset or having a temper; he referred to all mood changes as "mania." Because of intractable mood and behavior problems, he was tried on a variety of medications and had frequent hospitalizations, with no apparent benefit. He eventually rejected the diagnosis of bipolar disorder, left the group, and stopped all medication. One year later, he was attending Alcoholics Anonymous (AA) and had no further hospitalizations, although his difficult behavior persisted.

In this case, it appears that the diagnosis of bipolar disorder may have been inaccurate and was not useful as a predictor of response to treatment interventions or management. In fact, it may even have been counterproductive, providing a language that diverted attention from substance abuse and characterological issues.

Maintaining the Group Structure

In several of the bipolar multifamily groups, some members have initially challenged the structure of the meetings. They have wanted to skip the "chatting" phase, shortcut the problem-solving format, or use the meeting to discuss problems and issues not related to the illness. This may be a consequence of the increased energy and emotional tone of the families, the very factors that make the structure essential to the effective functioning of the group. Therapists new to the format may have difficulty withstanding the pressure to modify it, but we have found that the structure is crucial; poor attendance and dropouts can often be prevented or corrected by returning to the original structure and content.

Sometimes the challenge to the structure is an expression of a tenuous working relationship between the group leaders and the family. In this instance, a few additional joining sessions may increase the strength of the alliance enough to allow the family to give the group a chance. At other times, the problem may lie in the group leader's beliefs about therapy and change. For example, a leader's belief in the therapeutic benefit of self-expression may lead to allowing monologues and expression of feelings to take precedence over problem solving, or a leader's interest in exploring personal therapeutic issues may dilute the group's focus on illness-related topics. In this case, a supervisory review of psychoeducational principles and practices will often serve to redirect the leader's efforts.

Psychiatric Conditions in Family Members

Perhaps because individuals with bipolar disorder tend to marry more often than those with schizophrenia, the effects of assortive mating[404] are often apparent. In a number of couples, the nonbipolar spouse also has had a psychiatric condition requiring attention. The husband of a woman with bipolar disorder suffered from chronic depression himself and was a recovering alcoholic. A man with bipolar episodes revealed that his wife had experienced delirium tremens during a recent hospitalization for surgery. Several spouses had personality disorders, some with paranoid features, that significantly interfered with their ability to participate effectively in the groups. This may be workable when the spouse acknowledges his or her difficulties, but when this is not the case, the problems cannot be addressed within this model, with its focus on illness in one identified individual.

CONCLUSIONS

Psychoeducational multifamily group treatment has proven to be very useful for families and individuals struggling with bipolar illness. As in the groups for schizophrenia, the model has benefited affected individuals and family members, and the group facilitators as well.

In general, affected individuals who participated in the groups behaved less angrily over time and were better able to manage symptoms and episodes. Group attendance also resulted in fewer hospitalizations for many individuals. For some individuals, episodes were less debilitating when they did occur, possibly because everyone moved more quickly to get help in response to early warning signs. A number of affected individuals noted that the group allowed them to appreciate their family's experience: "I had no idea what my family had to contend with."

Family members were often able to shift over time, from attending the group for the sake of the affected individual to attending for their own benefit. There was generally a drop in tension in the group when this occurred. Family members reported that the greatest contribution to an increased sense of confidence in their ability to cope with the illness came from the repeated experience of being listened to respectfully by group members and facilitators. Their confidence in the individual's ability to manage the illness over the long haul grew as they saw him or her participate actively and appropriately in the group, and contribute to the problem-solving process from the perspective of his or her personal experience of the illness. However, family members were able to benefit from the program even if the affected individual did not attend.

The group leaders reported that it generally took them about 2 years to master the techniques of adhering to a peer relationship, problem-solving, illness-management format. They discovered, as did leaders in the schizophrenia groups, that their experience with this model affected all of their clinical work. Group leaders found themselves becoming more participatory and less hierarchical, seeing their role more as consultant than therapist. They became more interested in the family's and individual's experience of illness and more respectful of, and empathic with, their efforts to cope with it. They learned in the groups that each person's struggle with illness is different, that what works for one person will not necessarily be helpful for another. Group leaders also learned that individuals and family members are ultimately responsible for managing their illness and that professionals, while very important allies, can only help them in this task.

ACKNOWLEDGMENTS

We wish to thank Judith Redwine, RN, MSW, and Kit Perry, MSW (Brunswick, Maine), and Eileen Stewart, MSW (Bronx, New York), who facilitated the groups on which this chapter is based and contributed significantly to the development of the model.

Chapter 13

Multifamily Group Treatment for Major Depressive Disorder

GABOR I. KEITNER, LAURA M. DRURY,
CHRISTINE E. RYAN, IVAN W. MILLER,
WILLIAM H. NORMAN, AND DAVID A. SOLOMON

Major depression is one of the most common psychiatric disorders. The illness interferes with biological, psychological, and social functioning. It disrupts a person's ability to sleep, eat, concentrate, have adequate energy, and experience pleasure. Psychological symptoms include feelings of guilt, worthlessness, hopelessness, and a tendency to interpret events from a negative perspective. Social functioning is also significantly impaired. Not surprisingly, depression exerts a major influence on significant others in that patient's social field. Family relationships and interactions particularly are adversely affected. Furthermore, the way in which significant others respond to the patient's illness has a clinically significant impact on the symptomatology and course of that illness. Understanding both biological and psychosocial parameters that influence the course and treatment of depressive disorders will reinforce efforts to develop cost-effective treatments.

FAMILY FUNCTIONING AND THE PHASES OF DEPRESSION

A variety of studies have consistently shown that an episode of major depression is associated with significant difficulties in many areas of family life. Communications in the family, the ability to resolve problems, and appropriate role functioning are particularly disrupted. There is evidence to suggest that families of depressed patients experience more difficulties than do families of patients with other psychiatric disorders.[405-407] Particular areas of concern include financial worry, chronic marital disharmony, social isolation, loss of social status, chronic tension, and fears of recurrence.[408] Key symptoms of depression, namely, worrying, irritability, nagging, anxiety, and anergia, are especially upsetting to relatives because they appear to be an extension of normal behavior and seemingly under the patient's control. Florid symptoms are more easily attributed to the illness.[409] Patients with comorbid conditions have even more problematic family functioning both during the acute episode and at 6-month follow-up than do patients with pure major depression.[410] This functional impairment may be more crippling than that brought about by chronic medical illnesses.[411]

Studies suggest that family functioning improves as the depressive episode remits, but that families of patients with major depression still experience more problematic family functioning at remission than do control families.[412-416] Family dysfunction during the acute episode does not appear to be just a reaction to the acute stress brought about by the intensity of the illness but may represent more enduring interpersonal problems.

Family functioning and social support influence the course and outcome of major depression. Ongoing family conflicts consistently predict poorer long-term outcomes.[417] Patients whose family functioning improved over the course of the depressive illness had a significantly shorter time to recovery than patients whose families did not improve.[416] The size and supportive nature of the social network also predicts the course of depressive illness.[418] Patients with a close confidant and less family conflict showed better outcomes in brief therapy than those lacking such support.[419] For women in particular, the quality of support received from a spouse is a very strong predictor of posthospital symptom course. Women without supportive marriages are less likely to recover.[420] Spouses' positive response to the depressive illness are associated with rapid recovery rates, whereas conflictual relationships predict a slow recovery.[421]

Residual family dysfunction is significant not only for delaying recovery but also in potentially inducing relapse. It is not only related to a lower chance of recovery from the depression by 1 year[422] but is also associated with a more episodic and chronic course 5 years later.[423] High levels of criticism are strongly related to the likelihood of relapse.[424-426] Depressed patients tend to relapse at lower levels of criticism than do patients with schizophrenia. Marital distress, in combination with perceived criticism, is particularly related to a tendency to relapse.

Evidence from a series of studies over the past 10 years suggest that there is significant psychosocial impairment in patients with chronic depression, affecting interpersonal interactions with spouses, family members, and friends; vocational functioning, including housework; social leisure time/recreational activities; sexual functioning; and life satisfaction.[427] The psychosocial impairment in chronic depression is comparable to that of patients with episodic major depression[407, 428] and as dysfunctional as that which occurs during the acute episode of major depression.[427] Chronic depression has been found to have greater impact on marital life than chronic physical illness (rheumatoid arthritis, cardiac disease).[411]

We do not know the causal sequence between depression and problematic family functioning. It is likely that there are mutually reinforcing patterns of interactions between patients' vulnerability to depression and families' ways of coping with the illness. Patients' vulnerability to depression may include genetic predisposition, early life experiences, personality variables, current life events, or persistent family conflicts. Regardless of the etiology of the episode, the patient's family and/or significant others have to respond to, and deal with, the depression. If the family and the social support system respond effectively, the depressive illness may be relatively brief and may remit more readily. Conversely, if the family is unable to respond adequately to the patient's illness because of its own difficulties, then the illness may be more prolonged, with the patient less likely to recover and more likely to relapse into subsequent episodes. A family's ability to cope with the illness is influenced by a variety of factors, including socioeconomic level, composition, current stresses, assortative mating, and overall functioning.[429] Patient vulnerability and family coping skills are seen as mutually reinforcing forces; the latter may act to lengthen the depressive illness, facilitate recovery, or confer protection against relapse.

PHARMACOTHERAPY, FAMILY THERAPY, GROUP THERAPY, AND MULTIFAMILY GROUP THERAPY

Pharmacotherapy of even a short duration (6 to 12 weeks) has been found to lead to significant improvements not only in depressive symptoms but also in social functioning.[427, 433–438] The greatest improvement in social functioning was found in patients most responsive to pharmacotherapy. In virtually all these studies, better psychosocial functioning was associated with better response to drug therapy and less residual psychosocial impairment at the completion of pharmacotherapy. Patients with high levels of psychosocial impairment prior to pharmacotherapy did not respond well to the medications, in terms of symptom improvement, and continued to experience psychosocial impairment. In addition, in spite of improvement, social/family functioning at the end of 12 weeks of pharmacotherapy was still worse for the depressed population than for the nonclinical controls.[427, 430] Although helpful for a subpopulation of depressed patients, pharmacotherapy still does not adequately address the psychosocial aspects of the illness.

Because of the predictive value of family factors on the course of a depressive illness, there has been increased interest in the use of family interventions on a routine clinical basis. However, only five studies have investigated the efficacy of family or marital treatments for depressive disorders. Four of these five studies reported that marital/family treatment alone for depressed outpatients produced response rates equivalent to pharmacotherapy or individual treatment.[405, 436–438] The one published study with an inpatient sample[439] did not find significant treatment effects for family intervention. Perhaps methodological differences, patient populations, or both, contributed to the different findings. Thus, while there is strong evidence that family treatments for depression are useful, it is not yet conclusive.

Our search of the literature revealed 23 studies[440–462] of the efficacy of group therapy for depression that were published in peer-reviewed journals between 1977 and 1990. Overall, the results of these studies indicate that (1) group treatments for depression are more efficacious than no treatment or waiting-list controls, and (2) the efficacy of group treatments appears comparable to individual treatments for depression. There appears, therefore, to be evidence for some effectiveness of group treatments of depressive disorders.

To date, the only previous multifamily group treatment for depression has been the model developed by Anderson.[387, 399] Although this multifamily approach has been used clinically at the University of Pittsburgh for many years, the only empirical data that have been collected on this model are comparisons of participants' satisfaction with the group.[399] This study indicated that patients and families were very satisfied with the treatment and believed that they obtained significant benefits. However, despite the fact that this intervention has been incorporated into several long-term studies of depression,[463] there has been no study of the potential effects of this multifamily treatment on outcome or course of illness in major depression.

CONDUCTING MULTIFAMILY GROUP
TREATMENT FOR DEPRESSION

The following section describes guidelines and procedures used in conducting multifamily psychoeducational groups for patients with mood disorders who participated in a 5-year National Institute of Mental Health–sponsored research study. While our study focused on patients with bipolar disorder, the multifamily group component was made up of patients with both unipolar and bipolar illness. Patients with both diagnoses were combined in order to ensure a critical mass of patients and families for the effectiveness of the format, and also because we felt that there was a significant overlap in the themes of remission and relapse between unipolar and bipolar forms of mood disorders. Additionally, both unipolar and bipolar patients had a common experience in the depressive phase of the illness, and we assumed that a certain percentage of unipolar patients might eventually experience an episode of mania.

The first section provides an overview of (1) the basic goals, assumptions, and rationale of the multifamily group intervention; (2) the group's structure, including family group size and composition; and (3) the therapists' roles, training, and experience. The second section details the format, content, and procedures of the individual screening session and the six multifamily group sessions. The final section is a discussion of common themes and issues of concern that emerged from conducting 12 waves of multifamily group interventions composed of 68 families and 170 individuals.

Much of the material is drawn from previous descriptions of psychoeducational groups. In particular, material has been borrowed from Basco and Rush,[464] Holder and Anderson,[387] Yalom,[465] and Gonzalez and colleagues.[466]

Overview of Goals and Structure

The mood disorders multifamily group intervention has several goals. First, the group helps patients and family members become knowledgeable about the signs and symptoms of depression and mania. Second, the group promotes relationships and increases understanding of the effects of the illness by sharing information, support, and its members' own perspectives on family interactions. Third, patients and family members gain insight and learn new coping strategies in dealing with different phases of the patient's illness. Finally, patients and families have a better understanding of how they can work with each other, and with mental health professionals, in dealing with a difficult and chronic illness.

Although patients and families come to the group with different levels of understanding of mood disorders, the majority of patients and families agree to group participation following the patient's recent hospitalization or because he or she is experiencing an exacerbation of manic or depressive symptoms. In fact, we have found that the intervention is most acceptable and useful for persons who are motivated by immediate and pressing needs.

The intervention itself consists of two major components: (1) an initial 60-minute screening session involving the therapist, the patient, and his or her family member(s); and (2) six multifamily group sessions conducted by two experienced psychotherapists. Each group meeting is approximately 90 minutes long and meets for 6 consecutive weeks.

The group therapists balance the presentation of educational information about depression and mania with guided discussions in which patients and family members share their personal experiences and concerns in coping with the illness. The first three sessions are more didactic in nature, and the last three sessions are more interactive and interpersonal.

Family Composition

A core feature of this program is that both the patient and family members attend the sessions. All family members of the household over the age of 12 are expected to attend. While complete attendance in large families, or families with adolescents, is sometimes difficult, all family members are strongly encouraged to attend. Minimum attendance includes the patient and spouse or, if the patient is an adult child living at home, the patients and his or her parents. Children below the age of 12 are excluded due to (1) their potential lack of attention and capacity to disrupt the sessions, (2) their potential limited understanding of the topics to be discussed, and (3) potential inhibition of discussion among adult family members when a young child is present.

While the concept "all family members" refers to persons living together, other family members who live nearby and play important roles in the patient's life may wish to attend the group sessions. It is our experience that group discussions regarding day-to-day interactions with a patient with a mood disorder are most meaningful to those who share significant amounts of time with the patient. While using the criterion of "living together" should be followed in most cases, the therapist can make exceptions on individual bases.

Patients attending the group sessions should be sufficiently improved from the acute episode to be able to profit from the group. Therefore, patients in a depressive episode should be able to concentrate sufficiently to follow and tolerate group discussions of affective symptoms with other family members. Patients with a manic episode should be sufficiently improved, so that they do not disrupt the group process and can take appropriate redirection by the therapists.

Group Composition

A minimum of four families seems to be necessary to ensure adequate activity and group discussion. However, more than 18–20 people is an upper limit, above which the opportunity for each family member to participate is significantly diminished. Groups of five to six families, or 12–14 people, are optimal.

As noted earlier, we typically include both patients with bipolar disorder and patients with major depression in our groups. While families of patients with major depression usually do not have experience with manic symptoms, we have found that the heterogeneity within the broader category of mood disorders often facilitates focusing the group on the family issues that are common to both disorders. Differences between bipolar disorder and unipolar major depression also serve to highlight both the commonalities and heterogeneity within affective disorders.

We have also found that the best group dynamics occur when there is a mixed composition. Too many manic patients in the group may promote chaos, and too many depressed patients may inhibit a lively discussion. To ensure that members do not feel isolated, there should be more than one family representing each illness.

Therapists

Because of the relatively large number of people participating in each group and the multiple levels of interaction involved, two cotherapists are necessary to monitor and lead the discussions effectively. In addition, two leaders are needed in case a patient or family member becomes upset during the session and requires immediate attention. Therapists should be experienced in working with psychiatric patients, families of patients, and also in group process and therapy. Therapists should be knowledgeable about current issues and treatments of major depression and bipolar illness, including the biopsychosocial model of mood disorders.

The therapists should not advocate the efficacy (or lack of efficacy) of any specific approach to treatment. Also, in order to promote frank discussion within the group sessions, the therapists should not be otherwise involved in the patients' treatment. Our multifamily group therapists include a psychologist and a social worker, each with over 10 years of experience.

Clinical Procedures

The group therapists should meet before each session to discuss the content of the session and the division of tasks between the therapists. They should also meet immediately after the session to review and assess group members and to plan future agendas and strategies. This debriefing is particularly important if a crisis occurred with either a patient or a family member during the group session.

The occurrence of a crisis situation is not uncommon in multifamily group settings, especially for patients with mood disorders. A total of six crisis situations arose in the 12 waves of group interventions (72 meetings), five involving patients and one involving a family member. A crisis situation may consist of an individual becoming very upset and/or disruptive during a group session or a patient voicing psychotic/suicidal thinking. While disturbing, a crisis situation can also be very instructive to group members. However, it is extremely important for the therapists to assume full responsibility for the safety of both the group and the distraught individual.

Screening Session

The screening session is an individual meeting between the patient, family member(s), and one of the two cotherapists. This session serves several purposes. First, it serves to introduce the family to the therapist. Since many families are reluctant to attend a multifamily group, this initial family meeting allows the therapist to explain in detail the group and its procedures, and to address any concerns that the patient or family members have about the intervention.

Second, it provides an opportunity to assess the family's and patient's knowledge about mood disorders; coping skills and methods employed to deal with the illness; and the family's interpersonal style, communication pattern, and personal resources, including social support, for coping with the illness and stressful events. It is equally important for the therapist to gather information about the family's strengths, including sources of enjoyment and pleasure, as well as outside social and community resources.

In addition, the screening session begins to build an alliance between the therapist and family. Finally, this session allows the therapist to assess the appropriateness of the family and the patient for the psychoeducational group.

Outline of Screening Session

The therapist who will be meeting the family reviews the patient's medical records and any notes from the referring therapist regarding the patient and family member(s). The session progresses as follows:

1. Begin the session by welcoming the family. Ask family members to introduce themselves. Ask about each member's expectations concerning the program.
2. Discuss the rationale and purpose of the program. Present structure, rules, and format. Ask members about questions and concerns.
3. Address administrative issues—meeting times and places, fees (if any), feedback mechanisms to psychiatrist and/or primary therapist. Emphasize the importance of regular attendance of all family members.
4. Ask the patient and family member(s) if they have ever participated in a group format before. If yes, ask what their experience has been in a group. Ask about other kinds of treatment the patient had, his or her reaction to it, and the outcome.
5. Discuss some of the potential benefits of participating in the group, including the opportunity to develop relationships with members of other families, to generate better skills or enhance existing coping skills, to gain increased emotional and social support, and to learn more about the illness. Stress the fact that the patient and family member(s) will also learn how to communicate more effectively with each other.
6. Whether or not they have participated in a group, ask if they feel comfortable talking in a group setting in general, and if they are able to talk about themselves specifically.
7. Discuss how it will feel to get feedback from both therapists and other group members, and whether they are willing to learn how to give feedback.
8. Talk about the commitment to attend every session from the perspective of building group trust and group cohesion, and developing a common language to facilitate group discussion.
9. Determine the willingness of both the patient and family members

to take responsibility and participate in group discussions, and to allow other group members to participate as well.

At this point the therapist needs to make a judgment about the appropriateness of the family for the psychoeducational group. To do so, he or she draws on all information gathered from his or her review of the medical records, any notes from referring therapist(s), and the 60-minute screening session. It is a clinical decision made by the experienced therapist. If the family is judged to be inappropriate, then the therapist should discuss reasons for this decision frankly with the family, offering the possibility of participation in a later group and/or making a referral, if indicated.

If the therapist is not clear about the appropriateness of the multifamily group for the patient and his or her family members, then he or she voices these concerns directly in the screening session. If the therapist still feels ambivalent, he or she can postpone the decision until after it is discussed at the team meeting with colleagues, or with the referral source. Once the decision is made, the therapist notifies the patient and family members, and provides alternate referrals, if necessary.

10. Remind the family about meeting time, place, and fees. Make sure they have phone numbers to reach the therapists. Give the family a written information sheet about the group, including all administrative information.

Psychoeducation Group: Session 1

There are several goals of the first multifamily group session. The first session orients the families to the multifamily group. Roles of the therapists and group members are explained and introductions are made. The session both elicits information from the families and provides then with information concerning the signs and symptoms of depression and mania. The first session also begins to develop group cohesion, group trust, and a common language and knowledge base for members to use during discussions.

Preparation

Cotherapists review available information about each family and share perceptions of each family from the screening sessions, specify the tasks and role of each cotherapist, and give everyone a name tag (including therapists)color coded by family, with easily readable lettering.

Outline of Psychoeducation Group

1. The group therapists introduce themselves and welcome group members to the first group session. The therapists go over the purpose of the group and briefly describe the format of the first session.

2. The group members introduce themselves, identifying why they have come and what they hope to learn or obtain from the group. Members who have a mood disorder identify themselves; others identify themselves as family members.

3. One therapist presents administrative information and group guidelines. The guidelines include rules regarding the following:

   a. Confidentiality. The group is confidential and participants are cautioned to protect the confidentiality of what is shared in the group.

   b. Issues of safety. Although all patients have a prescreening interview where it is determined that the patient is stabilized and able to participate in the group, occasionally patients experience an exacerbation of symptoms that requires immediate intervention by the group leaders. It is explained to the group that, at such a time, the leaders will take appropriate measures to ensure the safety of the patient and of the group.

   c. Respect for others' opinions. Everyone wants a chance to talk, but one person talks at a time, and others listen until he or she is finished.

4. Group leaders present an overview that includes both the content and goals of each of the six sessions. The overall goals of the program are (a) to provide current information concerning mood disorders to the patients and families; (b) to focus on the way the disorder affects day-to-day family life and patterns of family behavior that develop in response to the disorder; and (c) to develop strategies for coping more efficiently with a mood disorder. Since there are no "right" answers about how to handle difficult issues, patients and families can help each other by sharing their experiences.

5. Group members and one leader are seated in a semicircle, while the other leader stands at a chalkboard in front of the group and records signs and symptoms of depression and mania generated by the group discussion. The majority of those who come to the group have experienced crises and hardships as a result of one family member having a mood disorder. Thus, they already come with a lot of knowledge about the day-to-day effects of the illness. However, members often feel alone and discouraged in managing the illness.

As group members discuss their experiences and the symptoms of depression and mania, group trust develops and members feel less alone. Members also learn that many of their experiences with mood disorders are shared by others. This exercise enables members to begin speaking in a group and empowers families by acknowledging their experience and the fact that they can both contribute to the sessions and learn from them.

Participants are given handouts listing depressive and manic symptoms, along with guidelines to assess the severity of symptoms. Members also learn how to monitor change on a continuous basis, so that they can take note of subtle improvements. Initial phases of the illness are discussed, along with factors that contribute to relapse.

6. The therapist uses the information offered by the group and expands on it by discussing the distinction between normal mood variations and the symptoms of mood disorders. These distinctions help families distinguish how much of the patient's behavior may be due to the disorder. The importance of identifying symptoms early in the onset of the episode, as well as reactions to environmental stress, is emphasized, since early intervention may prevent a full-blown episode.

7. Summary and wrap-up. The therapist summarizes the session by drawing on the group's contributions to establish a common knowledge base and language for future discussions.

8. At the end of Session 1, the following brochures published by the National Depressive and Manic–Depressive Association are distributed and members are asked to read them for the next group session: *Dealing Effectively with Depression and Manic Depression* and *A Guide to Depressive and Manic–Depressive Illness: Diagnosis, Treatment and Support.*

Psychoeducation Group: Session 2

In the second session, the therapists use the two brochures distributed at the end of the previous session as a springboard for a group discussion of concerns and experiences with mood disorders. The group addresses issues concerning living with a family member who has a mood disorder, the problems associated with the disorder, and potential coping strategies.

Preparation

Review the previous session and identify potential issues that should be addressed in this session. Specify the tasks and role of each cotherapist. Arrange for handouts at the end of the session.

Outline of Psychoeducation Group

1. Checking In. Each subsequent session begins with a "check-in" to determine how the week has been for group members. It is sometimes useful to check directly with each person to make sure that no one is overly anxious or feels threatened or hurt by something that was said. Each person should feel that his or her concerns are heard and appreciated. The therapists ask the group to summarize the previous session and discuss any impressions or reservations about the first group session. *A check-in and summary of the previous group session becomes part of the beginning of all group sessions to follow.* This becomes particularly important when a crisis situation has occurred in the previous session.

2. The group therapists facilitate group discussion of the two brochures that members read for homework. These brochures are used as a springboard for group discussion of members' concerns and experiences with mood disorders. Members share the impact that the illness has on patients and families, as well as the strategies for coping. The following points should be included:

   a. The purpose of the next several sessions is to discuss the challenges, concerns, and stresses faced by families with a member who has a mood disorder.

   b. Families respond to this challenge as best they know how. In spite of this, family members often feel uncertain or even guilty about the way things have turned out. As these meetings progress, many different feelings about the disorders are expressed and shared by others. Different families try different ways of coping with the problems they face. We hope that sharing these solutions may help members learn from each other.

Therapists should take care that group members discuss solutions and their effectiveness. This process is not a formal evaluation of what is "right" or "wrong"; rather, it is one way to expose patients and family members to a range of solutions and new ways of addressing problems that may have worked for others.

3. Therapists ask each family to discuss some of the problems that occur when a family member becomes ill. Then they ask other participants to comment on their experience with the problems. If not volunteered by the group, the therapists may include the following potential problem areas (taken from Holder & Anderson[387]):

- Agitation
- Lack of reasonableness
- Behaviors that appear willful
- Apparent lack of caring for others
- Increased need to control relationships

- Oversensitivity
- Unresponsiveness
- Inability to function in normal roles
- Unpredictable behavior
- Dangerous or violent outbursts

4. Therapists also discuss economic issues and systemic barriers to long-term treatment. An example of the former is how role conflicts arise with concerns over patients' excessive spending sprees during a manic episode, when bank accounts are shared, or job incapacity or loss when patients are depressed. The latter issue becomes important when insurance and financial limits are reached due to the costs associated with the patient's mood disorder.

5. Therapists ask group members to discuss their concerns when the patient is not ill. These should also be listed on the board and discussed by all group members.

6. There is a general discussion of strategies for coping with these problems: "What are some of the things you have tried that have helped with this issue?"; "What things haven't worked?"

7. Summary and wrap-up. Remind group members that discussion will continue.

8. At the end of Session 2, members are told that a psychiatrist will attend the next group session and present an overview of mood disorders. The following readings on medication and treatments are distributed to be read for homework: *Lithium Treatment of Manic Depressive Illness: A Practical Guide*[470] and *A Guide to Depressive and Manic–Depressive Illness: Diagnosis, Treatment and Support.*[468]

Psychoeducation Group: Session 3

The purpose of Session 3 is to provide information concerning pharmacological treatments for mood disorders and to give group members the opportunity to discuss their concerns with a medical expert on mood disorders. The psychiatrist gives an overview of affective illness, its treatments, and obstacles to effective treatments. The brief presentation is followed by a question-and-answer period.

Preparation

Review the previous session and identify potential issues that should be addressed in this session. Specify the tasks and role of each cotherapist, and confirm attendance of the psychiatrist.

Outline of Psychoeducation Group

1. After checking in, patients and their family members often have questions about depression or bipolar disorder that have not been addressed. A psychiatrist joins the group in order to provide some basic information related to genetics and childbearing, and to answer any questions about the disorder. Important points that can be covered in the brief presentation include prevalence, age of onset, and risks of heritable transmission.

2. The bulk of the hour is spent in answering questions about etiology, course of illness, and treatment options. Topics include discussion of different types of medications, their indications and side effects, with particular emphasis on lithium, anticonvulsant, and antidepressant medications; interaction of illicit drugs and alcohol with psychotropic medications and symptoms of mood disorders; potential misconceptions about psychotropic medication use, including issues of addiction and dependence; and issues of compliance with medication treatment and the typical results of noncompliance.

During this session, the psychiatrist emphasizes several important points about the pharmacological treatment of mood disorder:

- There are many new, effective antidepressants (e.g., selective serotonin reuptake inhibitors) with better side-effect profiles.
- Three standard mood stabilizers are lithium, valproate, and carbamazepine.
- Alternative mood stabilizers include verapamil and other calcium channel blockers, lamotrigine, gabapentin, thyroid hormone, clozapine, and other atypical neuroleptics.
- In addition to mood stabilizers, many patients with bipolar I disorder benefit from treatment with neuroleptics, antidepressants, and benzodiazepines.
- Electroconvulsive therapy can be helpful for patients who are not responding to medication.
- Maintenance treatment is the best way to prevent recurrent episodes of mania and major depression.

- Compliance is crucial.
- Alcohol and street drugs will interfere with the prescribed action.
- If a medication regimen is not effective or is causing significant adverse side effects, it is important for the patient and the family to keep working with their physician and not to abandon drug or psychosocial treatment.

3. Summary and wrap-up.

Psychoeducation Group: Session 4

In the fourth session, the discussion focuses on group members' reactions to the presentation by the psychiatrist and any remaining questions or clarifications concerning medications. The discussion also continues with the previous topic of coping strategies and introduces feedback mechanisms and the notion of taking responsibility for one's actions.

Preparation

Review the previous session and identify potential issues that should be addressed in this session. Specify the tasks and role of each cotherapist and arrange for handouts at the beginning of the session (e.g., "Guidelines for Patients and Families Living with an Affective Disorder"[469]).

Outline of Psychoeducation Group

1. After checking in, discuss the previous session's topic of medication. Stress the importance of compliance as well as communication between the patient, family members, and psychiatrist. Go over issues of "ineffective" doctors, second opinions, and changing physicians.

2. Group members share coping strategies for medication and compliance problems. This continues the previous week's discussion of living with a family member who has a mood disorder and how to deal with problems that arise.

3. The group leaders refer "Guidelines for Patients and Families Living with an Affective Disorder."[469] Group members take turns reading each guideline aloud, followed by group discussion of that guideline. Members share their reactions to the guidelines and suggest their own successful strategies when dealing with problems arising from the illness.

4. Therapists use the guidelines and group reactions to remind members about the amount of information and experience they already have in living with someone who has a mood disorder. In addition to empowering the group, the therapists use the discussion to begin to focus on feedback mechanisms and taking responsibility for one's actions. Points to cover in this discussion are as follows:

a. Emphasize how previous sessions have used the firsthand experience of the patients and family members to discuss issues, how important the information is that the group members already possess, and how that information was harnessed by the group to learn from and to support each other.

b. Therapists then guide the discussion toward the premise that behavior can affect others—the idea is true for both the patient and family members. Lead group members to understand how one person's behavior is partly responsible for how others treat and react to them. Draw on both patients' and family members' experiences to provide examples.

c. After hearing a few examples of a specific reaction to a specific behavior, therapists suggest that some behaviors can be modified, and that one's behavior can be separated from one's intention. At this point, the therapists use the examples to demonstrate these ideas.

5. In response to a reported behavior, the therapist asks, "What were you trying to do? What was your intention?" The therapist then asks the group for feedback: "How was the individual coming across?" The question goes back to the individual: "Is that what you were trying to do?" The group and the individual use these exchanges to show how one thing was intended but the behavior may have suggested something else.

6. Summary and wrap-up. Remind group members that they will continue to practice techniques for giving and receiving feedback.

Psychoeducation Group: Session 5

The fifth session is used to raise the awareness of how patients and families differ in both their perspectives and experience of affective illness. The "fishbowl" technique[469] helps patients and family members better understand and empathize with each other. The feedback mechanisms introduced in the previous session are put into practice in this session.

Preparation

Review the previous session and identify potential issues that should be addressed in this session, paying special attention to previously identified affective issues within each family. Specify the tasks and role of each cotherapist.

Outline of Psychoeducation Group

1. After checking in, therapists give an overview and rationale of the "fishbowl."

   a. It is important to understand that different people in the family have different perspectives and opinions about things.

   b. Therapists make the structure and different roles clear to the group members.

- Patients form a small circle with one therapist.
- Family members and the other therapist form a circle around the outside of the patients' circle (a circle within a circle).
- The task for the patients in the inner circle is to discuss *among themselves* what it is like to have an affective illness.
- The task for the families in the outer circle is to listen and mentally "put themselves in the place of someone who has affective illness." They are not allowed to talk, only to listen.

2. At the conclusion of the patients' discussion (which lasts about 20 minutes), the patients share their experience in discussing their illness with others who have affective illness. Similarly, family members then discuss their observations and insights about what it must be like to have an affective illness.

3. The format is then reversed, and the family members become the inner circle, while the patients form the outer circle. At the conclusion of the family members' discussion of what it is like to be a family member coping with affective disorder, patients relate their observations and reactions about what it must be like to be a family member.

4. The group as a whole then discusses reactions to the "fishbowl" exercise. Group members typically report that this exercise has not only heightened their awareness of the other person's experience but it has also been a powerful experience.

5. Summary and wrap-up. The therapists summarize the important is-

sues that emerged and how patients and family members have different perceptions of the effect that affective illness has on others.

Psychoeducation Group: Session 6

The sixth session focuses on summarizing the main themes and important issues that have been addressed throughout the five previous sessions. It offers group members the chance to provide feedback to the therapists. In addition, practical issues are discussed and a member of a local mental health support association is invited to attend the session.

Preparation

Review the previous session and identify potential issues that should be addressed in this session. Specify the tasks and role of each cotherapist and verify attendance of the advocate.

Outline of Psychoeducation Group

1. After checking in, group members share what the overall group experience has been like for them. Members give feedback about what has been helpful to them and suggest what needs to be improved for future groups.

2. As the group comes to a close, it is important that members be given information about both continued support that is available in the community and follow-up with their mental health provider. Members typically voice concerns about the termination of the group and the loss of the support system that they have developed over the past 6 weeks. A member of the local Manic–Depressive Disorders Association (MDDA) joins the group for the sixth session, explains how the MDDA is a national, self-help group for patients and families coping with affective illness, and invites members to attend weekly MDDA support groups.

3. Other topics of concern to group members are discussed:

   a. How to access the professional care system when a crisis evolves.

   b. Use of managed care, what buzzwords to use, how to "talk the talk."

   c. From a legal perspective—what patients and family members can and cannot do when a member is in crisis.

    d. What strategies to use to make treatment more accessible for the patient.

    e. Insurance issues—what is and is not covered in the changing health care environment.

    f. What to do when patients and/or family members would like a second opinion or to change clinicians.

4. Summary and wrap-up. Therapists should leave group members with a feeling of empowerment about how much they know, how much they've learned over the past 6 weeks, how they can take responsibility for their actions, and how they have learned to use feedback mechanisms to communicate better and to modify some of their behavior.

5. Finally, therapists should remind the group of the importance of getting the family involved, especially as these illnesses tend to have a remitting and relapsing course.

DISCUSSION

This chapter combines psychoeducational treatment techniques with family therapy techniques in a multifamily group format. Psychoeducation and family therapy can be seen as addressing distinct aspects of real and potential family problems in mood disorders in a complementary way. The psychoeducational approach is aimed at helping families cope with the increased stress associated with the presence of a mood disorder in one member of the family. This approach targets common problems and specific family stresses by informing group members about biopsychosocial aspects of the illness, and by offering and discussing solutions to problematic patient behaviors. However, the psychoeducational intervention does not address the more heterogeneous family dysfunctions that are found in many families and that may be exacerbated when one member suffers from a mood disorder.[405]

    Family therapy specifically addresses dysfunction associated with the families' long-standing interaction patterns and responses to the patient's disorder. Our clinical experience and research data suggest that a substantial proportion of families with a depressed member have significant difficulties that require changes in the basic family system and pattern(s) of interactions. These changes are less likely to be accomplished by psychoeducation alone. Psychoeducational and family therapy interventions are both potentially useful for patients with mood disorders and their family members. In an attempt to find common problems and solutions between the two methods, we looked for themes or clinical issues that cut across the two treatment strategies. We were able to identify five recurrent areas of concern throughout the six sessions, areas that were explored using both multifamily group and family therapy techniques.

Common Themes and Concerns

Illness Stages and Coping Strategies

With the help of the group therapists, patients and family members discuss key stages of a mood disorder and various coping strategies. For example, in the early stage of the illness, many patients and family members are aware of prodromal signs and symptoms that can serve as a warning for the onset of an episode. The patients and their families are helped to identify the warning signs and symptoms, and whether there is a particular pattern or seasonality to the illness. The middle stage of the illness, often very difficult for families, is a frequently discussed topic in the group setting. Therapists can help families discuss their frustrations and sense of helplessness when patients need help but refuse it, while not being sick enough to meet criteria for involuntary hospitalization. Families discuss how fearful, angry, and helpless they often feel when the patient refuses to get help. Advocacy and support groups (National Depressive and Manic–Depressive Association/National Alliance for the Mentally Ill) are noted as useful resources.

Even when an episode resolves, residual symptoms often remain.[470] Therapists guide patients and family members through discussions of what they can realistically expect in the aftermath of an episode. Throughout these discussions, the therapists continue to validate for family members the limitations of what they can do and how upsetting it must be to watch an episode worsen.

Collaboration with Mental Health and Other Professionals

When and how to intervene effectively to be of help to the patient is a major concern for families and patients. Both patients and families need to establish trusting, collaborative relationships with the patient's psychiatrist, mental health professional, and/or mental health agency. Group leaders stress that patient–doctor confidentiality must be respected by the family; however, patients are encouraged to give permission for the family to be involved in their treatment, when appropriate. Families also discuss practical issues such as how to access emergency medical help and assistance from police; how to deal with state mental health laws, insurance, and managed care claims; and how to negotiate and overcome frustration when working with these professionals.

The Patient in Crisis

A universal concern for group members is the patient in crisis. Occasionally, a patient exhibits acute symptoms of depression or mania during the group session. Although it is upsetting and frightening to witness a patient in crisis, the therapists' immediate interventions can help the group members to discuss their own feelings/reactions about what happens in the group, to share their fears and sense of not knowing what to do, and to relate how they experience similar situations within their own families. Discussion also affords the group the opportunity to discuss effective interventions and coping strategies before dealing with a patient in a crisis situation at home. Specifically, patients and families are encouraged to develop a "safety net" of effective strategies for dealing with the illness, and to do so while the patient is euthymic and between episodes.

Difficult Family Interactions

It is important for patients and families to understand that a mood disorder is a family illness in the sense that it has an impact on both patients and family members. Patients and families must work together to cope effectively with the illness. A common concern expressed by patients is that families are too controlling. Patients feel that family members are hypervigilant and watch them constantly. Patients report that they cannot have a "bad day" or "be up and happy" without family overreaction—fear of the start of a manic or a depressive episode. While some patients report that families "overreact and are intrusive and controlling," other patients complain that families do not understand the illness and are hurtful, with comments such as "Snap out of it," "Pull yourself up," "Try to be more positive."

On the other hand, family members are often concerned that they are on the front lines when a patient decompensates and they have little access to the mental health professionals providing treatment to the patient. Families feel they are "left out of the loop." They complain that patients often have little idea of how their mood disorder affects those around them. Families report that they would welcome the patient's self-determination and need to be in charge of his or her life; however, often when called upon to intervene in a crisis, they then become the recipient of the patient's hostility for "taking over."

During multifamily group sessions, verbal exchanges between a patient and a family member can be highly charged. The therapists use these opportunities as a learning experience for the entire group to discuss effective and ineffective communication patterns, and to show how to handle the "fallout" that accompanies mood disorders. Group members learn to identify their own and other's interpersonal styles, as well as how their styles get in the way of what they are trying to communicate. The therapists invite the group to give feedback.

Empowerment and Responsibility

Many patients and family members already know a great deal about mood disorders and their effect on the family system. The therapists draw on this knowledge and the families' experience, as well as additional input from invited experts and assigned readings, to share and discuss successful coping strategies. In doing so, the therapists stress individual responsibilities, interpersonal feedback techniques, and individuals' knowledge and power to modify some behaviors.

CONCLUSIONS

The optimal treatment of depression has yet to be defined. Pharmacotherapy, psychotherapy, family therapy, and group therapy each have a role to play for many patients at some point in their illness. None of these treatments are effective for all patients. Their effectiveness for any given patient ranges from 20 to 80%, depending on the severity of the depression. The more severe the depression, the more likely it is that some combination of these treatment options should be provided simultaneously. The multifamily group format is a welcome addition to the currently available treatments for depression. It not only combines family therapy and psychoeducational group therapy, but it is also synergistic and complementary to pharmacotherapy. The psychoeducational component of the model serves to improve the patient's compliance through knowledge, empowerment, and support for the family. The family therapy component of the model engages families in the treatment process and encourages them to recognize, to address, and to improve dysfunctional interactions. The role of the family is significant in determining the course of the depression and the patient's response to treatment. The psychoeducational group format taps into both a broad social support network and a large reservoir of knowledge and experience in dealing with depressive disorders.

Additionally, the multifamily group format should prove to be cost-effective in the long run. It can cut down on the necessity for other forms of psychosocial treatment; it has economies of scale that, by enhancing compliance and knowledge about the illness, and ways of coping, have the potential to speed recovery and minimize relapse. As with other therapies, the ultimate use of multifamily group treatments for depression will depend on its perceived effectiveness in community settings and on the availability of research studies supporting its clinical and economic efficacy. Although multifamily group therapies have been shown to meet these goals in the treatment of schizophrenia, studies of its value in mood disorders are just getting under way. The results of these studies are not yet available; nonetheless, there is sufficient clinical experience with multifamily group therapy to justify expanding its use for depressed patients and their family members.

Chapter 14

Multifamily Psychoeducational Treatment of Borderline Personality Disorder

CYNTHIA B. BERKOWITZ AND JOHN G. GUNDERSON

Since 1970, there has been a remarkable surge in the quantity of literature and research pertaining to borderline personality disorder (BPD). In the early literature, BPD was conceptualized as a type of personality organization that was differentiated from psychotic and neurotic organizations. It later took on an identity as a specific syndrome that was considered to be an atypical form of schizophrenia. It has also been considered an atypical form of depression, posttraumatic stress disorder, and bipolar II disorder. Currently, BPD is recognized as a distinct personality disorder, having both a specific course and specific risk factors in its etiology. As BPD has taken on this distinct identity, there has been growing interest in understanding the deficits specific to the disorder that should be the targets of treatment, and in developing treatments that are relevant to these deficits. The psycho-educational treatment approach described here represents a contribution in this effort.

The development of psychoeducational multifamily treatment of BPD is prompted by four factors:

1. The need for novel psychosocial interventions in this disorder.
2. The success of multifamily psychoeducational treatment of schizo-phrenia.

3. The need for more effective family interventions in this disorder.
4. The emergence of a deficit model of BPD.

Dialectical behavioral therapy (DBT) was developed by Linehan, Heard, and Armstrong[471] as a disorder-specific treatment of BPD, focusing on the diminution of the self-destructive behavior that is the major cause of morbidity in BPD. It is the only psychosocial treatment of this disorder that has been subjected to a controlled outcome study. Linehan and colleagues established the effectiveness of this cognitive-behavioral treatment of BPD and set a precedent that encourages others to follow in the pursuit of empirically evaluated, disorder-relevant psychosocial treatments. It has contributed to the validation of the conceptualization of BPD as a meaningful diagnostic entity by establishing the effectiveness of disorder-specific treatment. Furthermore, it has alerted clinicians to the value of cognitive-behavioral interventions in the treatment of the disorder. Now, as clinicians struggle to improve treatments in a health care climate that provides diminishing resources, there is a dire need for increased development of cost-effective psychosocial treatments that also have established efficacy via empirical testing. When treatment models have had their efficacy established empirically, the overall costs of treatment usually will diminish along with the morbidity of the condition.

The effectiveness of multifamily psychoeducational treatment of schizophrenia has alerted us to its potential value in the treatment of BPD. The development of psychoeducational treatments grew out of recognition that factors in the family environment, specifically, expressed emotion (EE), influence the course of the illness once it is established. The controlled outcome study by McFarlane and colleagues[313] has provided empirical evidence that the treatment can alter the family environment and significantly decrease the risk of relapse in patients with schizophrenia. By educating families regarding the handicaps in their ill relatives, clinicians can teach them to adjust their responses to illness to accommodate for the handicaps specific to the disorder. Furthermore, the treatment has established the effectiveness of eliciting families' participation in treatment by calling upon them to be *members of the treatment team*, providing disorder-relevant interventions that can alter the course of the disorder. The multifamily group model of the treatment achieved a dramatic improvement in relapse rates over the single-family model, bringing the relapse rate from 25.6% to 16.3%.[313] These results alerted us to the power of the multifamily group model to produce change within families. Although the assumptions in McFarlane's model are specific to the treatment of schizophrenia, they are also relevant to many major mental illnesses, as is evident in the value of the model in treating depression, bipolar disorder, and obsessive–compulsive disorder. The success suggests that the model may be effectively applied to the treatment of BPD. Clinicians who treat individuals with BPD are highly aware that the recurrent crises that mark the course of the illness often occur in response to interactions between the individual with BPD and relatives. This pattern strongly suggests that a treatment targeted at altering the family environment could positively influence the course of BPD.

Another factor prompting the development of this treatment is the previous experience with family treatments for BPD. In the 1970s and 1980s, clinicians often undertook ambitious and intensive psychodynamic family therapies in which all family members were encouraged to voice their emotions. These treatments usually included a borderline patient and his or her parents or spouse. Typically, the patients wished to have their families hear their accusations of mistreatment in the presence of a clinician who could provide support and validation. Such meetings often ended with angry flight by the patient, if he or she felt that the family was supported by the clinician, or by withdrawal of parents who could not tolerate the intensity of anger. Families of people with BPD shared the same sensitivity to interpretation as other families of the mentally ill—they experienced it as criticism. As a result, family therapy often did not last very long.

Previous family treatments of BPD developed within an intellectual climate in which the families were often vilified. The early literature on the etiology of BPD characterized the families as overinvolved and separation-resistant, with dependence-generating mothers. A study in 1981[472] found that the families were more commonly *underinvolved*. Subsequent literature documented high rates of neglect and hostile, conflictual family environments. Later, the literature documented a 75% incidence of traumatic experiences, including physical and sexual abuse and abandonment.[473] This literature led to a revised view of parents as the cause of BPD and to their frequent exclusion from treatment. As a result, clinicians often failed to recognize and draw upon whatever strengths existed within the families. Such vilifying views of families failed to take into consideration that the patients often remained highly dependent on their families, and that their families in turn could serve as an influential source of strength in coping with BPD.

The goal of the current treatment is to alter the environment within the family of the individual with BPD and thereby improve the course of the illness. This chronic disorder is rarely cured. It is marked by recurrent crises, often in response to stresses such as separations from important others, increased responsibilities, recurrent traumas, or interpersonal conflicts, as so often encountered in families of patients with BPD. If the recurrent crises of suicidality, self-mutilation, disabling depression, recurrent substance abuse, and eating disturbances could be prevented, the quality of life for these individuals could improve significantly. To design a treatment with this goal, we must first discern what factors in family environment influence the course of the disorder.

The literature gives sparse assistance here. The vast majority of literature regarding family environment and BPD focuses on aspects of the childhood environment that could lead to the development of the disorder in adulthood. Few studies address family process—that is, the structure, communication patterns, and attitudes—in families of adolescents and adults who have already developed the disorder. Among the few studies available, none are longitudinal studies that determine whether particular aspects of the family environment predict risk of relapse. So we must make use of the literature at hand, along with clinical experience and suggestive findings from work with other disorders, to hypothesize which factors in the family environment would be useful targets for treatment.

The first hypothesis is that regression and crisis in the individual with BPD may result from feeling alienated from the family. Young and Gunderson[474] examined both attributions that adolescents with BPD perceived in themselves and attributions that their parents perceived in them. They then compared the data from this group to data from families of adolescents with other personality disorders. Adolescents with BPD saw themselves as being significantly more alienated than did adolescents with other disorders. Meanwhile, their parents did not perceive them as feeling especially alienated. Overall, adolescents with BPD had significantly different perceptions of themselves than their parents' perceptions of them on dimensions including alienation, narcissism, ego weakness, isolation, antisocial traits, and cognitive compromise. The discrepancies in the perceptions themselves demonstrate the adolescents' alienation. For alienated adolescents, suicidal gestures and self-mutilation may serve as desperate messages about their internal state, dramatic messages that cannot be denied, messages that are more likely to elicit worried concern than alienating anger.

The findings of Young and Gunderson[474] suggest that alienation in the family environment is a useful target for intervention and indicate that psychoeducation may be a powerful intervention if it can diminish alienation. In particular, family members may need to be taught that the suicidal or self-destructive behaviors of the individual with BPD may arise from a strong sense of alienation. If relatives can be induced to feel curiosity about the inner experiences of the self-destructive individual, that curiosity may effectively diminish the patient's alienation and need for self-destructive behavior.

A second hypothesis regarding factors in the family environment lead-ing to crisis in the individual with BPD is suggested by the literature on schizophrenia and mood disorders. The role of EE has been examined ex-tensively in both schizophrenia and in mood disorders. A review of this subject is found in Chapter 2 of this book. While studies of the role of EE in BPD have not yet been published as of this writing, they have been un-dertaken by both Jill Hooley and John Vuchetich, the latter study in associ-ation with development of the current treatment. The interest in the role of EE in this disorder follows logically from the nature of the disorder. Clini-cians working with patients who have BPD know all too well that the fre-quent crises that mark the course of this disorder often occur in response to family interactions (conflicts, hostilities, criticisms, etc.), the stuff of which EE is made. Furthermore, the established role of EE in multiple psychiatric disorders, including schizophrenia,[232] major depression,[425, 475] and bipolar disorder,[366] suggests that it could be relevant in understanding the course of BPD as well. We therefore hypothesize that EE in the family may be a risk factor for worsening psychosocial functioning in the individual with BPD.

If EE in the family environment is in fact a variable that predicts the course of the disorder, the question remains as to what family processes the variable would be measuring in the families of people with BPD. EE is an operationalized variable that is used to classify families in simple, dichoto-mous terms, as high or low EE. Yet the factors measured—criticism, hostil-ity, and emotional overinvolvement—may represent complex interpersonal processes. Hooley and colleagues[476] have written about the nature of EE in families of patients with depression. They hypothesize that high EE occurs when families attribute the unwanted behavior of a member to weakness of character rather than to illness. When relatives regard the behavior as being under willful control, they are likely to attempt to change it. The expected result is an increase in nagging, criticism, and other attempts to coerce the individual into change. Hooley[476] writes, "High levels of EE may also be marking high levels of social control" (p. 183). If, instead, relatives can see the unwanted behavior as a symptom of an illness, their expectation of change in response to nagging may diminish, and their attitude may be-come more supportive, tolerant, cool, and calm.

A parallel hypothesis can be made regarding what EE represents in families of people with BPD. Again, families may attribute willfulness and a bad attitude to the suicidal gestures and fits of rage they witness. Here, the parallel to patients with major depression or schizophrenia falters. The behavior of a person with BPD does not simply represent the expression of uncontrollable symptoms that are easily conceptualized as biological. The problem is located within the realm of character by our current diagnostic system. Families must maintain the belief that the behavior can be brought under conscious control in order to give the individual responsibility for her behavior. However, families may fail to understand *how difficult* it is for the individual to change. They may lack understanding of the intense and unconscious emotional forces that motivate the behavior, emotional forces that may be as powerful as a biological disposition to depression. If they could understand the intensity of these emotional forces, they could see the futility of labeling, blaming, and nagging, and take a calmer, more controlled approach, one that still calls upon the individual to change but provides a supportive, noncritical context that helps to bring about that change.

The question remains as to why individuals with BPD may be vulnerable to the effect of EE. In the case of schizophrenia, evidence indicates that there is an impairment in attention, arousal, and gating of stimuli[49] that leaves the patient vulnerable to psychosis when exposed to EE. A parallel hypothesis can be made about BPD: that individuals with this disorder are also handicapped in their ability to tolerate emotional stimulation, but for very different reasons. The development of the current treatment coincides with the emergence of a deficit model of BPD. Once regarded as a disorder caused by psychological conflict, increased knowledge of its definition, etiology, and treatment have led to BPD being reconceptualized as a disorder involving deficits. Three deficits can be recognized in patients with BPD: (1) affect and impulse dyscontrol, (2) dichotomous thinking, and (3) intolerance of aloneness. We hypothesize that these deficits impair the ability of the individual with BPD to tolerate painful emotional stimulation. If families can be educated to view individuals with BPD as *handicapped* in their ability to tolerate the usual emotional stimulation in the home, they may then become motivated to respond to the individual in new ways that are consistent with therapeutic goals.

DEFICITS IN BORDERLINE PERSONALITY DISORDER

The first deficit, *affect and impulse dyscontrol*, is a modification of the concept of unintegrated rage that appeared earlier in the literature. Kernberg[477] wrote of a basic temperamental disposition toward excessive aggressivity. The centrality of affect and impulse dyscontrol in BPD suggests that a neurobiological basis for the disorder might be found. Subsequent empirical support for this hypothesis has been presented.[478, 479] This evidence underscores the medical basis and seriousness of the disorder. The deficit model potentially makes the characteristic dyscontrol of BPD less likely to evoke anger and more likely to evoke a sympathetic response in families and in the public at large. Although neurobiological theories about this deficit can evoke unrealistic hopes of a dramatic biological intervention, the possibility that improved interventions of this kind can eventually be developed is a perspective that many people find useful. It is important in the course of psychoeducation to present this perspective to patients with BPD and their families, but to caution them that biology alone cannot fully explain this disorder.

The second deficit, *dichotomous thinking*, is a reconceptualization of the defense mechanism of splitting. It refers to the tendency to think in all-or-nothing, black-and-white terms about self, others, problems, or situations, and represents a pervasive, distorted thought process characteristic of BPD. This deficit emphasizes a distorted cognitive process as a central characteristic of BPD. The traditional term, "splitting," has emphasized the related inability to integrate one's love and hate for the same person, to experience ambivalence. It is hard to tolerate intense ambivalence about oneself and others. As with all human abilities, some individuals are going to be able to do this better than others; it is hypothesized that this ambivalence poses a more extreme challenge to those individuals who develop BPD.

The third deficit, *intolerance of aloneness*, derives from the theoretical contributions of multiple psychoanalytic theorists, including Modell,[480] Masterson and Rinsley,[481] Adler and Buie,[482] Gunderson,[483, 484] and Bowlby.[485] This deficit refers to the extreme anxiety—often including the sensation of no longer existing—that occurs in the absence of close physical proximity to a significant other. Intolerance of aloneness has been linked to many of the central diagnostic criteria of BPD. Fear of abandonment in individuals with BPD is linked directly to their manipulative, self-destructive behavior, mood lability, impulsivity, and inappropriate anger. Patients and their families can readily recognize this deficit. It underscores the unrealistic nature of the individual's expectations within interpersonal relationships. Awareness of this deficit highlights for families the difficulties that the individual experiences during any experience of separation or rejection. Most importantly, education regarding this deficit can help families to understand that, for individuals with BPD, any attainment of independence brings with it fears of being abandoned by their supports. Such fears can be intense and lead to a crushing relapse.

RATIONALE FOR PSYCHOEDUCATIONAL MULTIFAMILY TREATMENT OF BORDERLINE PERSONALITY DISORDER

The following rationale explains the basic principles of the current treatment, which borrow heavily from the previous work of Anderson, Hogarty, Falloon, Leff, and McFarlane in the development of psychoeducational treatment, but also incorporate emerging concepts of BPD, particularly the deficit model. These basic principles provide a blueprint for the structure and goals of treatment.

1. *BPD is characterized by deficits of (a) affect and impulse dyscontrol, (b) intolerance of aloneness, and (c) dichotomous thinking. These deficits result in intense and maladaptive reactions to interpersonal experience.* This first principle gives families a rationale for altering their family environment. If individuals with BPD have deficits in their ability to cope, it follows that they would benefit from an environment that could help them cope with those deficits.

2. *The deficits render individuals with BPD handicapped but not disabled. This means that they can be held accountable for their actions, but that change occurs very slowly and with great difficulty.* The catchphrase "handicapped but not disabled" captures the struggle families face between giving individuals with BPD responsibility for their behavior and accepting the reality of the extreme difficulty in changing.

3. *BPD is an enduring disorder characterized by recurrent crises. Crises lead to impairment of psychosocial functioning that may be preventable. Crises may resolve and remit in the absence of stress.* This principle delineates the specific goal of the treatment, which is to diminish crises rather than to cure the disorder. The disorder is regarded as chronic. Cure is not the goal of the current treatment. We hypothesize that stress in the family environment may significantly influence the course of the disorder.

4. *Families can influence the course of illness in that they can either diminish the stresses that cause relapses or inadvertently create them.* This statement about the role of the family focuses on the here and now, not on etiology. It does not vilify families for their role in the etiology of the disorder. It does give families responsibility for their role in the perpetuation of crises that mark the course of the disorder once it is established, calling upon them specifically to make the home environment calmer and to protect the individual with BPD from stress.

5. *Living with an ill relative has negative consequences for the family.* A major goal of the current treatment is to diminish stress within the family,

independent of the goal of improving psychosocial functioning in the patient. In the current health care climate, in which funding for intensive treatment of severe mental illnesses is quite limited, the family plays a vital role in maintaining the stability of the patient. A treatment that eases the family's burden may improve the well-being of each member considerably and allow the family to maximize its caretaking effectiveness.

6. *Family members will want to use education to change their behavior, if they believe they can help an ill family member by doing so.* Some families may be resistant to change because they believe that change must come from within the ill relative. When angry and hurt family members expect change to come from an internal locus of control in the individual with BPD, they do not establish boundaries and limitations within the family that would motivate the individual to change.

7. *Stress within the family may have at its root alienation between the individual with BPD and family members.* Alienation may be diminished by greater familial understanding of the internal experience of the patient and by improved communication. Thus, a psychoeducational treatment must focus on giving families a new understanding of the affects and motivations that underlie behaviors typical of BPD.

This rationale is notable for its neutral stance toward the role of the parents in the etiology of the disorder. The psychoeducational approach begins with the idea that families have a very disturbed and disturbing member. This approach is simultaneously sympathetic to the problems that such an individual creates for the family and sympathetic to the difficulties facing the individual with BPD. It does not focus on issues of development or etiology. The approach not only moves parents away from issues of their possible causal role in the occurrence of the illness, but it also leads them away from blaming and criticizing the individual with BPD.

This neutrality may arouse criticism given that many of the individuals with BPD have, in fact, reported trauma or neglect inflicted by a family member. If the treatment focuses on the individual's illness but takes a neutral stance toward the family's role in its etiology, will patients experience denial in the treatment environment that may retraumatize them? The concern is a legitimate one for a subgroup of families who have entered our treatment.

We believe that there are strong arguments to support our "neutral" approach. First, we do not exempt parents from any causal role in the etiology of the illness, as is typically done in psychoeducational approaches to schizophrenia, bipolar disorder, or major depression. Instead, we emphasize that there are many factors—inborn, developmental, and familial—that put individuals at risk for development of the disorder. Our approach is intended to be sobering but does not vilify parents. We urge families to move away from a preoccupation with this question of causation, so that they may devote their energies to the here and now. In the families who present for treatment, the individual with BPD continues to have significant involvement with and dependency upon the family. Therefore, the family needs to devote its energy to the present, not the past, in order to care for the individual. Furthermore, we do not believe our approach is biased toward parents. Remember that just as we move away from blaming parents, we also move away from blaming the individual with BPD, even though— just as parents may have blamed their children—borderline patients can be extremely destructive to other members of the family. The feelings of anger and guilt that are aroused by issues of blame are not constructive when dealing with the present situation and recurrent crises.

Relevant to this issue is the high frequency with which these patients have reported physical, emotional, or sexual abuse by their parents. When physical or sexual abuse is recent or ongoing, it is unrealistic to expect parents to participate in treatment. This is not true for what borderline patients call emotional abuse, and it is sometimes possible to involve parents who were abusive during the patient's childhood.

Our neutral approach to causality often enables us to form an alliance with parents who are highly sensitive to criticism. As with other mental illnesses, the parents of individuals with BPD often feel significant guilt for possibly causing the illness. Treatments that expose them to their offspring's blaming or other forms of vilification can be intolerable. In traditional treatments that have exposed parents to their offspring's blaming, parents often left treatment, obviously rendering it ineffective. A more neutral stance allows treatment to occur.

THE ROLE OF THE MULTIFAMILY GROUP IN TREATMENT OF BORDERLINE PERSONALITY DISORDER

While the multifamily group has the obvious practical advantage of diminished cost in the treatment of BPD, it also has significant therapeutic advantages. As in the treatment of other major psychiatric disorders, the multifamily group can be a powerful intervention for producing change in families. The mechanisms of the multifamily group directly address the problems that typically face the families of individuals with BPD, including the need for improved clarity of communication and directness, diminished hostility, and reduced overinvolvement.

In our pilot study of the families presenting for this treatment, we found that patients with BPD and their families agreed that communication was a major problem facing them. The multifamily group improves communication in the family in two primary ways. First, the process of the multifamily group may improve the clarity of communication. Family members may be vague, disorganized, or secretive in their patterns of communication. The multifamily group provides a social structure in which members call upon each other to clarify their meaning in the course of normal conversational exchange. Group members, after direction from the group leaders, learn to encourage each other to focus on one issue at a time, in an organized manner, and discourage free ventilation about multiple conflicts. When an angry group member ruminates on multiple issues in close succession, another group member is likely to refocus that person gently on the primary issue that the group has decided to discuss. Group members who may be secretive about family issues are encouraged to speak more freely by the open sharing of other group members.

The second benefit of the multifamily group is to improve the directness of communication within the family. Often, the relatives of an individual with BPD feel that they must avoid discussing stressful topics around that individual. The prospect of any direct confrontation brings fear of triggering the angry tirades that are typical of this disorder. Thus, relatives must muster considerable courage in order to handle conflicts in a direct manner. This may occur safely within the multifamily group, where the social atmosphere encourages direct communication yet discourages intense expression of emotion. More importantly, families offer each other strong support to endure the fear of facing anger.

The multifamily group may significantly diminish the levels of hostility and criticism in the family. Several mechanisms lead to that result. The multifamily group greatly diminishes the sense of burden and isolation experienced by families. Many individuals are prevented from sharing their troubles with families and friends by feelings of shame and stigma. The social networks of families with a member who has BPD have not been studied, but the families in our study appear to be very isolated in their struggle with this condition. Many come to see the group as a refuge that greatly diminishes their sense of stress. As the support in the group modulates the impact of crises on the family, it is expected that the family members will be able to take a calmer, more deliberate, thoughtful, moderate, and less hostile approach to their relative with BPD. The multifamily group members also serve a powerful modeling function for one another. Group members may vary considerably in terms of their attitudes and styles of expressing emotions. Those who have greater empathy and understanding for the feelings of the individuals with BPD may demonstrate their attitudes to others. Members who can remain calm in the face of criticism and angry outbursts are often admired by other group members. Members trade "war stories" and receive praise for calm, self-possessed "courage under fire."

The term "overinvolvement" is vague and may in families of people with BPD have a very different meaning than it does in families of people with schizophrenia. In families of individuals with BPD, overinvolvement takes distinct forms. First, families may struggle with enduring but unrealistic expectations of the individual. Often, people with BPD demonstrate periods of high-level functioning, along with considerable creativity and intelligence, yet overall, their psychosocial functioning may be severely impaired. Families may ally with and encourage the individual's plans to attempt new responsibilities that are beyond her reach. For example, they may support a plan for an individual to return to school full-time, even if she has not held a job or taken a college course in years. The support of the group may help these families to accept the degree of disability in the person with BPD and thus be more realistic with their support and expectations.

A second distinct form of overinvolvement takes the form of a crisis orientation in the family. Family members may give attention and support in connection with an individual's rages, threats, or hospitalizations. For example, parents may respond to their daughter's hospitalization by visiting frequently and providing home-cooked meals. In families in which the individual with BPD has been traumatized, parents often wish to make up for this past traumatization by providing extra support at times of distress. The result is to reinforce regression and crises as a means of gaining much-needed attention. The support of the group may greatly reduce feelings of guilt that motivate this type of overinvolvement. Furthermore, the positive feedback obtained from fellow sufferers may enable relatives to demonstrate "tough love," that is, to make decisions that may incur angry responses from the relative with BPD. The following case report illustrates this point.

A mother of a young woman with BPD felt immense guilt about her daughter's condition. When the daughter was 4 years old, the mother had become critically ill and required many months of treatment in an intensive care unit. During this time, hospital policy prevented the daughter from visiting the mother. As the daughter became suicidal in later years and required frequent hospitalizations, the mother wished to compensate for the past injury by visiting the daughter often in the hospital and by using any other means possible to express her empathy and concern. During her participation in the multifamily group, the mother experienced a gradual lessening of her guilt feelings as other group members supported views of the illness that were less blaming toward parents. One day as she left the group with her son and continued the discussion, her son complained of the mother's relationship with the daughter: "You're always chasing her." The mother began to feel angry about the role she had taken on. She decided to confront the daughter, who at the time was hospitalized. With the assistance of hospital staff, she explained that she was weary and exhausted by her own tireless attempts to heal the daughter through constant visits and would no longer visit her while she was in the hospital. The daughter expressed rage but, in the following months, improved considerably. She decided that hospitalization was regressive and avoided it successfully. The daughter was able to live at home again after many years of living in supervised settings. She maintained part-time work.

The case example demonstrates ways in which the multifamily group provides benign yet powerful interventions from fellow sufferers that can greatly reduce feelings of guilt and encourage parents to diminish over-involvement in their offspring's crises. In cases in which parents do experience extreme guilt, similar interventions on the part of professionals might be taken as criticism, for example, "You are enabling your daughter's regression." The multifamily group can provide these interventions in a manner that is supportive and constructive, diminishing the conflicted motivations and interpersonal behaviors that arise from guilt.

STRUCTURE OF THE PSYCHOEDUCATIONAL MULTIFAMILY TREATMENT

The psychoeducational multifamily group treatment of BPD follows the same three-stage structure as that used in the treatment of schizophrenia. Treatment begins with a joining phase, followed by a psychoeducational workshop. Families then join a multifamily group for an extended period of biweekly treatment.

Joining

The joining phase of treatment involves establishment of a working alliance with the relatives of the individual with BPD. Families are typically referred for treatment at a point of crisis. The therapist meets with the relatives as long as is needed to reach the following goals:

1. Establishment of expectations, commitment, and rules regarding the treatment.
2. Development of an emotional alliance between the clinician and family.
3. Establishment of the diagnosis of BPD.
4. Formulation of hypotheses about family interactions that may be problematic.
5. Establishment of an understanding of the family's frustration and anger with the illness and the mental health system.

Families are provided with a description of the treatment structure and philosophy. Our study of compliance with the treatment[486] indicates that families who discontinue treatment prematurely do so most often within the first 4 months of treatment. Therefore, relatives are typically asked to commit to at least a 4-month period of treatment. We reassure families of our supportive and nonblaming stance toward their role in the illness. This approach distinguishes our treatment from past, more traditional treatments in which family members may have felt criticized.

Often, the parents share the interpersonal sensitivity that the patients with BPD experience. Therefore, it is crucial to the success of the treatment that clinicians establish an affective alliance with relatives. To achieve this purpose, there should be a minimum of three joining sessions. The therapist provides considerable empathy for the feelings of the relatives, as well as support for their role in influencing the future course of the disorder. The clinician's stance recognizes the strengths of the relatives and their potential contribution to the improvement of the patient's health. This recognition can improve the relatives' sense of confidence and thereby enable them to endure a potentially stressful social situation in the multifamily group.

Often, when families are referred for treatment, they have not been told of the diagnosis of BPD, because great secrecy and stigma continue to surround the discussion of this condition among mental health professionals. We speak of the diagnosis matter-of-factly describing the criteria and applicability to the ill relative. In our experience, families are relieved by this approach. They learn that the problems that have caused them so much frustration and confusion are well known to professionals. They are comforted to hear that the etiology, course, and treatment of BPD have been studied extensively. This open and empathic discussion diminishes the sense of stigma usually associated with the diagnosis.

The joining sessions provide an opportunity for the therapist to take a careful history of the relationships within the family and thereby develop hypotheses concerning which family interactions may exacerbate the recurrent crises in the individual with BPD. The development of these formulations at the joining stage will be greatly useful in the multifamily group, enabling the therapists to focus group interventions on the modulation of any dysfunctional patterns of family interaction.

The joining phase provides a critical opportunity for therapists to allow families to ventilate about the frustration, fear, anger, and confusion they have experienced while caring for the person with BPD. During the multifamily group, such free expressions of feeling will be discouraged by the highly structured format and treatment philosophy of reducing EE. Therefore, the joining phase gives the therapist the chance to express empathy for the family's struggles and to enable family members to express their rage and distress in a forum where it is fully accepted by the treaters, even though they may subsequently suggest that it be avoided; that is, only after accepting their pain and anger will the therapist present family members with a model suggesting that, *for practical purposes* (not from a judgmental, moralizing stance), hostile criticism must be modulated and avoided whenever possible.

The Psychoeducational Workshop

Following the joining phase, families are invited to attend a half-day psychoeducational workshop that begins with didactic teaching about BPD, followed by provision of coping guidelines, and concludes with an introduction to the problem-solving method.

The psychoeducational workshop typically includes approximately 20 relatives of individuals with BPD. The first half of the workshop presents current knowledge of BPD. Families are given a series of short talks on subjects including diagnosis, etiology, course, and treatment of the disorder. We then introduce the three deficits: affect/impulse dyscontrol, intolerance of aloneness, and dichotomous thinking. The atmosphere is informal. Bagels and coffee are served and participants are given the opportunity to ask questions and share comments. Many people realize for the first time that they are not alone in their struggle with the disorder. As families gain knowledge, they also gain some sense that the condition's manifestations are predictable and treatable. Thus, the educational experience may significantly diminish their sense of anxiety.

The subject of etiology must be given special care. We tell families that multiple etiologies are possible for this disorder, that risk factors include traumatic experiences, neglect, neurological deficits, temperament, and developmental experiences. We stress the view that no single factor is likely to act in isolation to cause the disorder, and that multiple risk factors most likely work in combination. In this way, we acknowledge the possibility that the family may play a role in the etiology but do not focus on it to the point of aggravating feelings of guilt and shame. We emphasize the likelihood that multiple factors work in conjunction to create the disorder, and that knowledge is still incomplete and evolving.

In the workshop, we explain to families that they can help to prevent crises in their relative with BPD by adopting new coping methods. We present the hypothesis that hostility and conflict within the family may be intolerable for the individual with BPD, due to the deficits we have described, even though it may be useful and necessary for other family members. We then encourage families to respond to the individual with BPD in ways that may at first seem artificial to them but will take the deficits into consideration.

In the second half of the workshop, families are given the guidelines shown in Table 14.1 for coping with BPD.

The first set of guidelines regarding goals warns families that the individual with BPD may fear abandonment as she takes on increasing responsibility. The assumption of greater independence in work or self-care may lead to the fear that family members will assume she is better and withdraw their support. Such fear in the individual with BPD may lead to rapid regression soon after progress is made. Therefore, families are reminded to acknowledge these fears in the individual and show empathy by avoiding "You can do it" reassurances.

The second guideline calls upon family members to modify their expectations. Individuals with BPD tend to "swing on a pendulum," alternating between assumption of responsibility in great leaps and subsequent regression into a state of crisis under the stress of the new responsibility. In order to diminish crises, families must not encourage plans that involve resumption of responsibility too rapidly.

TABLE 14.1. Family Guidelines for Borderline Personality Disorder

Goals: Go slowly
1. Remember that change is difficult to achieve and fraught with fears and setbacks. Be cautious about suggesting that "great" progress has been made or giving "You can do it" reassurances. "Progress" evokes fears of abandonment.
2. Lower your expectations. Set realistic goals that are attainable. Solve big problems in small steps. Work on one thing at a time. "Big" or long-term goals lead to discouragement and failure.

Family environment: Keep things cool
3. Keep things cool and calm. Appreciation is normal. Tone it down. Disagreement is normal. Tone it down, too.
4. Maintain family routines as much as possible. Stay in touch with family and friends. There's more to life than problems, so don't give up the good times.
5. Find time to talk. Chats about light or neutral matters are helpful. Schedule times for this, if you need to.

Managing crises: Pay attention but stay calm
6. Don't get defensive in the face of accusations and criticisms. However unfair, say little and don't fight. Allow yourself to be hurt. Admit to whatever is true in the criticisms.
7. Self-destructive acts or threats require attention. Don't ignore. Don't panic. It's good to know. Do not keep secrets about this. Talk about it openly with your family member and make sure professionals know about these events.
8. Listen. People need to have their negative feelings heard. Don't say "It isn't so." Don't try to make the feelings go away. Using words to express fear, loneliness, inadequacy, anger, or needs is good. It's better to use words than to act out feelings.

Addressing problems: Collaborate and be consistent
9. When solving a family member's problems, ALWAYS:
    a. Involve the family member in identifying what needs to be done.
    b. Ask whether the person can do what's needed in the solution.
    c. Ask whether they want you to help them "do" what's needed.
10. Family members need to act in concert with one another. Parental inconsistencies fuel severe family conflicts. Develop strategies that everyone can stick to.
11. If you have concerns about medications or therapist interventions, make sure that both your family member and his or her therapist/doctor know. If you have financial responsibility, you have the right to address your concerns to the therapist or doctor.

Limit setting: Be direct but careful
12. Set limits by stating the limits of your tolerance. Let your expectations be known in clear, simple language. Everyone needs to know what is expected of them.
13. Do not protect family members from the natural consequences of their actions. Allow them to learn about reality. Bumping into a few walls is usually necessary.
14. Do not tolerate abusive treatment such as tantrums, threats, hitting, and spitting. Walk away and return to discuss the issue later.
15. Be cautious about using threats and ultimatums. They are a last resort. Do not use threats and ultimatums as a means of convincing others to change. Only give them when you can and will carry through. Let others—including professionals—help you decide when to give ultimatums.

In guidelines 3, 4, and 5, we advise families to take steps that will ease tension in the family environment. These measures include improving social connections. Relatives are reminded not to allow illness and problems to become the sole focus of family interactions.

Guidelines 6, 7, and 8 regarding management of crises advise families on ways to diffuse tension and improve safety when facing demonstrations of extreme rage and self-destructive behavior. Families are advised to attend carefully to all demonstrations of self-destructiveness. These acts are regarded as cries for help that will escalate if given either too much or too little attention.

In guidelines 9, 10, and 11 families are advised to use open negotiation as the primary means of mediating disputes and solving problems. Many families live in an atmosphere of secrecy, in which they feel afraid to negotiate management of a problem openly with their ill relative. These guidelines encourage them to speak with the ill relative, with other family members, and with professionals in order to create a family atmosphere of direct communication in which all members act in concert with one another.

The final set of guidelines encourages limit setting without creation of undue hostility. Families are advised to avoid protecting individuals with BPD from consequences of their actions. Too often, parents wish to protect offspring from the consequences of actions such as stealing, but by so doing, they inadvertently allow the behavior to continue. Relatives are advised to avoid use of ultimatums as a means of convincing others to change. Such ultimatums are often forms of coercion that produce hostile responses and are rarely taken seriously by those who give or receive them.

At the conclusion of the workshop, families engage in a sample problem-solving session. Thus, families are given an opportunity to interact as they will in the subsequent multifamily group.

The Multifamily Group

Our multifamily groups consist of approximately six families. It is usually parents who seek this assistance in dealing with BPD in a daughter. The preponderance of female patients in our groups is not surprising given that approximately 75% of patients with the diagnosis of BPD are female.[5] As in other psychoeducational applications, the "family" often consists only of the mother. We have made aggressive attempts to encourage the presence of daughters in the group. Their attendance has been poor, probably due to their extreme interpersonal sensitivity and subsequent difficulty tolerating the group situation. Many people with BPD are offended by the diagnosis and refuse to participate in the discussion of it.

The multifamily group meets biweekly for at least 1 year and includes approximately six families. It follows a structure very similar to that used in the multifamily groups described in Part II of this volume. Meetings begin with mandatory social chatter, followed by review of the most recent problems facing each family. One problem is selected for the group to solve together using the brainstorming method. The family whose problem has been discussed is then given a task to complete in the coming weeks.

Multiple aspects of the group format convey the message to families that problems can only be solved gradually. First, the group intends to meet over an extended period of time. Second, leaders' support in the development of enduring social relationships between members indicates to families that leaders are interested in the long-term functioning of the group, not simply in conveying a body of information. Third, problems are solved in small steps. Although the families often face complex crises, the focus in the group is on smaller, more manageable problems. For example, if a woman with BPD is hospitalized after a severe suicide attempt, the group would not ask how to diminish her suicidality but might consider the question of how often her parents should visit her in the hospital. The message of taking a gradual approach to problems steers families away from a crisis orientation, in which they may desperately hope to see a rapid return to normal functioning in the individual with BPD. When families can give up this crisis orientation, the pressure they feel may diminish considerably.

The early discussions focus on reinforcement and explanation of the guidelines, as well as the concept of deficits in BPD. Families are helped to apply the deficit model to the understanding and management of their relative's behavior. As the educational material is emphasized, families are meanwhile discovering that they share common experiences of facing self-destructive behavior, poor psychosocial functioning, and extreme rage in their relative with BPD. These cognitive and supportive aspects of the early group interventions may greatly ease families' sense of burden and provide a rapid diminution of anxiety in the family members.

As the group members review the recent events in their families, leaders must address not only the common issues facing them but also the unique situations in each family. Common themes include the extreme interpersonal sensitivity of the individual with BPD; management of self-destructive behavior, including self-mutilation, substance abuse, starvation, and purging; management of displays of rage; responses to apparent lack of motivation to resume work or education; and development of patterns of direct communication. Leaders address these issues by reinforcing educational material, strategically selecting problems for the group to solve, and encouraging exchange of common experiences between group members.

STAGES OF CHANGE IN THE PSYCHOEDUCATIONAL MANAGEMENT OF BORDERLINE PERSONALITY DISORDER

In the early months, as families join multifamily groups, they are often unrealistically hopeful that they will be able to grasp some simple lessons that will result in significant change. They are wary about other families but have hopes that the group leaders will provide useful answers. In line with these expectations, the leaders are often more active during this stage. They actively promote adherence to the guidelines, advising families to keep them on the refrigerator door or under their pillows, and they refer to them frequently during discussions. In addition, during this phase, the group leaders offer didactic asides. For example, they may review facts about issues such as diagnostic criteria or expectable course. The leaders also actively introduce exercises during this stage.

The first exercise involves communication. Handouts describing three simple steps to confrontation are provided and discussed. Family members are asked to provide sample situations from their personal experience in which confrontation was necessary. Group members then role-play the "how to" of the confrontation.

A second exercise involves instruction about attributions. Families members are taught how to alter the usual meaning they might attribute to behaviors to conform to understanding of deficits in the individual with BPD. For example, when people with BPD say they "hate" someone, this usually means that they feel rejected. Saying that they "don't need someone" means they believe that being needy is unacceptable. This task increases the empathy of family members for the their relative and may diminish her alienation. Conversely, the leaders describe the most common ways in which patients with BPD misattribute feelings and motives to their parents.

It is during the middle stage that families are most apt to drop out. The hope for rapid change has diminished, questions about the suitability of the diagnosis or exercises for their specific issues have been revived, and the awareness that they need to change patterns within their relationship is unwelcome. Attendance issues need to be addressed, especially the question of whether, or how, to have the relative with BPD come to the meetings.

Within the multifamily group meetings, the format now more exclusively rests on problem solving. Each family describes a current situation and can expect the other families to offer suggestions. When the group concludes that a family should adopt responses that are unwelcome to the member with BPD, this creates tension: The family members either adopt responses that feel uncomfortable or they defy the input from the group. The leaders try to diminish such problems by underscoring the fact that changes occur slowly and by directing positive reinforcement to families that are more receptive to suggestions. Leaders also try to model ways of relating, for example, being tolerant when suggested changes are adopted, resolving open disagreements about what topic to focus on, or accepting criticism without becoming defensive. In general, this is the stage in which the group members "come together," developing cohesion and a good working knowledge of each other's situations.

In the late phase, the group functions quite smoothly. Attendance is regular and the problem-solving format is predictable. Now families feel bolder, more confident in giving feedback to each other. Some will have made changes in which they take pride. Others have persistent, difficult-to-solve problems that everyone can recognize. The leaders' roles are seldom directive. Rather, they are facilitators of processes that the members can confidently undertake.

As for termination, the date for ending the multifamily group has been set well in advance, but the time devoted to termination per se is relatively brief. The leaders invite members to review what they have learned and to anticipate remaining issues. Similarly, family members are invited to comment on the progress of others. Sometimes this is a time for group members to remember pivotal or humorous incidents during the group's life, or to vent emotional statements about guilt or angry feelings toward the family member with BPD and receive great empathy from others. The leaders themselves are more open and frank in discussing their experiences within or outside the group, thereby further leveling professional distance. Families are encouraged to make ongoing use of the relationships they have formed with one another in the course of the group, and to join self-help groups and remain proactive about the needs of other families with problems like their own.

TREATMENT OUTCOME

The psychoeducational multifamily treatment of BPD has been studied in a pilot project involving two multifamily groups. Each of the families consisted of a mother or two parents with a daughter having BPD. The data yielded in this project must be viewed with great caution because the sample size is small. Data are currently available for eight of the participating families. The effectiveness of the psychoeducational multifamily group can be assessed using two types of data: patients' level of functioning, and families' perceived burden.

The present data describing parental change includes parents' subjective ratings of the helpfulness of the treatment. In our study, 66.7% of participants felt that the multifamily group helped them to modulate angry feelings; 66.7% felt less burdened. All the participating families felt that the multifamily group improved their communication with their daughters, and 75% felt that the improvement was "very great." All the participating families felt that the treatment improved their knowledge of the disorder. Of parents, 91.6% felt that the treatment had helped them to set limits. All (100%) of the participating families felt supported by the group.

Responses to a problem identification form showed that parents' concerns shifted over time. After 1 year of treatment, parents' concerns about suicidality, unpredictability, and impulsivity diminished, while concerns about independence, resistance to suggestions, and separation increased. This shift reflects a diminished crisis orientation, correlated with diminished occurrence of crises. As crises subside, the focus of the family moves to the psychosocial functioning of the individual with BPD. Concerns about separation may reflect parents' increased sensitivity to their daughters' intolerance of aloneness.

Data comparing the number of self-destructive acts occurring in the year prior to treatment and in the first year of treatment show a downward trend. While statistical significance cannot be established due to the small sample size and the large amount of variability in the data, these initial results are encouraging and indicate that a controlled outcome study of the treatment is worthwhile.

CONCLUSIONS

The psychoeducational multifamily group treatment of BPD represents a novel application of a treatment form that has been found to be highly successful in the management of schizophrenia. While the evidence supporting its effectiveness is preliminary, it indicates the need for further study of this treatment method. The data available suggest that patients are experiencing improved communication and diminished hostility within their families. Thus, the treatment may be creating an altered, specially adapted environment within the family that is responsive to the needs of the individual with BPD. We predict that further study will demonstrate the benefit of the altered family environment in terms of the patient's overall psychosocial functioning and diminished length of hospitalizations.

The reports of the families in our study indicate that the treatment has greatly reduced their sense of burden and isolation. While this change in the family is most likely experienced by the patient as diminished tension, its immediate benefit to the family is also very important. Parents have a greater sense of confidence and well-being, as well as increased ability to carry on in their caretaking role.

It is our hope that the psychoeducational approach will bring the diagnosis of BPD into more public usage. At present, it tends to be used privately among clinicians and is rarely shared with patients, thus enhancing the stigma it bears due to the connotation of *a difficult patient.* We believe that this is often due to clinicians' countertransference (i.e., the meaning that they attach to the diagnosis). As clinicians use the diagnosis more openly and matter-of-factly, it can lose that stigma and become a more familiar concept for use by families. Its use may lead patients and their relatives to discovery of a body of knowledge about the disorder that will help them to feel less overwhelmed and more in command of their troubles. Parents who have completed treatment in our groups have been invited to join a new relatives' support/advocacy organization: the New England Personality Disorders Association (NEPDA). NEPDA joins Treatment and Research Advances (TARA), a similar organization based in New York City. Like the National Alliance of the Mentally Ill (NAMI), these new organizations will function to improve public knowledge of BPD and support for research and new treatments. We hope that these organizations can foster development of similar groups elsewhere. These, in turn, may coalesce into a national organization to champion the needs of individuals with BPD.

Chapter 15

Multifamily Behavioral Treatment of Obsessive–Compulsive Disorder

BARBARA VAN NOPPEN AND GAIL STEKETEE

Obsessive–compulsive disorder (OCD) is recognized as one of the most common anxiety disorders. The role of psychosocial factors in the pathogenesis and treatment of OCD has been overshadowed by advances in understanding the neurobiology of the disorder and promising pharmacological, behavioral (primarily exposure and response prevention), and newer cognitive treatment strategies. Despite the success of standard treatment, persistent problems, such as failure to seek or stay in behavioral therapy, lack of compliance, and poor treatment outcome, may in part be due to psychosocial factors.

Family variables have been identified as predictors of OCD treatment outcome in the literature.[487–490] For example, relatives' perceptions that the OCD patient is malingering or can "just stop," as a matter of will, play a particularly potent role in outcome.[491] This investigation of family factors and outcome reveals that poor social and familial functioning, anger, and criticism predicts fewer gains at 9-month follow-up. Thus, psychoeducation about OCD and the reduction of critical responses to behavioral symptoms are important family factors in the course of illness and, possibly, treatment outcome for OCD. Clinical investigation of family members' responses to OCD symptoms and of their impact on the symptoms can lead to the development of family behavioral interventions that may prove fruitful for both the patient and the family.

In addition, as the cost of health care spirals upward, clinical researchers are challenged to explore alternative methods of applying exposure and response prevention that may be cost-effective. We have developed a type of family behavioral treatment modeled after individual behavioral treatment (IBT) that is time-limited and utilizes a group modality. Multifamily behavioral treatment (MFBT) includes patients and their significant others in a 20-session intervention (12 weekly and 6 monthly sessions) over a period of 9 months. Preliminary findings reveal efficacy of MFBT comparable to standard individual behavioral therapy.[492] Furthermore, reductions in OCD symptoms for patients who complete MFBT have been maintained at 1-year follow-up. MFBT is a unique intervention that offers families and patients the benefits of didactic psychoeducation, support, communication skills training, problem solving, in-group exposure, and response prevention with participant modeling and family behavioral contracting. In this chapter, we discuss MFBT in detail via a clinical example.

DIAGNOSIS AND PREVALENCE OF OBSESSIVE–COMPULSIVE DISORDER

Currently, OCD is characterized by recurrent obsessions or compulsions that provoke distress and interfere with a person's routine social/occupational functioning.[5] Obsessions are intrusive thoughts, images, or impulses that the person perceives as inappropriate and that cause marked distress; compulsions or rituals are repetitive behaviors or mental acts performed in response to an obsession and aimed purposely at preventing a dreaded consequence or reducing discomfort. It is important to recognize that compulsions can be covert mental acts, such as praying, reviewing events, counting, or repeating words or phrases, to neutralize anxiety or feared outcome. DSM-IV includes a "poor insight type" OCD, which refers to persons who do not recognize the unreasonableness or excessiveness of their obsessions and compulsions. However, a history of insight at some point during the disorder is required to distinguish OCD from delusions. Not surprisingly, lack of insight can be especially troubling to family members.

Once considered a rare illness with a poor prognosis,[5] OCD has been determined to be the fourth most common psychiatric disorder,[493] with a lifetime prevalence rate of 2.5% (about 1 in 40 persons).[494] OCD is among the most severe of the anxiety disorders and often results in crippling effects on social and occupational functioning. Reporting that 41% of patients who belong to the Obsessive–Compulsive Foundation were unable to work due to OCD symptoms, Hollander and colleagues[495] found that people incurred an average loss of 2 years' wages. Furthermore, 84% of respondents had lowered their career aspirations, and 82% had difficulty maintaining relationships because of symptoms. In addition to the adverse effects of OCD on sufferers, the strain on family members as a result of the demands of OCD is striking.

OCD rarely occurs in isolation and is most commonly found in concert with other anxiety and affective disorders, including social phobia, panic disorder, and depression.[496] Family studies have suggested a shared genetic vulnerability for other anxiety disorders,[497] as well as for depression. Not surprisingly, when OCD is complicated by other comorbid conditions, family burden can increase, along with confusion about how to manage multiple problems.

THE FAMILY AND OBSESSIVE–COMPULSIVE DISORDER

It is interesting that a surprisingly high percentage of adults with OCD do not marry, as indicated by the majority of epidemiological and psychopathology studies. Some studies have reported that as many as 60–70% of patients are single,[491, 498, 499] although other studies have found much lower figures. Compared to the national norms showing that 73.2% of men and 80.6% of women marry,[500] Steketee and colleagues[501] noted that 37% of their sample of 75 adult patients had never married, and 25% continued to live with their parents. Even among studies with higher marriage rates, it appears that men may be especially prone to remain single. Several studies have reported that approximately 65% of men in their samples are unmarried compared to 25–40% of women.[502–504] Perhaps this is related to the earlier onset age of OCD in males, who typically experience symptoms in early to midadolescence compared to females, whose onset occurs on average during the late teens or early 20s.[505]

The effects of OCD symptoms on the family are mostly anecdotal and descriptive. For example, out of anger and frustration over trying to accommodate his wife while seeing the symptoms of OCD get worse, one husband spoke about dumping a can of garbage on the bed. He was sick of having to conform to the rules about what was clean and what was "dirty." He had been allowed to sit in only one chair, on only one end of the couch, to use only "his" pillow and not to touch his wife once she was "clean" and got onto her side of the bed. Unable to fully understand what was happening, one spouse placed his hands around his wife's neck and shouted,

"What is wrong with you? Why can't you just be normal? Everyone else cooks eggs and meat and doesn't worry about poisoning. I don't get it!"

Fearful of what would happen if she were to stop participating in rituals, a wife of 12 years told of how she stayed awake until 3:00 A.M. doing laundry because her husband only had three outfits he would wear; his coat, the towels he sat on in the car, and the one pair of underwear he felt comfortable in "had" to be washed every day. Though she was exhausted, she was trying to "help" him to cope.

Situations such as these leave clinicians wondering why adult family members elect to remain in a home where they feel have no control over their life and large areas of living space. Indeed, some family members choose to leave under these circumstances. While these cases may seem to represent extreme circumstances, OCD rarely leaves the family system unaffected. Often unwittingly and unknowingly, family members are inexorably pulled into the patient's pathology.

Impact of Obsessive–Compulsive Disorder on Family Functioning

Research findings suggest that OCD may occur in families with a significant degree of unhealthy functioning, but it is unclear whether OCD symptoms adversely affect family functioning or compromised family interactions exacerbate anxiety symptoms. When family members of 50 patients were assessed using the Family Assessment Device (FAD)[506] to measure family problem solving, communication, roles, affective responsiveness, affective involvement, behavior control, and global functioning, 52% scored in the unhealthy range of functioning on at least one of these dimensions of family functioning.[507] In a pediatric population, Hibbs and colleagues[488] reported that nearly half of fathers and three-fourths of mothers of children with OCD exhibited high levels of criticism and/or overinvolvement with their children's symptoms.

Consistent with some of the examples we described earlier, Calvocoressi and colleagues[508] found that 88% of spouses or parents accommodated to the family member's symptoms. This was associated with poor family functioning, rejecting attitudes toward the patient, and family stress. Thus, OCD can have an adverse effect on family interaction and the quality of family life. As a result of a family member's OCD symptoms and the family's often inadvertent involvement in those symptoms, many families become dysfunctional. Of the 34 family members surveyed in the Calvocoressi study, nearly one-third reassured the patient three or more times per week. A similar number participated in compulsion-related behaviors or took over activities that were the patient's responsibility. Likewise, family and leisure-time routines and activities were modified to accommodate the demands of the person with OCD. These changes in family behavior and expectations seemed designed to manage the patient's distress and potential anger. However, accommodation to OCD led 35% of family members to experience moderate distress and 23%, severe or extreme distress.

Another large survey on the effect of OCD on family functioning was conducted by Shafran and colleagues in British Columbia.[509] The investigators recorded the reactions of 98 family members (67% spouses or partners, 17% parents, 16% child, sibling, or other) of volunteers who scored high on obsessive–compulsive symptoms. Ninety percent of respondents indicated that the symptoms of OCD interfered in other family members' functioning. In addition, 20% reported "severe" interference in their functioning. Thus, it appears that living with OCD often leads families to try to reduce obsessive–compulsive fear and anxiety symptoms by taking on extra responsibilities that in turn disrupt individual family members' functioning and the homeostasis of the family. By accommodating to the demands of the OCD, family members who may be trying to reduce conflict and discomfort may in reality be facilitating the disorder and fueling feelings of frustration, anger, burden, and guilt.

Family Responses to Obsessive–Compulsive Disorder

Clinical experience suggests that the family support system ("family" refers to all significant others), particularly family responses to obsessive–compulsive symptoms, may play a critical role in the prognosis and outcome of treatment.[492] Family responses to obsessive–compulsive symptoms seem to fall on a continuum of behavioral interaction patterns, ranging from families who give in to and assist in compulsions and avoidance, as discussed earlier, to those who completely oppose obsessive–compulsive behaviors.[507] According to this conceptualization (see Figure 15.1), enmeshed families lie on the accommodating end of the spectrum, demonstrating few boundaries, poor limit setting, and avoidance of conflict. At the other end are antagonistic families, who are rigid, demanding, intolerant of symptoms, and highly critical; such family responses tend to generate feelings of loss of control and increased anxiety in the patient. Most families lie between these extremes, often oscillating inconsistently in their responses to symptoms. In some cases, one family member is usually antagonistic, while another is understanding and indulgent of obsessive–compulsive

```
Antagonistic - - - - - - - - - - Accommodating
Rigid - - - - - - - - - - - - - Enmeshed
Demanding - - - - - - - - - - - Lack of boundaries
Intolerant - - - - - - - - - - - Poor limit setting
Critical, hostile - - - - - - - - - Avoids conflict
```

FIGURE 15.1. The continuum of family response patterns in OCD. From Van Noppen and Steketee.[584] Copyright 2001 by the American Psychiatric Press. Adapted by permission.

demands. In other cases, individual family members may fluctuate in responses that are sometimes intolerant and sometimes yielding. Not surprisingly, both patient and relatives in these families end up feeling confused and uncomfortable.

Some of these strong negative or inconsistent reactions may derive from the stress that OCD puts on both the patient and family members, and accompanying guilt, blame, and social stigma. Parents of people with OCD, in particular, seem to experience strong guilt reactions.[509, 510] Preoccupation with the patient's needs, feelings of burden and loss, and increased isolation as families remove themselves from usual social contacts are some of the unfortunate family effects of OCD. Tynes and colleagues[510] stressed the importance of the attitudes of those around the OCD patient as contributory to the severity of the illness. Many people do not understand patients' inability to control their symptoms and become angry about the obsessive–compulsive intrusion into their lives. They suggested that severely negative or rejecting reactions are likely to exacerbate anxiety and depression, as well as obsessions and compulsions.

BEHAVIORAL AND FAMILY TREATMENTS

The psychosocial treatment of choice for OCD is behavioral therapy that includes exposure for obsessions and response prevention (prevention of rituals), otherwise referred to as ERP. This treatment has been conducted mainly in an individual format, with a growing body of literature reporting benefits using a group modality.[492, 511] Exposure and response prevention are based on early findings that obsessions increase anxiety and compulsions reduce it. Not surprisingly, behavioral therapy based on this model has proven very effective for those who receive adequate ERP treatment.[512] However, despite the wealth of data supporting the efficacy of ERP in the treatment of OCD, refusal, premature dropout, noncompliance, and persistent symptoms detract from positive outcomes. Furthermore, OCD carries with it considerable costs for patients, family members, and society. In a recent survey of the practices of 42 behavioral therapists, Turner, Beidel, Spaulding, and Brown indicated that OCD treatment requires significantly more hours and longer duration (median = 6–12 months) than other anxiety disorders.[513] A report by Hollander et al. estimated that lifetime hospital costs for OCD are in the $5 billion range, and lifetime indirect costs for lost wages are at $40 billion.[495] Thus, it is clear that development of alternative efficacious and cost-effective treatment methods is warranted.

Family Factors Predicting Treatment Outcome

Relatively few studies have examined whether family functioning variables or attributes (such as those discussed earlier) affect treatment outcome. For example, clinical wisdom suggests that family accommodation to obsessive–compulsive symptoms and critical responses from family members impede patient gains, but there is limited research to support these impressions. Several early reports shed light on the effects of familial environment on treatment outcome and maintenance of gains. Hafner[514] noted that after returning home to conflictual marriages, women patients with OCD had relapsed. Hafner and colleagues also reported that spouse-aided behavioral therapy produced gains for a sample of five women.[515] Consistent with findings for persons with schizophrenia that relapse is associated with time spent with parents who are critical or emotionally overinvolved, Hoover and Insel[516] found that 10 of their patients who were living with parents relapsed slightly upon returning home after behavioral therapy. In contrast, separation from their parents contributed to further improvement. These anecdotal reports have been partly supported by later empirical studies of family variables that seem to predict immediate and long-term treatment benefits.

   With respect to the marital context, patients in distressed marriages benefited from behavioral treatment and did not differ in outcome from patients who reported having good marriages.[517, 518] These two studies support earlier findings that, for OCD and phobic conditions accompanied by marital distress, exposure-based treatment results in benefits for both anxiety and marital problems.[519]

   Proposing a model for relapse in OCD, Emmelkamp and colleagues[520] hypothesized that patients who lack coping skills or social support, or who experience criticism in the face of stressors, are likely to relapse. They recommended involving spouses or family members in treatment that emphasizes empathic listening skills and communication training, and the use of group treatments for the OCD clients who have problems with social interaction. This report implies that people with OCD could be affected by components of expressed emotion (EE), similar to findings that have been widely published for schizophrenia and affective disorders.[521] Consistent with this model, Emmelkamp and colleagues found that the combination of EE ratings, avoidant coping style, and life events and daily hassles significantly predicts relapse. This and other studies[491] also indicate that the immediate family environment is a more important influence on treatment outcome than broader social support.

Consistent with Emmelkamp and colleagues' report, Steketee[491] found that poor social and family functioning, and household interactions characterized by anger and criticism, predict fewer gains in OCD symptoms at 9-month follow-up. Perhaps relatives' criticism and expressed anger increase patients' feelings of anxiety and guilt, leading to a reduction in the capacity to fight urges to ritualize in response to obsessions. The result, an increase in obsessive–compulsive symptoms, generates more criticism and expressed anger, and evokes a vicious cycle. Patients' and relatives' attitudes about OCD symptoms may also influence outcome. Relatives' beliefs that OCD patients are malingering is also strongly associated with poor outcome.[491]

Preliminary findings obtained by Chambless and Steketee[522] from an ongoing trial of family variables as predictors of behavioral treatment outcome in a sample of patients with OCD and agoraphobia revealed that patient-perceived criticism and relatives' hostility predict or tend to predict poorer outcome both after treatment and at follow-up, particularly for the OCD sample. Furthermore, OCD patients with more emotionally overinvolved relatives (perhaps similar to those we consider to be accommodating) dropped out of treatment prematurely and showed less benefit at follow-up. Surprisingly, observer-rated criticism that was not hostile predicted better outcome, suggesting that nonhostile criticism may be an important motivator for some patients during exposure therapy.

These findings on family variables suggest that addressing family overinvolvement or accommodation to obsessive–compulsive symptoms, patients' and relatives' beliefs, and family communication and functioning during therapy might improve behavioral treatment outcomes. In addition, because patient-perceived criticism and relatives' hostility proved to be predictors of relapse, strategies that reduce these factors may be useful adjuncts.

Models for Behavioral Family Therapy

Early efforts of the pioneers of behavioral family therapy were based primarily on the application of operant conditioning to problems that could be relatively clearly defined in stimulus–response terms.[523–525] Focusing on the interpersonal environment of a family, Stuart developed the idea of contingency contracting. Building on the principle of reciprocity, Stuart's intervention maximized the benefits of positive behavioral exchange between family members. He extended the ideas of homeostasis and "quid pro quo" developed by Jackson, who applied these concepts to describe balance and behavioral exchange as social phenomena.[526] Stuart's work incorporated written contracts, and family members learned to utilize positive reinforcement. Most of his treatment centered on marital discord, but the principles he set forth continue to be used by behavioral family therapists.[492]

Jacobson took the behavioral ideas one step further by incorporating cognitive strategies.[527] He suggested that techniques such as relabeling negative attributions, changing unrealistic expectations, and creating realistic, positive expectancies for change were all important in successful behavioral family therapy. This work undergirds the psychoeducational approaches of many forerunners in family therapy.[178, 528] Similar strategies aimed at cognitive change in family members are also evident in writings on support groups for OCD.[529]

Because family members can serve as modifiers (reinforcers or extinguishers) of OCD symptoms, the origins of which lie in biological, psychological and, to a limited extent, family processes, we developed a behavioral family model that capitalizes on this. As discussed earlier, excessive family accommodation reinforces symptoms, and produces frustration and negative family attitudes and behaviors. We hypothesize that including family members in treatment is beneficial, because educating partners and families about OCD symptoms and the principles of exposure treatment alters negative attitudes, increases expectancy and cooperation during treatment, and provides a rationale for altering problematic family behavior. Furthermore, relatives who are practiced in behaviors that inadvertently reinforce OCD symptoms must deliberately learn alternative responses, which usually means behavioral contracting that enhances recovery and reduces risk of relapse. A form of communication skills training, behavioral contracting assists families in utilizing clear communication to negotiate expectations and contingencies for explicit situations that are consistent with ERP. ERP often seems counterintuitive to patients and families until they are provided information and in-session experiences that result in symptom control. Behavioral contracting also serves to encourage self-instruction without the assistance of a therapist.

Family Support Groups for Obsessive–Compulsive Disorder

Support groups for OCD patients and their families provide an opportunity for educating and involving family members in treatment of patients. Early application of this was utilized by Marks and colleagues[530] who instituted a mixed patient and relative group that met every few weeks, while the patient participated in individual behavioral therapy. The benefits of combined patient–family or family-only support groups have also been reported by Black and Blum,[531] Cooper,[532] and Tynes and colleagues.[529] Usually including a psychoeducational component, as well as social support for participants, these groups are designed to instill hope, to alleviate fear, and to provide assurance to patients and their family members that they are not alone. The content of family group discussions typically included the exploration of strategies for managing difficult problems such as patients' persistent reassurance seeking and requests that family members participate in obsessive–compulsive behaviors.[530] Educational topics, such as types of symptoms, etiology of OCD, treatment options, medications, complications, and relapse prevention, were included in the support groups containing both patients and their significant others.[529] Surveyed participants reported good satisfaction with these groups, although no outcome data about the effects of family support groups on patient symptoms or family responses have been provided.

Family-Assisted Treatment

Single-Family Interventions

In several studies, parents, spouses, or other family members have assisted in ERP therapy, mainly following instructions given by the therapist to encourage ERP and to resist participation in rituals. Benefits have been described for parental involvement in behavioral treatment of children,[533–535] and of adolescents and adults.[515, 516] The possible benefits of incorporating spousal assistance into behavioral treatment have also been investigated. In a large uncontrolled trial of 45 mostly OCD inpatients, Thornicroft and colleagues[536] reported benefits of teaching relatives to reduce their involvement in OCD symptoms and to monitor patient behavior, while encouraging self-exposure in a noncritical manner. OCD patients experienced a 45% decrease in symptoms at discharge and a 60% reduction in symptoms and concomitant improvement in functioning at 6-month follow-up for a smaller sample. Considering that this study was conducted with an inpatient population that scored in the extreme range on disability as a result of OCD symptoms, these gains are impressive.

Conducting two separate, controlled studies of the benefits of spousal assistance during ERP therapy, Emmelkamp and colleagues'[518, 537] comparison of this treatment and individual behavior therapy showed mixed results. In the first study,[537] spousal participation led to more benefits than individual treatment but did not persist. In a later trial, there were no significant differences,[528] although the spouse-aided group reported improvement in marital satisfaction. As in other studies examining spouse-assisted ERP, partners in these two trials followed the instructions of a therapist. This method differs from our multifamily behavioral treatment, in which the emphasis is on behavioral contracting. It is possible that the lack of formal training in family communication skills about patients' OCD symptoms in the Emmelkamp and colleagues trials might have reduced possible benefits, because in a later report, they particularly emphasized the need for empathic communication in family treatment of OCD.[520]

Mehta's[538] controlled study of family assistance during behavioral treatment for 30 OCD patients produced more favorable conclusions regarding family-assisted ERP. Patients in the family assistance treatment group benefited significantly more than those who received no family participation, and were more likely to maintain their gains than individually treated patients, who relapsed more. Especially effective were the nonanxious, firm family members. It seems clear that some types of family intervention may positively influence patients' outcomes.

Multiple-Family Group Treatment

A potentially valuable contribution of multifamily behavioral therapy (MFBT) compared to single-family behavioral therapy is the opportunity for reduction in perceived isolation, enriched opportunities for problem solving, and emotional distance from the OCD, enabling family members to respond to the symptoms in a less personalized manner. A sense of community and social support often develops through the course of the MFBT, as families share quite private stories with one another. Another result is a lessening in feelings of shame and stigma, which encourages family members to take a more proactive role in treatment and join with the patient to combat the OCD. The presence of other families with similar problems provides an opportunity for patients and families to learn effective negotiation of agreements and to adopt symptom management strategies modeled by other members of the group. Additional potential benefits of multifamily intervention are reduced therapist burnout and greater cost-effectiveness of treatment, particularly if gains are better maintained.

Recently, Van Noppen and colleagues[492] tested the value of MFBT. This intervention was specifically aimed at both reducing obsessive–compulsive symptoms, and changing dysfunctional patterns of communication between family members that seem to fuel symptoms. The family group treatment incorporated psychoeducation, communication, and problem-solving skills training, clarifying boundaries, social learning, and in vivo rehearsal of new behaviors, in the context of ERP with therapist and participant modeling. This uncontrolled trial[492] examined the effects of this format for 19 patients and family members treated in four groups. Patients experienced significant reductions in obsessive–compulsive symptom severity and similar reduction in scores on a measure of family functioning (FAD). Among MFBT patients, 47% were clinically significantly improved (reliably changed and scoring in the nonclinical range on OCD symptoms) at posttest, and 58% achieved this status at 1-year follow-up. Results from MFBT were comparable to those achieved by individual behavioral therapy. Overall, then, the multifamily intervention was quite effective, although some patients did not show strong gains, and there is clearly room for improvement. Efforts to identify family variables that played a role in treatment outcome yielded some findings of interest. Poorer family role functioning and communication predicted less benefit on obsessive–compulsive symptoms and was associated with more disability. From this research, then, it appears that MFBT is another therapy option in which family assistance might enhance outcome for patients.

Although our multifamily intervention is similar to methods described by McFarlane in this volume and by Falloon,[539] it utilizes interventions that are specifically aimed at reducing obsessive–compulsive symptoms and changing the dysfunctional patterns of communication that seem to fuel symptoms. This family group treatment incorporates psychoeducation, communication, and problem-solving skills training, clarifying boundaries, social learning, and in vivo rehearsal of new behaviors, in addition to in-group observation of the application of exposure and response prevention with therapist and participant modeling. An illustration of the MFBT method is given below.*

---

*From Van Noppen and Steketee.[584] Copyright 2001 by the American Psychiatric Press. Adapted by permission.

FEATURES AND PROCEDURES
OF MULTIFAMILY BEHAVIORAL TREATMENT

The key practical features include the following:

1. Four to six families (we recommend no more than 16 total participants), including patient and significant others who are in considerable daily contact with the patient; "family" can include homo-
   sexual as well as heterosexual couples, stepparents, second-degree
   family members, and so on.
2. Co-leaders are optimally trained, at least one of the leaders should
   have an advanced degree in social work, psychology or certified
   counseling, and experience in clinical work with individuals, families, and groups, and proficiency in cognitive-behavioral therapy,
   with experience in populations with OCD.
3. Sessions are 2 hours long and typically meet in the late afternoon or
   early evening. The key clinical procedures include the following:
   a. Each patient and family undergoes a pretreatment screening by
      phone with the therapist(s) to determine their appropriateness
      for the group and readiness for treatment. Following this, two
      intake sessions are scheduled.
   b. At the 1½-hour intake sessions, pretreatment forms are com-
      pleted, symptom severity and family response styles are deter-
      mined, goals of the group and behavioral therapy principles are
      discussed, and pretreatment concerns and questions are ad-
      dressed.
   c. Treatment: 12 weekly sessions, six monthly group follow-up ses-
      sions, providing: education about OCD and reading of self-help
      material, education about families and OCD, *in vivo* ERP plus
      homework and self-monitoring, homework discussion with fam-
      ily group feedback and problem solving, and behavioral con-
      tracting among family members and communication skills train-
      ing.

MULTIFAMILY BEHAVIORAL TREATMENT:
A CLINICAL EXAMPLE

Kim, a 28-year-old secretary and mother of a 2-year-old daughter, described
symptoms of OCD that dated back to childhood. She sought treatment fol-

lowing severe exacerbation of her symptoms during her first pregnancy. Kim was referred for MFBT after a partial response to clomipramine and pimozide and 6 months of unsuccessful psychotherapy elsewhere. Kim reported that her primary fears had to do with extreme worry that she would contract cancer from various "substances" even when they could not be seen. In response to these fears, she was washing her hands over 100 times a day, avoiding any situation or object that would trigger the worry about cancer. In addition, out of fear of "additives," Kim had restricted her diet to only one brand of "natural" ice cream and "natural" granola. Kim also spoke about feeling that she "had to sit with clenched fists to be sure" she was not making blasphemous gestures to God. She had given up on doing laundry, grocery shopping, and cooking, because every task "took too long." Kim described "piles of clothes on the basement floor that have been there for 3 years, and some were starting to mold" due to her avoidance. When asked about her husband's response, Kim said that he would "give in" to her requests to "keep the peace." She involved him in extensive reassurance-seeking rituals, usually more than 50 times a day, although she stated that she wanted to stop her "strange behavior" because it was "tearing" her family apart. However, Kim "really believed" she could die from the "cancer germs." She had begun to involve her daughter, Lilly, by washing the child's hands so frequently that she had protested against it. Kim's husband Joe "gave up" trying to get Kim to cook. Sneaking food into the house created such an "uproar" that he resorted to taking Lilly to his mother's house for most suppers.

The beginning of Kim's obsessive–compulsive symptoms dated back to the age of 8, when she felt she "had to touch certain things" in her room to ward off fears that people close to her would die. She described a life riddled with magical thinking and ideas that she "had" to perform actions a certain way to prevent "bad things" from happening. For example, she would open and close the refrigerator in a certain way, touch the floor and then touch both eyes, walk up and down steps with the right foot leading, say ritualized prayers at bedtime, and get in and out of bed. She hid most of her rituals from others. Despite her worries, she was able to manage without seeming peculiar. The aggressive fears, mental rituals, and undoing behaviors became a hidden way of life for her until her pregnancy, when she began to make "unreasonable" demands on her family; Kim became withdrawn and showed apparent decline in her occupational functioning.

Joe had viewed Kim's worries as just part of her personality, and their life appeared quite "normal" to others. Joe worked as a computer programmer, and Kim landed a good job as a secretary at a large company. Shortly after they bought their own home, Mary, Kim's sister, with whom she was very close, was diagnosed with ovarian cancer. To make it easier to receive chemotherapy, Kim insisted that Mary move in with her and Joe. Kim was wonderful to Mary during this time, sharing everything she owned. Mary's cancer remitted and she moved back to live with their mother. Two years later, Kim became pregnant and began to express fears that she and the fetus would contract cancer from Mary, or from anything Mary had touched. Because Mary had been living in Kim's house, nearly everything seemed "contaminated."

To avoid conflict, Joe went along with all of Kim's requests, no matter how extreme. For example, he complied with the demands of OCD: taking specific routes to the grocery store, so as not to drive by "asbestos" contaminated areas; buying dairy items at the back of the case, so they were not exposed to "radiation"; not using certain dishware, spices, and foods that had been used by Mary; and not sitting on certain "clean" chairs.

Much of this history and detailed description of Kim's obsessive–compulsive symptoms were obtained during the first two 90-minute information-gathering sessions. Kim attended the first of these sessions alone. It was clear that despite her strong conviction about her beliefs, she was eager to change behavior that was generating conflict in her marriage and distressing her daughter.

At the second information-gathering session, Kim and Joe appeared eager to learn more about OCD and how to handle it. Joe spoke about feeling as though "Kim's demands were controlling everything." He gave up trying to convince her not to be afraid, because nothing seemed to work. Joe reported that "lately, Kim was going too far by involving Lilly." The therapist spoke about MFBT offering this kind of help to family members. Besides problem solving with other families dealing with OCD, Joe would learn a specific technique, behavioral contracting, to begin to set some limits on his participation in the compulsions. Also, the more that Kim and Joe could learn about OCD, the more they would be able to control it. Hierarchies were established based on the severity of Kim's fears (see Table 15.1). Together with the therapist, the couple planned treatment to confront each trigger. Kim and Joe were asked to read Chapters 1–4 in *When Once Is Not Enough* by Steketee and White,[540] before the group began and were encouraged to call the therapist if they had any lingering questions.

Multifamily Behavioral Treatment Session 1

At the outset of this co-led MFBT group, anticipatory anxiety ran high. Kim and Joe were among a total of seven couples/families. As people arrived, we distributed name tags. Once everyone was seated in the circle, the formal

TABLE 15.1. Kim's Fear Hierarchies

Situation	Discomfort (1–100)	Treatment session
Hierarchy 1. Fears of contamination: cancer from sister and cigarettes		
Holding unopened cigarette pack	45	1
Touching makeup sister used	50	1
Touching mug sister used	50	1
Touching doorknobs (general)	55	2
Holding opened cigarette pack	55	2
Holding "clean" ashtray	60	3
Holding clothes worn by sister	70	4
Touching "dirty" clothes (basement)	85	5
Touching cigarette filter	90	6
Using cup served by a smoker	90	6
Stepping barefoot on a cigarette	95	7
Touching cigarette to lips	95	7
Hierarchy 2. Fears of contamination: cancer from "chemical" contact		
Microwaving food	30	1
Pumping gasoline	35	1
Touching sand in sandbox	35	1
Touching Sweet 'N Low	40	2
Holding batteries	40	2
Touching sand at beach	65	5
Walking barefoot at beach	70	5
Eating food items "scanned" at checkout	75	6
Drinking soda	85	7
Eating chicken	100	8

group began. We asked each person to introduce him- or herself and indicate what he or she hoped to get out of the group. This facilitated participation and began the foundation for trust and group cohesiveness. The themes at the beginning of this and other MFBTs included: "What should I do when my daughter is in the shower for 3 hours? Can that really be OCD?", "How do other families deal with the rituals?", "What is OCD?", "How can each of us cope with it effectively?"

A quick review of the "ground rules" clarified group expectations about the time frame of the group, the meeting place, confidentiality, and notification of absent group members. Group members were encouraged to contact the leader(s) to discuss any feelings or issues that arose as a result of their group experience. The proposed agenda for the 12 weekly sessions and 6 monthly check-in sessions was outlined. After this, a handout entitled "What Is OCD?" (definition of obsessions and compulsions, theories of etiology, course of illness, common coexisting disorders, and treatment) and the Yale–Brown Obsessive–Compulsive Scale (YBOCS) Symptom Checklist were distributed. The information was reviewed, and the checklist served as a springboard for patients and family members to disclose about the obsessive–compulsive symptoms and behaviors typically hidden in shame.

Families talked about the bizarre symptoms in an atmosphere with little social stigma. Meeting others with OCD who were "normal people" seemed to quiet family members' fears that maybe their loved one was going crazy. The group provided the first real opportunity for several family members to learn about the content of the patients' obsessions and the extent of the rituals.

A stress–diathesis model of OCD's pathogenesis was presented. In addition to genetic factors, familial and cultural factors were discussed as important in the development and expression of OCD. Some moments of silence occurred in the group as the excitement of comparing stories died down, and it appeared that, in these silences, many family members were trying to come to terms with the illness.

The leaders left time for patients to select ERP homework challenges in a "go-round" fashion, with patients taking turns one at a time. Kim chose to begin with all of the items lowest on her hierarchies. Homework forms were distributed. The session formally ended with the therapists' encouragement that the first week is a trial time to begin practicing ERP. If patients did not sense a decrease in their distress, they were encouraged to modify the exposure challenge and stay with one item until the discomfort diminished. Family members were reminded that one of the goals of MFBT is to learn to be involved in the OCD as little as possible except in life-threatening or dangerous situations. Family members were instructed to keep their involvement to a minimum but to make no drastic changes in their responses to the demands of OCD until they learned to utilize behavioral contracting. The leaders asked all patients to bring any of the items in their hierarchy to the next session, so that these could be used therapeutically.

Multifamily Behavioral Treatment Session 2

The second session began with a review of what was covered or accomplished in the group the previous week. Patients reported on the homework they completed during the week, and the therapists collected homework, verifying that patients completed it as assigned. Patients reported on their levels of anxiety during the exposure homework and, if anxiety declined, discussed this and noted that prolonged exposure made this possible.

The majority of this session was dedicated to the description of behavioral therapy and ERP techniques. The techniques of direct and imagined ERP *in vivo* and imaginal exposure were described. Examples were given and each patient was asked to practice by choosing an exposure homework task.

As each patient selected his or her homework, the group leader translated the task into a form that could be rehearsed in the group; the therapist and other group members participated in the exposure challenge. Kim, along with all the other group members, was asked to touch the doorknobs in the room. As they did this, it was difficult for other patients who feared contamination for reasons other than cancer. Patients with severe obsessions joked that they wished they had this problem instead of their own—a common remark made in such groups. Observing so many people unaffected by the task led Kim to comment that it helped to see how easily most people touched doorknobs. This process led her to question her behavior and beliefs.

The leaders asked Kim to take out the cigarette pack, batteries, Sweet 'N Low, makeup, and mugs that she had been avoiding and pass them around the group. Every 10 minutes, Kim was asked, "What is your level of anxiety or discomfort from 0 to 100 right now, as you focus on what you're doing?" Other group members were asked the same question. The unreasonableness of the fears, resultant anxiety, and compulsive behavior was identified by the therapist as a hallmark of OCD. Because the fear could not be reasoned with, why try? This universal problem was identified as another symptom of the OCD: reassurance seeking that, like checking or washing, leads to more of the same. As patients and families experienced this in the group, the therapists encouraged symptom identification and the rehearsal of dismissal, distraction, and redirection. Kim began to develop better insight into her OCD and how she had grown to rely on Joe to answer "the unanswerable." The strategy of ERP started to make sense as her confidence grew through education, exposure, homework, and the support and feedback of the group.

At the end of the second session, the therapists instructed patients to continue the exposure from that day's session and practice any other homework items at least 1 hour a day, preferably all at once rather than split into segments. Patients were reminded not to leave the exposure situation until their anxiety had declined noticeably and to record their distress levels on their homework form.

Multifamily Behavioral Treatment Session 3

The group began in its usual way, with each patient reporting on homework task results. Joe added that he noticed a big improvement in Kim's outlook and that she seemed more willing to take risks. For example, they went out to eat pizza for the first time in 8 months and Kim stepped on a cigarette butt, drove behind a bus, touched the doorknobs, sat with her hands open, and did not perform any rituals. The group was tremendously supportive of Kim.

At this session, the therapists presented a brief videotaped lecture to the group on the neurobiology of OCD. This tape provided information on medication and the interplay between behavioral therapy and biological processes in the treatment of OCD. Following the discussion of this tape, the therapists asked each patient to select exposure items with a discomfort level of approximately 50 to 60.

After about 60 minutes of *in vivo* or imaginal exposure, the group's attention was shifted to focus on the "Guidelines for Living with OCD" (*Learning to Live with OCD*[495]):

1. Learn to recognize the signals that indicate a person is having problems.
2. Modify expectations during stressful times.
3. Measure progress according to the person's level of functioning.
4. Don't make day-to-day comparisons.
5. Give recognition for "small" improvements.
6. Create a strong, supportive home environment.
7. Keep communication clear and simple.
8. Stick to a behavioral contract.
9. Set limits, yet be sensitive to the person's mood.
10. Keep your family routine "normal."
11. Use humor.
12. Support the person's medication regimen.
13. Make separate time for other family members.
14. Be flexible!

As the group members took turns reading aloud, the therapist asked the families which of the responses described them. Kim and the other patients reassessed their behavioral homework task with family guidelines in mind and added another challenge.

Multifamily Behavioral Treatment Session 4

The first three sessions provided patients and families with a clearer understanding of OCD. The next step was to learn how, as a family, to cope more productively with the symptoms using cognitive and behavioral techniques. This fourth session was designed to prepare families for the family contracting in the following sessions that forms the essence of family collaboration in the treatment of OCD. As usual, each patient reported on his or her homework during the week, with family members commenting on their roles or observations. Kim and Joe said they felt discouraged. When they went away for the weekend, Kim was "afraid that the condo was sprayed with pesticide." She "stayed in the same clothes all weekend, didn't let Joe bring their suitcases out of the car, didn't allow Lilly to play on the floor, felt like the makeup was ruined," and that she was "back to square 1." Joe knew he had to be firmer and despite bickering, insisted that Kim try. The group gave Joe positive feedback for doing this and confronted him about his "tendency to give in too much."

The therapists introduced the concept of behavioral contracting, emphasizing the following points:

1. One at a time, each family identifies problem areas as a result of the demands of obsessive–compulsive symptoms: How does OCD impose on others? Do family members participate in rituals? Is criticism directed toward the patient by family? Do family members take over the patient's tasks and responsibilities? The problems are to be defined in very clear, specific, behavioral terms.
2. The group leaders guide the family to focus on one problem area and define it (as in the earlier example).
3. Family members utilize feedback from the group to explore behavioral response options and the possible consequences of each.
4. With principles of behavior therapy in mind, the family members select the best response options.
5. The leaders facilitate a negotiation process between family members. This consists of direct dialogue of behavioral expectations among the family members, interspersed with group comments, suggestions, and feedback. At this point, the family creates a contract that establishes the behavioral therapy goal for the patient and the behavioral responses for family members.
6. The family, with the assistance of the group, assesses whether the solution is reasonable.

7. When possible, the family rehearses the behavioral contract during the treatment session.
8. The group members evaluate the contract, adding suggestions based on observations of the family's ability to carry out the plan.
9. If necessary, family members negotiate any modifications in the planned contract before moving on to the next family. All exposure homework is written on the homework sheets, with contracts recorded in the space provided.

With feedback from the group, Kim and Joe negotiated a behavioral contract: Kim was to use the makeup several times a day and touch the "contaminated" clothes to her "clean" clothes, then wear the touched garment. Kim agreed to this and to resist reassurance seeking from Joe. Also, she was to hold Lilly or let the child touch the "contaminated" clothing. Joe raised the possibility that Kim would want to wash her hands, Lilly's toys, and anything else that came into contact with the "contaminants." Others in the group quickly responded that this would "defeat the purpose" and urged Kim to resist these compulsions.

Other group members participated in the negotiation process to assist Kim and Joe in arriving at a behavioral contract that seemed satisfying and feasible. Other spouses coached Joe to be consistent and stick to the agreement. Although the contracts are meant to provide expectable guidelines for behavior in any given situation, they should be amenable to renegotiation and modification as needed. All families left the session with a behavioral contract to practice and homework forms to record the progress. As in the proceeding sessions, each patient committed to individual exposure homework as well as the family contract.

Multifamily Behavioral Treatment Sessions 5–11

During these sessions, the 2-hour group meeting was devoted to *in vivo* and imaginal exposure and response prevention, practice in family contracting, self-monitoring distress levels, and homework planning. Family responses to OCD were discussed in greater detail, and greater disclosure about symptoms emerged. Group interaction became highly personalized as family members described the interpersonal conflict that intruded in their attempts to manage the obsessive–compulsive symptoms. Each session began with the go-round of patients and families reporting on the previous week's exposure homework and behavioral contract.

Families were supported by the therapists and group members in their efforts "to help." In each of the sessions, the therapists asked which family wanted to initiate the contracting first. After hearing about the success Kim and Joe had using their contract, a woman with a 20-year OCD history decided to reduce unnecessary hand washing anytime she entered the house or touched anything she suspected of being "contaminated." She asked her husband to go about his business without accommodating her and to avoid "hovering" around her. This cross-family modeling appeared to be a therapeutic factor in the MFBT.

The question "How much should I push?" was a pervasive family concern. The therapists noted that using force or ultimatums in the midst of rituals would likely lead to frustration and anger, resulting in more conflict and possible physical violence or destructive acts. Families were advised not only to encourage resistance and discourage avoidance as much as possible but also to recognize mounting tension, often manifested as an increase in obsessive–compulsive symptoms, as a warning signal to "back off." No family in this group required crisis intervention and interruption of behavioral family contracting.

Throughout the later sessions, there was a growing emphasis on independent initiation of ERP challenges and behavioral contracting with less therapist involvement. The therapists continually stressed the importance of self-instruction and patients' and families' ability to utilize the techniques on their own. By Session 11, the therapists ensured that each family had reviewed its gains and the symptoms that need more intensive work. With feedback from other group members, therapists highlighted the symptomatic improvement, wealth of knowledge, and understanding gained through the MFBT.

Multifamily Behavioral Treatment Session 12

The last weekly session began with the go-round and practice of ERP and family behavioral contracting. Throughout this session, families and patients asked, "What will we do now?", "Does this group have to end?", "Can't we extend it? We just got to know each other." The therapists addressed feelings of sadness and loss as part of the termination of the group. Kim and Joe spoke about how much they would miss the encouragement and coaching from the group. Kim, like other patients, was well aware of the importance of consistent practice of the strategies but feared she would not continue to be so diligent without the accountability to the group. Joe responded that, with the behavioral contracting and his better understanding, she did not have to worry, because he would not let her "get away with as much." Through the MFBT, Joe had simultaneously learned to communicate understanding and to set limits. Kim described a contract they made that when they were in public and she got into "an OCD thing." Joe would gently squeeze Kim's hand and wink at her as a "signal" that she was being unreasonable. This worked very well, because there were no hostile, critical comments made toward the patient. Joe spoke for other family members in the group when he said that before the MFBT, "I thought I knew about OCD, but now I not only understand it intellectually, I understand it emotionally, too."

CONCLUSIONS

Clinical research has clearly demonstrated that behavioral treatment that offers a combination of exposure and response prevention is effective in reducing obsessive–compulsive symptoms. Despite these promising findings, a large number of patients refuse or drop out of treatment, remain symptomatic following treatment, or experience a loss of benefits once therapy has ended. In addition, the cost of providing individual behavioral treatment has spiraled upward. Family treatment offered in a group modality appears to be a promising alternative to labor-intensive individual behavioral treatment. MFBT is a 12-session treatment for groups that meet weekly and includes psychoeducation; exposure, with modeling and response prevention; and homework assignments. Six monthly group sessions follow the active phase of behavioral treatment to help consolidate gains and encourage independent problem solving in relation to obsessive–compulsive symptoms.

Our clinical impressions and recent research findings suggest that MFBT may offer hope for patients who have not benefited from standard, individual treatment, and who are living with family members. Families of OCD patients commonly participate in symptoms in some fashion, and their responses are often countertherapeutic. MFBT incorporates families into behavioral treatment by teaching family members and patients to negotiate contracts. The goal of this treatment is to encourage patient exposure and anxiety reduction, to educate and model reasonable interactive responses within families, and to extract family members (and others) from the patient's compulsions in a supportive manner. Such efforts are likely to enable patients to consolidate their gains and to establish a family environment that is supportive and firm, without being punitive or overly indulgent. Clearly, further study of MFBT is warranted. This could prove to be crucial in this era of stringent managed mental health care. Mobilizing natural support systems and offering families an opportunity to resume healthy functioning is certainly a worthy goal to strive for as we enter the 21st century.

Chapter 16

Application of Multifamily Groups in Chronic Medical Disorders

SANDRA GONZALEZ AND PETER STEINGLASS

As detailed in previous chapters, psychoeducational multifamily groups represent one of the more exciting currently available interventions for treatment of the major mental disorders. In this chapter, we discuss another potentially important use of these interventions as a means to assist families facing the challenges of severe or life-threatening chronic medical conditions. While the use of multifamily interventions with chronic medical illness has developed more slowly than the analogous work utilizing such groups with schizophrenia and bipolar disorder, an interesting story nonetheless is beginning to emerge. This is the story that we tell in this chapter.

Just as is true for families struggling with major psychoses, families who must face chronic medical illness also experience profound challenges. Clinical reports are consistent in describing families' pressing need for psychosocial support attendant to the diagnosis, course, and treatment of illnesses such as diabetes, asthma, AIDS, end organ disease (with or without transplantation), and cancer.[126, 541-544] Families not only experience tremendous stresses secondary to the challenges associated with major medical illnesses but also play a major role in the ongoing treatment of severe medical conditions, particularly in the current atmosphere of medical cost containment.[545] Parents, spouses, or adult children of severely ill patients shoulder the largest share of symptom assessment, medical decision making, and treatment collaboration—demands for which they are usually ill-prepared.

These issues arise for families at virtually every stage of medical illness. During the peridiagnostic period, family members often find themselves precipitously immersed in a foreign medical culture, left to decode a new language, to decipher an unfamiliar social order (the medical hierarchy), and to develop a new set of social ties that is crucial to the adequate treatment of the ill member. Later on, as the chronic stage of illness sets in, families experience anxiety and depression at the potential loss or severe limitation of the ill family member. In addition, families often have difficulty balancing illness needs with the normative demands of family life during the chronic phase. Finally, for illnesses that move on to a terminal phase, families struggle with decisions about stopping aggressive treatment and initiating palliative care. They are often left on their own to struggle through such discussions and decision making, because medical care professionals often neglect the psychosocial aspects of chronic illness management.

This mounting anecdotal evidence and preliminary empirical data regarding the tremendous psychosocial and economic costs of chronic medical illness borne by non-ill family members[545–549] suggest that a family-based intervention should be considered a standard component of the comprehensive treatment of chronic medical illnesses. Furthermore, multifamily groups appear to be ideally suited to address these family stresses and vulnerabilities. Thus, it is no surprise that a number of clinicians and investigators have been experimenting with their use in medical settings.[469, 550–554] Additionally, initial reports indicate that these groups have had a positive impact, especially in their ability to improve the functioning of non-ill family members, by helping families combat the sense of isolation they often feel in their struggles with chronic illnesses, and by increasing collaboration between families and health care professionals.[469, 541, 555]

In spite of the initial positive response to multifamily groups for chronic medical illness, these interventions have been more difficult to implement than multifamily groups for the major mental disorders. There have emerged a number of obstacles to their routine inclusion in chronic illness management protocols. These obstacles can be attributed to two features of most medical treatment settings: the dominant influence of the biomedical model in these settings and in medical education in general, and the lack of training of treatment staff for interacting constructively with families of medically ill patients. For example, although many clinics and hospitals now offer educational programs and support groups for families, these interventions frequently separate patients from other family members and rely on staff with limited training in family systems approaches. This mismatch between the biases of the biomedical model and those of family-centered health care underlies some of the difficulties encountered in establishing multifamily interventions in medical settings. These issues are described below.

MEDICAL VERSUS PSYCHIATRIC MULTIFAMILY GROUPS

We begin our discussion of the use of multifamily groups in medical illness settings by describing some differences between the use of these groups for the major psychoses (the topic of the previous chapters in the book) and their application in medical settings. These differences have to do with (1) the empirical research and conceptual bases that inform medical versus psychiatric intervention with multifamily groups, (2) the very different cultures that exist in medical versus psychiatric settings, and (3) the primary objectives of each multifamily group intervention (i.e., to influence clinical course of the illness vs. improving the well-being of all nonpatient family members). In combination, these differences have challenged the implementation of multifamily group interventions in medical settings, making it more difficult to design a practical chronic illness version that would address the needs of families and that would find acceptance in treatment settings that are predominantly influenced by the biomedical model.

The details are as follows.

Obstacle 1: The Biomedical Bias of Medical Settings

Although, historically, the treatment of the major mental disorders has almost always included psychological and milieu modalities to reduce or prevent symptoms, the shift to family-focused interventions grew out of research documenting the profound effect of social and emotional environmental stressors on the exacerbation or reduction of symptoms in these disorders.[556] The effectiveness of multifamily psychoeducational interventions in reducing stress and symptoms in conditions such as schizophrenia and bipolar disorder has dramatically altered the course of these illnesses and has led to the inclusion of these interventions in the routine standard of care.

In contrast, the data about the impact of family psychosocial variables on medical outcomes are more preliminary,[546, 557, 558] making it less widely accepted in medical settings. Although some preliminary reports link psychosocial interventions to improved medical competence,[555, 559] at this point most clinicians find it easy to downplay the role of family psychosocial factors in the face of often ravaging and predictably progressive disease processes dictated by biomedical factors. Furthermore, even when psychosocial needs are included in treatment planning, the focus remains on the individual patient. With the exception of those conditions that demand family involvement (e.g., family participation controlling environmental allergens for asthma patients, or the need for a family donor for a transplant procedure), the family is not seen as a true partner in medical treatment planning or illness prevention. Thus, because a family intervention such as multifamily group therapy does not treat the illness itself, it is rarely included in treatment protocols as part of standard care.

Furthermore, it is likely, although not yet firmly established, that the multifamily group intervention may have its greatest impact on non-ill family members and only secondarily impact the index patient through more timely provision of appropriate care. The fact that family support is not perceived by the health care system as a core component of treatment for severe medical conditions has an impact on the family's own expectations regarding the psychological and social costs of a member's chronic illness or disability. While consistently voicing the need for support and guidance, families simultaneously see these services as luxuries that must be forgone in the face of the often overwhelming demands of treatment. This in turn completes a confusing circle by supporting the medical team's perception that family group attendance is difficult, if not impossible, to sustain, and is therefore a poor use of staff time.

Obstacle 2: Demonstrating the Multifamily Group's Effectiveness

As documented in previous chapters, an impressive body of empirical research has established a key role for psychoeducational multifamily treatments in managing the course of mental disorders. A comparable body of research does not yet exist for medical conditions and disabilities, and researchers conducting outcome studies of multifamily groups for medical illness have faced formidable challenges. In particular, it has been difficult to define and operationalize meaningful outcome variables for assessing the impact of these interventions. For example, few would argue that exacerbation rates in illnesses such as diabetes, asthma, or cancer are *primarily* tied to specific psychosocial variables (analogous to the role of expressed emotion in schizophrenia). Rather, they would point to nonspecific stress factors as possibly important, factors that are much harder to operationalize for research purposes. Furthermore, individual variation in severity of illness, toxicities of treatments, and development of complications are confounding covariates, making it more difficult to tease out the primary impact of the multifamily group intervention.

Medical cost savings constitute another currently popular outcome indicator that has proved useful in assessing the benefit of this type of intervention in treating the major mental disorders (see, e.g., McFarlane et al.[171]). Linked as it is to exacerbation of symptoms and complications, this outcome has not been useful in assessing the efficacy of multifamily group intervention in chronic illness for two reasons. First, the costs of treating these medical conditions are influenced primarily, although not exclusively, by biological factors that are largely outside the realm psychosocial influence. Even when psychosocial interventions improve the quality of life or sense of well-being in the patient, the illness course (and therefore the cost of treatment) may remain unaffected. Second, when cost offset is the outcome, typically, only the medical utilization of the index patient is measured. In future evaluation of the cost-effectiveness of multifamily group intervention in chronic illness, the health care utilization of all family members may prove to be a more useful outcome. The increased use of health maintenance organizations by entire families may provide the data necessary to assess the overall effectiveness of family interventions in containing medical costs.

Obstacle 3: Convincing Families to Participate

A third difficulty for conducting research of the medical multifamily groups is recruitment of participant families. Variation in illness course often puts family support needs in direct opposition to research requirements. As we describe later in the chapter, the multifamily group format researched to date typically has been a structured, six- to eight-session intervention requiring the attendance of all household members (except for very young children). Coordinating schedules and arranging babysitting while ensuring that treatment needs will be met often add another burden to the family. Because family members have not yet experienced the benefits of the intervention, they are reluctant to commit precious family time to yet another illness-related activity.

This is true particularly during the acute, postdiagnosis period in the illness journey, when family stress is often highest, and when new families might benefit most from the input of more experienced families. In response to these illness demands, more recent efforts to provide psycho-social interfamily interventions have assumed varied forms (telephone contact between primary caregivers, monthly or bimonthly group meetings, and even Internet chatrooms), many of which are not easily incorporated into systematic research protocols, much less into controlled clinical trials.

Taken together, these obstacles have meant that most research on the benefits of multifamily group interventions for medical conditions is anecdotal or relies on very small sample sizes (typically, 20–40 families). Outcome variables have focused primarily on perceived improved family functioning, individual satisfaction, and psychosocial adjustment of individual members, all of which can be strongly influenced by the processes and complications of the disease. Given the dearth of supportive empirical evidence, family interventions have not found their ways into standard treatment protocols. That, in turn, makes it extremely difficult to collect such confirmatory data. Yet despite these difficulties, there remains a strongly held intuitive view that interfamily psychosocial and psychoeducational support is crucial for families dealing with severe chronic medical illness or disability.

Thus, in summary, this contrasting picture for medical versus psychiatric conditions means that multifamily group models developed in the psychiatric arena are unlikely to be transportable "as is" to the medical setting. Instead, new models have evolved that target the needs and well-being of nonpatient family members as much as those of the index patient. Although these models assume that improved functioning of the whole family should in turn lead to improved functioning of the index patient (perhaps even including a positive impact on adherence to treatment and on illness course), research support for this assumption is still in its early phase.

THEORETICAL FRAMEWORK

In this section we briefly describe the clinical model that has formed the basis for our approach to multifamily groups. Four core concepts underlie our family-systems-based model: (1) that chronic illness or physical disability profoundly affects every member of the family, and the family as a unit; (2) that as the chronic illness increasingly comes to dominate family life, with a predictable tendency toward excessive family resource (financial, parental attention, time) allocation to illness management; (3) that, with rare exceptions, all family members experience emotional and social isolation, both within the family and with extended family and friends; and (4) that there is an interaction between "family style"—problem solving, affective style, communication, organization—and the illness, reciprocally affecting the family's premorbid identity and management of the illness or disability.

These four processes contribute not only to the family's sense that life is dominated by the demands of illness management but also lead to an array of secondary consequences that reshape many aspects of family life. To address these underlying processes, our multifamily group model is specifically designed to (1) bring these issues to the surface for examination and (2) help families develop new strategies for containing the impact of the illness on their lives without undermining good clinical care. We have described this overarching goal as "finding a place for the illness in the family, while at the same time keeping the illness in its place"[469] (p. 80).

Each of these concepts is described below.

The "Familiness" of Chronic Illness

Our first assumption is that the family as a functional unit is profoundly altered by the occurrence of life-shortening or disabling disease in one member.[560] Every aspect of family and individual life is touched by these conditions. Employment and educational pursuits of adult members may be diverted by the need to care for a sick spouse or child, or to ensure the continuity of health care insurance coverage. This impact is even more profound when the principal family breadwinner becomes ill or disabled and his or her key family role is relinquished. During illness exacerbations, children are often separated from parents for extended periods of time and cared for either outside the home or by less familiar caretakers. Infants' or toddlers' normative attachment may be disrupted, with the appearance of corresponding symptoms.

Individual developmental milestones are frequently affected as when a non-ill child is expected suddenly (or over time) to take on adult responsibilities or always to behave properly. At the same time, the ill family member may be infantilized beyond the absolute requirements of the illness or, conversely, be required to demonstrate a premature (or not really possible) return to normalcy in the postacute period. Similarly, well members may be expected to take on attitudes and responsibilities that exceed their capacities. Late adolescents may delay leaving home or limit educational pursuits to assist ill parents or siblings with practical or emotional support. Disruption of age-appropriate social development in both ill and non-ill children is often observed, as when extracurricular activities are limited or when school-age children or teens are reluctant to bring friends into an illness-dominated home. And in addition to these often-profound alterations in the life course of all family members, there is frequently the belief that non-ill family members are not permitted to experience, let alone express, any of the expected negative affects—anger, sadness, neediness—that would attend these alterations in lifestyle.

Further exacerbating, or even precipitating, these developmental issues is the highly stressful experience of the family's immersion in the illness-specific medical culture of the treatment delivery system. When illness onset is acute, this immersion is precipitous and disorienting. When onset is gradual and insidious, ambiguous symptoms must be decoded and a number of specialists selected, consulted, and evaluated. Once a diagnosis is obtained, spouses or parents are expected to acquire a new and complicated vocabulary and to learn a basic body of knowledge about the condition. Sometimes the treatment team provides the information, but often the family must do its own research with the aid of illness-related advocacy groups.

In addition to the basic information about illness, patients or family members must acquire and process information about current, state-of-the-art treatments, some of which is not easily available. Families dealing with medical conditions quickly realize that all options will not be routinely offered and that they must know which treatments to request. They also learn that all possible symptoms and treatment side effects will not be described in advance, leaving each family to develop a system for monitoring and prioritizing physical changes and problems. In most families, one or more adult members take on the job of case manager, overseeing and integrating input from a number of medical specialties. Persistent uncertainty and the worry that some important or time-dependent intervention is being missed exacerbate the burden for spouses or parents.

Beyond medical information processing and treatment management, family members are also required to learn the formal and informal organizational structure of the medical system in which treatment is sought. Information about the accessibility and competence of different treatment providers—physicians, nurse practitioners, technicians, and aids—is learned through many interactions. If the patient's medical condition requires repeated hospitalizations, the family must navigate a second social and professional system. A family's successful negotiation of the treatment team hierarchy, particularly when there are many trainees from different disciplines, can have a profound impact on the treatment experience. The demands for constant vigilance, and for decoding and responding to communications from various specialists and other staff, are typically profoundly confusing and exhausting for adult family members, who become the primary care providers and de facto case managers.

In addition to burdens and disruptions in the lives of individual family members, the family as a functional unit is affected by chronic medical conditions. Family routines such as mealtimes, children's morning and bedtime routines, and parents' participation in school activities are typically interrupted or permanently altered by the intrusion of a chronic illness or disability into family life. The work that supports family life—food shopping, preparing meals, housecleaning, gardening, and doing laundry—is done differently in response to illness demands. Often, family rituals and celebrations may change, and shared recreational activities are temporarily or permanently forgone. In short, the characteristic, shared, repeated activities of family life, the experiences that make up the fabric of a family's self-concept and unique identity, are disrupted and altered. The starting point of all multifamily group interventions is this overarching notion that every family member, as well as the family as a functional unit, is profoundly affected by the presence of chronic illness or disability.

Disproportionate Allocation of Family Resources

A key marker of the profound impact of medical illness on family life is the focus of family resources on the patient and the illness. This overallocation of resources—parental attention, time, space, money—to the illness, a second issue that dominates most of these families' lives, is addressed in the multifamily group intervention. During the acute, peridiagnostic period, the family appropriately interrupts its normal functioning to focus time, attention, and effort on the patient's illness or disability, assessing symptoms, acquiring information, and providing hands-on care. This is particularly true when illness or disability, such as cancer or head injury, is initially understood to be potentially fatal. This "all-out" family response is typically required by the presentation of acute, often life-threatening symptoms, and by the requirements of the diagnostic workup and acute treatment procedures.

Once families have negotiated the acute diagnostic and treatment phase, however, there is a tendency for family members' lives to remain dominated by illness concerns. Early in the chronic phase, the family's persistent and often exclusive focus on illness management appears to be driven by the belief that the ill member can be restored to health and to former levels of functioning through family vigilance and action, such as the pursuit of remedial services. Typically, after diagnosis, it takes the family 2 years to understand and integrate the chronic nature and permanence of the illness or disability. Families struggle with the dawning understanding that family life and development has been forever altered by the occurrence of the injury or disease. During this time, the family devotes much attention to figuring out which of the patient's deficits can be remedied, even if herculean family effort is required, and when to initiate compensatory measures, such as altering the home environment or pursuing job retraining.

During the acute phase, and often long beyond, the family's other work—attention to non-ill children, professional or educational development of adults, restorative recreational activities, emotional needs of all members—remains on hold. The cost to all family members, particularly younger children, is tremendous. Symptoms of anxiety and depression, even if less than clinically significant, often appear in family members[561] and over time are incorporated into styles of personal functioning both at home and in the wider world. During this early, chronic period of illness, the overallotment of resources easily becomes reified, an undiscussed but expected family behavior that is difficult to acknowledge and alter. Even when spouses and parents acknowledge these unmet needs of non-ill family members, it remains very difficult to redirect attention and resources to other family needs, because such a redirection means withdrawing some of these elements from patient care. This shift is experienced as a lapse in vigilance that may lead to the patient member's demise. Strong but often unacknowledged affects such as guilt over patient needs not being optimally met, and unprocessed grief over the diminished capacity or potential loss of a loved person, tend to hold this illness-focused family pattern in place well into the chronic phase of illness.

Emotional and Social Isolation

A third characteristic of families responding to chronic illness or disability is some degree of social and emotional isolation. Family members experience this isolation in two ways: between the family and its own familiar social groups and within the family itself, as members are increasingly constrained from sharing negative affects elicited by the intrusion of illness into family life. Most parents and spouses find that, beyond the immediate diagnostic period, neighbors, friends, and often even extended family, are reluctant or unwilling to hear about the illness and threat to life or the stress and exhaustion of caregivers. When talking with friends or relatives, caregivers learn to emphasize positive aspects and minimize illness setbacks and their own sadness or worry. After the acute phase, friends are less likely to offer practical or emotional help. A consistent theme among adult family members is that no one really understands what it is like to have a seriously ill child or spouse, nor does anyone know what the family is going through. In addition, family members dealing with severe chronic illnesses are frequently annoyed when friends complain of minor stresses and difficulties, further distancing caregivers from important and restorative friendships and acquaintances. Whether individuals maintain contact with friends or retreat into the family's protective shell, the sense of being markedly different and isolated persists.

Practical aspects of patient care further disrupt the family's ties to friends and relatives. Restricted mobility, need for ready access to emergency medical care, dietary restrictions, or the need for specialized equipment all contribute to a family's (especially the primary caregiver's) reluctance to travel, visit friends, or attend social events. Exhausted by treatment regimens and schedules, parents and spouses are unable to use the little free time they may have to maintain social relationships, even when these efforts might be restorative. Children, particularly adolescents, may be unwilling to bring friends into a home that is focused on illness management, or where friends might encounter a visibly disabled parent or sibling.

In addition to isolation from friends and acquaintances, family members tend to become emotionally isolated from one another. Well children may feel constrained from expressing the need for more parental attention or from revealing the jealousy and envy they feel toward their ill sibling. The primary caregiver, who remains at the patient's bedside during long hospital stays or observes repeated painful and frightening treatments, frequently feels isolated, experiencing strong affects not unlike those associated with trauma.[562] Resentments over the loss of opportunities or of normal life cannot be expressed for fear of hurting the patient or appearing burdened by his or her needs. Although chronic conditions typically involve continued changes and limitations for the patient member, the caregiver's expression of grief over the loss of a healthy functioning spouse or child is limited by the social expectation that he or she express gratitude for the patient's survival. In many ways, a death in the family permits normal grieving in a way that is impeded by disabling chronic illness, in which the ill or disabled family member remains physically present although profoundly and permanently changed.

We should clarify that the presence of these difficult feelings in family members is not the problem. A more realistic scrutiny of the family predicament would lead to the understanding that such reactions are expectable, normal, and deserve empathy. However, non-ill members typically feel embarrassed or guilty about their feelings, because the ill member is presumably suffering so much more. The problem with this family dynamic is that, over time, the constraint on emotional intimacy within the family takes an expensive toll. Members bound together by the demands of illness and care are increasingly constrained from expressing overwhelming and confusing feelings. Withdrawal and avoidance, conflict over trivial issues, or a diminishing capacity to manage even simple family or illness routines have been noted in families where strong affects remain unexpressed.[560] Accordingly, the structure and process of the multifamily discussion group is uniquely geared to allow the safe expression of these feelings and to provide social connections with other families facing similar challenges.

Family "Identity"

The fourth core concept of our clinical model of families and medical illness is called "family identity."[563] Central to the multifamily group model we describe is an appreciation of the extent to which illness has become a central organizing principle for family life. It is through the concept of family identity that we (1) illustrate this process to families in our multifamily groups and (2) facilitate a more balanced adaptation to illness.

What we have conceptualized as family identity functions in the background of family life, only partially within the awareness of any one family member, much like an individual's personality or interpersonal style. Family routines, rituals, role assignments, shared recreational activities, outside social ties, and shared sense of humor are all individual strands that are woven intricately and uniquely together in the warp and woof of daily family life, creating the fabric of the family's own unique identity. This identity guides the family through both periods of disruption and times of quiescent normalcy. However successfully the family's identity worked prior to illness, the challenges brought on by a life-altering chronic medical condition—the overwhelming stress of medical management combined with the threatened loss of a family member—tax many areas of family functional style.

A family's preillness identity predicts many aspects of its response to the demands of the illness. A particular family may excel at information gathering, decision making, and the organization of medical care tasks. However, that same family may have great difficulty accepting the patient's deficits, asking for help from friends, or listening to a child's expression of jealousy or neediness. Families adapt most successfully when they learn to recognize their own preferred approach to different illness demands—handling feelings, gathering information, assigning tasks, asking for help—and to assess, without judgment, how well these preferred modes work. This family self-knowledge can then be used by family members to make illness-related decisions that build on family strengths as members anticipate and plan more realistically for more difficult tasks and transitions. While we have seen some marginally dysfunctional families pushed into serious clinical difficulty by the advent of severe illness, the vast majority of these families manage extremely stressful situations in the best way possible given their preillness strengths and proclivities.

In reconstructing a portrait of the preillness identity—in making explicit what had been implicit—the family comes to understand what parts of family life have been given up in the service of patient care. This allows the family unit to reevaluate its own strengths and uniqueness and to adapt coping strategies in ways that preserve the best features of family identity while it responds appropriately to illness demands. All families need to reclaim at least some aspects of their former identity and as much normalcy for all members as possible. This may entail relinquishing illness pursuits for periods of time in order to respond to other family needs, particularly those of younger children and of the primary caregiver, who is frequently the most depleted of all family members. The families that most successfully adapt to chronic illness are those that maintain or reclaim at least some significant and valued pieces of their preillness identity. One mother told us, "Before Sarah was diagnosed, my husband and I had planned to coach Mark's soccer team during the next season. After 6 months of intensive treatment, sleeplessness, and tears, soccer was the last thing on our minds. But when the time came, we felt we had to do it. We took Sarah to games in a wheelchair, so that both she and Mark could see that his life was important, too. Besides that, the team had a great season and our family had a great time."

THE MEDICAL DISORDERS MULTIFAMILY GROUP: STRUCTURE AND PROCESS

Multifamily supportive interventions for medical conditions have taken many forms and pathways over the years, from informal "waiting room" conversations between family members to parent-organized support networks, to structured, professionally facilitated psychoeducational interventions that are often the focus of research protocols. There are features shared by all of these supportive interactions: (1) They address the needs of non-ill family members; (2) they provide a shared, illness-related information base; and (3) they address the family's sense of isolation by providing connections to other families that are on the same journey.

At George Washington University Medical Center (GWU) in the mid-1980s, we began work on the design and implementation of a structured, time-limited, facilitator-led intervention developed specifically to address the core family systems issues associated with the chronic medical illness described in the previous section.[469, 564] In particular, the goal was to design a multifamily group that would facilitate family discussion and understanding of how the illness had invaded family life and distorted family priorities, and to devise strategies that would enable families to reclaim important aspects of their preillness family identity.

Over the ensuing decade, this version of a multifamily group intervention has been adapted for use with a wide range of medical conditions, including end-stage renal disease, Types I and II diabetes, adolescent and childhood cancers, autoimmune diseases, neurological disabilities, and chronic pain syndromes.[552] Detailed treatment manuals have been prepared for two different versions of our multifamily discussion group (MFDG)—the original GWU version[565] and a subsequent version developed as part of a collaborative project between the Ackerman Institute for the Family and the Memorial Sloan–Kettering Cancer Center, focusing on adolescent cancer patients and their families.[544] These manuals, along with videotapes of model MFDG sessions, have been used to train group leaders, both in our projects and at other sites.

This MFDG model, which we describe in more detail below, has five core features: (1) It is brief and time-limited (six to eight sessions); (2) it follows a highly structured protocol; (3) it incorporates a psychoeducational approach, one aspect of which is the establishment of a nonpathologizing attitude toward the efforts families have been making to cope with the illness; (4) it includes patient as well as nonpatient family members; and (5) it takes advantage of the structural richness of a multifamily group to create exercises that provide families with multiple perspectives on their illness experiences. In the earlier version of the MFDG, these exercises included several small group discussions complemented by opportunities to observe other group members talking about illness issues (what we called the "group within a group"). In a subsequent version of the MFDG, art techniques were added to afford families the opportunity to represent their experiences visually (in particular, having families create collages representing preillness vs. postillness family life).

However, although they contain many unique structural and conceptual aspects, our versions of a multifamily group share similar goals with most of the models that have been described in this volume and in the literature. The focus is on three different components—the first dealing with educational issues (including an opportunity for families to "educate" each other about their experiences with the illness); the second dealing with family social networks or social connections (especially how to overcome the sense of isolation that is almost universal in these families); and the third focusing on expanding the problem-solving and coping strategies families are using to manage illness-related demands.

The Educational Component

Most MFDG programs developed to date have been described as "psycho-educational" interventions. The "educational" aspects of these groups are based on the generally accepted notion that families benefit from being fully informed about the medical condition and its treatment. Groups may use medical experts to provide formal or informal presentations, schedule individual testimonials by patients or family members, or simply offer family members the opportunity to share their experiences with different diagnostic procedures, treatments, and medical personnel.

Belief in the importance of illness-related information motivates most families to seek out and attend multifamily support groups. In other words, most families are unlikely to begin with a perceived need for family psychosocial support or family-level intervention, particularly during the early phase (approximately the first year) of the illness journey. Even in a family that acknowledges the extreme stress associated with severe illness or disability, there typically persists the belief that the stress will be relieved most directly by additional or more appropriate medical or treatment information. Extremely well-informed families, while clearly acknowledging the permanence of a particular medical condition, often hold onto the notion that they have yet to discover some piece of information that will allow them to "fix" the illness problems. (This response is not dissimilar to that seen in families reacting to a diagnosis of schizophrenia or bipolar disorder in one of their members, as described in previous chapters.)

In reality, much information about most illnesses or disabilities comes to light only through informal channels mediated by interpersonal connections. Physicians are far from uniform in their approaches to treatment of many chronic conditions, and families may learn of alternative or auxiliary treatments only through contact with other families (or less frequently, with staff) from other medical centers. Parents who are told that their child's brain tumor is inoperable at one center will be encouraged by other parents to seek additional opinions and may even be directed to centers where difficult tumors have been resected in other children.

From another perspective, most medical conditions involve treatment by several different specialties, particularly during the chronic phase. An adult family member typically serves as the case manager, providing information and coordinating care among the various treatment teams. In multifamily group meetings, families remind each other of symptoms and systems that need to be monitored, and share information about treatments and successful outcomes in other patients. Recent observation by one of the authors (Sandra Gonzalez) of a parent-initiated support group for families coping with pediatric brain tumors illustrates this function. An ophthalmological surgery that corrected the vision of one child recovering from a posterior fossa tumor proved very successful for another child whose parents only learned of the procedure through the group, although their child had been receiving regular ophthalmological care.

In addition to the informal sharing of information among family members, many multifamily meetings include a more formal, didactic presentation by experts from key illness-related specialties. These presentations may focus on important auxiliary concerns such as nutrition, relaxation, special educational needs, employment support, and resources. In addition, these experts' presentations may provide informal, more personalized access to core treatment specialists such as oncologists, endocrinologists, radiologists, rehabilitation specialists, or surgeons. When the expert is someone other than the family's own treating specialist, family members feel freer to ask challenging questions and pursue worries or concerns that might otherwise be embarrassing.

A crucial educational component touched on in most interventions is the description and elaboration of milestones of the illness journey itself. Families learn about the expected course of the illness, focal concerns for both patient and other members at each phase, and the demands that each phase will likely make on family life. Unusual complications, timing of remedial interventions, and anticipation of exacerbations or setbacks are shared and discussed by families at different phases of the illness journey.

Another focus of family education in multifamily groups for chronic illness is information about family process and family dynamics in response to the stresses of illness management. The structured intervention used at GWU focused attention on the medical condition's invasion of family life and on the importance, in the long term, of attending to the needs of non-ill family members, even when those needs seemed less compelling than those of the patient. Families were encouraged to share perceptions about the way the illness had changed each member's life and to focus on the family group as a functional unit that had been altered by a serious illness. A case was made for the importance of studying one's own family group process in a way that is not typically required in the course of normal family life. Participants learned that this knowledge about their own family would enable them to respond more constructively to the demands of the illness.

In keeping with this core educational focus, the concept of family identity was introduced and defined using different media (adjective lists, art collages, group-within-a-group family discussions) depending on the target population. The goal was to help families identify their own unique patterns, preferences, goals, and values in the service of making explicit the family identity that would, under more normal circumstances, operate implicitly in the background of family life. Armed with this clearer picture of themselves as unique functional units, families were then prepared to make illness-related decisions that would preserve or integrate the most important, or treasured, aspects of the preillness family identity. Often these newly informed decisions involved reallocating family resources to address the needs of other family members or to reclaim some valued, "identifying" family activity, as described earlier in this chapter.

It is our understanding that the efficacy of the educational component of these interventions does not reside solely in the utility of the information shared but rather in its capacity to objectify, externalize, and normalize the emotional impact of life-altering illness on the family. The plethora of written and verbal information provided by health care teams at the diagnosis of a severe medical condition does not have the same impact. As described in more detail later in this chapter, the multifamily group, including its "educational" components, creates a context and a shared perspective for the emotional upheaval of the threatened loss of a family member. Family members "learn" that they are not alone in their "unseemly" feelings, their anger, fear, guilt, loss, and resentment. They learn that there is no single, right way to handle the illness in the context of all the family needs and obligations. They come to understand that even more information will have, at best, a limited impact on their handling of the illness and its treatment. Apart from its actual use in making illness-related decisions, sharing information promotes a sense of mastery of a frequently uncertain and unpredictable family experience. It appears that families, particularly the designated primary caregiver, derive great comfort (e.g., lowered anxiety and depression) from specific and detailed information about the illness journey and from the understanding that other families are on the same road.*

The Social Network Component

A social network (or social connections) component is another key element of virtually all multifamily groups for chronic illness. As described earlier, families coping with life-altering medical conditions all feel some degree of isolation from their familiar social groups, even when there is a large and supportive social network, an isolation that most studies have concluded impedes successful adaptation to illness.[126, 138] The multifamily group for chronic illness provides a social context in which other families share a key characteristic—the ongoing stress and formative challenges of managing a life-altering illness in one member. In this way, the groups invariably help families redefine what a supportive social context might look like for them.

This reframing process is accomplished in several ways. First, on the most apparent level, families share their stories with other families who can understand the pervasiveness of the medical condition's intrusion into family life. It has been our experience that, unlike typical therapy groups in which trust and cohesion develop slowly over many sessions, multifamily group participants connect with each other quite rapidly. It is not unusual during introductions at the first group meeting for participants to share their own illness stories with great emotion and strong, empathetic support from other participants. A typical statement from most group members is a variation of "Only another parent who's had a child with cancer can know what we've been through." It is this aspect of these groups, in part, that allows even short-term groups to be effective in helping families to process the ongoing stress and grief of severe chronic illnesses.

In addition, listening to the stories of other families helps participants to locate their own family experience on a continuum of illness severity and chronicity and of personal and family loss. We have come to understand that telling the family story in the presence of other, similarly afflicted families provides a meaningful context for the isolating experience of chronic illness. Most families' own friendship and extended family networks can no longer adequately provide this context. Furthermore, telling and retelling

---

*For a more detailed description of the content of the "educational" components of MFDG, readers are directed to the treatment manuals that are available upon request from the authors.

the family illness story, even in the midst of other, more structured group activities, allow families to rework the ongoing sense of loss and grief that inevitably accompanies the illness experience throughout its course.

Depending on the format chosen, multifamily groups may extend their social network effect in other practical and concrete ways. A telephone roster is often distributed at one of the early meetings, and families are encouraged to maintain their connections with other families outside group meetings or after group meetings have ended. One parent-initiated group developed a telephone network in which families dealing with similar diagnoses were connected with one another to share information and support. Groups may substitute a social event, such as a potluck supper, for one of the regularly scheduled meetings to promote social interfamily ties.

By providing an illness-related social context, multifamily groups may paradoxically enhance participants' connections to their own social networks (i.e., those outside the group). Disruption of social ties is a topic that is included in the formal agendas of most of these groups. During these discussions, families acknowledge frustrations with friends or relatives who ask insensitive questions about the patient or complain about their own problems, which seem so trivial when compared to the chronic illness. Sharing these perceptions and frustrations between families tends to normalize these reactions and dilute their isolating impact. By providing a social context for the illness experience, the multifamily groups reframe the family's expectations of relatives and friends, and promote the realistic use of available support and assistance. Families also share strategies for adapting family socializing to include the practical and emotional constraints of the illness and for arranging breaks for caregivers and other members to be with friends, temporarily away from patient care.

In adolescents, for whom the isolating impact of the chronic illness of a parent, sibling or self can be extreme, this paradoxical effect may be even more pronounced.[566] Teenagers typically want to keep all illness information out of their peer relationships in the interest of being "normal" and avoiding their friends' pity. Multifamily groups can provide teenagers an opportunity to share the illness experience with adolescents or children in other families, without contaminating relationships with their own peers. Teens are the least likely of all family members to pursue contact with other participants outside the group meetings. In providing a separate and protected forum, these groups may offer a unique opportunity for adolescents who are reluctant to discuss or hear about the illness anywhere else.

In addition to distancing themselves from their extended social networks, many families who deal with chronic illness also experience internal isolation, secondary to a prohibition against expression of emotions within the family. This drift toward emotional isolation within the family is a problem that is uniquely addressed by the very structure of multifamily groups. As the illness wears on in its chronic course and family members increasingly understand its permanence, feelings of frustration, anger, neediness, and disappointment build up within individual members. Sharing these feelings is constrained by the belief that such expression will harm the patient member either psychologically or physically. In group discussions, these emotional reactions to the illness are shared between individuals from different families rather than within a single family. This transmission across family boundaries allows feelings to be heard with less interpersonal threat than would be the case within an individual family. Because negative affects are acknowledged and shared among several families, they are understood to be normal reactions to severe stress rather than markers of personal or family inadequacy. In one of our early groups composed of retired couples, a wife of a man with severe heart disease described her group experience as follows: "I've talked about things here that I haven't said in 37 years of marriage."

In our version of a chronic illness multifamily group, a structured cotherapy approach called the "group within a group" was developed to utilize this feature of the MFDG. The goal was to emphasize the comparable relationships across families and have members in analogous family roles (patients, primary caregivers, adolescent children of ill parents, etc.) share their perspectives and feelings. A subgroup of analogous participants pulled chairs into the center of the room and "met" with one of the co-leaders to discuss their concerns. The other family members, along with the other facilitator, listened without speaking and then reflected in their own subgroup what they had heard expressed. This structured, interfamily exercise allowed members in different roles to express difficult feelings, share similar perspectives, and be heard, usually positively, by other members of their own families. Figure 16.1 is an illustration of the seating arrangements for the three-phase process followed in group-within-a-group intervention. This particular version is from the first session of our 6-week MFDG protocol, and starts with a small group discussion by each "patient" family member of the impact of the medical illness on family life.

In summary, the multifamily groups for chronic illness provide a shared social context and evolving social network within which families can locate themselves and their own illness experiences. Telling and updating the story of the family's own illness journey and having that story known by a group of knowledgeable others has a dramatically restorative

Phase One - Initial gathering as whole group

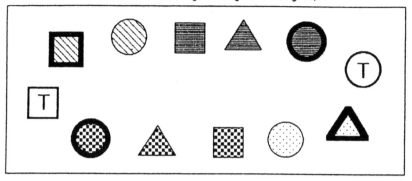

Phase Two - Patient subgroup

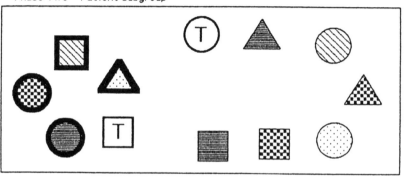

Phase Three - Observer subgroup

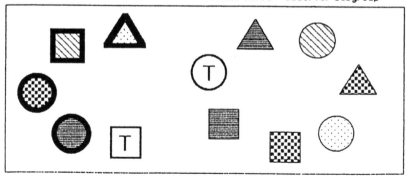

FIGURE 16.1. In this graphic representation, the sequence of group-within-a-group phases for Session 1 is illustrated for a four-family MFDG. The visual codes are as follows: family membership, cross-hatching design; index patients, heavy outlines; family roles: husbands, squares; wives, circles; children, triangles; co-therapists, Ts.

effect on members dealing with the ongoing demands of illness management. The link with other families who understand the burdens and losses associated with severe chronic illness helps families to orient themselves on their illness journeys and strategize their courses more effectively. Within and between participating families, the isolative affect of unexpressed feelings can begin to be addressed. Some groups, such as our MFDG model, address these issues more directly and intensely in a short-term (six to eight weekly sessions) format. Other, long-term family support groups with a changing membership may provide the same functions more diffusely over a longer period of time.

Problem-Solving Component

A third shared feature of all multifamily groups for chronic illness is some variety of family problem solving, in which each family in the group receives feedback from other participating families about how they are dealing with specific, illness-generated problems. As with the other two components, this group function may be implemented via a focused and structured activity or more informally, in the context of informational discussions.

For example, a family may learn during the educational component that it is important to reallocate family resources to meet the needs of all members while maintaining an adequate level of patient care. However, during problem solving, a particular mother may lament the fact that, since her husband's diagnosis, she no longer has time to read aloud to her toddler each evening. Participants from other families will ask questions to clarify the problem and then offer suggestions based on their own experiences about how to balance patient care with other family needs. The presenting family usually leaves the session with a plan to try out, then returns in subsequent sessions to review the results with group members. This method is shared by multifamily group models for other diagnoses (see Chapter 9).

Topics covered by the family problem-solving component vary greatly. Early in group life, families tend to focus on problems related to improving patient care and rehabilitation. Practical or logistical problems—such as obtaining hemodialysis while traveling, or rescheduling a radiation treatment so that a child may eat normally throughout the day—are often easier for families to address. On the other hand, issues that arise from and impact on family relationships often require facilitator guidance to receive adequate attention. Examples of these more difficult issues might include redirection of family resources from patient care to other family needs; caregiver stress and needs; differences between spouses in expression of feelings; and how to share patient care tasks. Facilitators encourage participants to seek and to share solutions to family problems by providing a framework that describes the different phases of the illness journey and locates expectable family problems on that continuum.

An example of a more structured approach to family problem solving is the strategy we utilize in the GWU version of our MFDGs. In the third and fourth sessions, after families have become familiar with each other, each family is offered the opportunity to present an ongoing illness-related family problem that had been difficult to resolve. The "target" family members begin by grouping their chairs in the center of the room and "meeting" with one of the co-leaders to discuss their particular issue. All other group members and the other co-leader remain silent but attentive on the periphery of the group, while the target family presents and clarifies its problem (including hearing from each family member about his or her own perspective on the problem). After an approximately 15-minute discussion, the observer members share their perceptions of the problem and propose different solutions while the target family listens. The exercise ends with an interactive summary, involving all participants, and a proposed trial solution.

In subsequent sessions, families report on the efficacy of different strategies and receive additional suggestions from coparticipants. Even when families cannot agree on a trial solution, these MFDG problem-solving experiences seem to help them view the presenting problem from new perspectives and begin relinquishing rigidly held rules and roles in managing patient care. This format is appropriate primarily for groups with consistent membership over 6–10 sessions. In groups where membership changes from session to session, a more informal problem-solving discussion seems necessary.

Summary

While all multifamily groups for medical illness tend to include some version of each of the three components discussed earlier, the time and emphasis given to each will depend on the membership, leadership, frequency, and longevity of a specific group. Where membership changes from meeting to meeting, family problem solving and some aspects of the social network component will be less effective.[551, 567, 568] Daylong intensive multifamily groups tend to emphasize the educational component and carry out individual family problem solving with the guidance of didactic materials.[550, 569] Clearly, the development of social ties and the opportunity for problem-solving feedback tailored to individual families require regular meetings (although not necessarily weekly) of a consistent group of participants over a number of months. The multifamily format works best when all family members over the age of 10 attend every meeting of a six- to eight-session intervention. Because younger children have difficulty understanding and attending to group discussion for the length of the whole session, this consistency and comprehensiveness of attendance have been the aspect of multifamily groups for chronic illness that is the most difficult to achieve.

Whereas families almost universally express the need for support when coping with chronic illness, arranging time, transportation, and schedules for all family members to attend regularly is extremely difficult, particularly in view of the additional demands on family resources created by the illness itself. This perennial difficulty emerges most noticeably in the effort to conduct multifamily group research where recruitment of participant families—those who can commit to attending regular weekly or biweekly meetings over a 2- to 3-month period—has been a major obstacle.[544, 570] With so many additional, stressful demands, families are extremely reluctant to add an activity that is not directly related to illness management. This understanding of the burdens and constraints faced by families with chronic illness has led to adaptations and modifications of early multifamily group formats to fit the needs and schedules of these overextended families. Modifications have included monthly rather than weekly meetings; drop-in meetings on inpatient services or regular outpatient clinics; computer "chat room" connections between individuals; parents-only groups for pediatric illnesses; and telephone network connections for families coping with similar conditions.[571-573] Testing the efficacy of these more diffuse interventions in systematic research protocols is the current challenge for research in this area.

FUTURE DIRECTIONS

Providers of medical-illness-oriented multifamily group interventions face challenges in both research and clinical arenas. While clinical reports, health care teams, and the families themselves consistently emphasize the value of such interventions,[560] thus far, few empirical research data have been generated to support their efficacy in improving the quality of life of patients and/or other family members.[555] This dearth of supportive research has been due, as outlined earlier, to the mismatch between the requirements of research protocols and the needs of overextended caregiving families. Recruitment of participant families—those who can ensure the attendance of all eligible members at six to eight sessions—remains a most difficult problem for conducting time-limited protocols. Furthermore, the efficacy of the intervention must be measured in terms of *all* family members, not just the index patient alone. The search for robust markers of improved family and patient functioning will probably include subjective measures of patient and family satisfaction with medical care as well as overall health care utilization by all family members. This latter variable has become more possible to assess in recent years, with health maintenance organizations providing a broad range of health care services to entire family groups over extended periods of time.

Timing multifamily supportive interventions to coincide with family needs and demands at different phases of the illness course will improve participation in these interventions. It is clear to us that families are much less likely to commit time and energy to multifamily groups during the acute or early phase (within 2 years of diagnosis) of illness, even when they are experiencing severe stress. During this phase, the demands of treatment are new and typically frightening and time-consuming. Family members, particularly primary caregivers, want to talk to someone who has been through the experience and can "show them the ropes." Building an ongoing relationship with one or two members of the treatment team and consulting another family with the same diagnosis and treatment plan are experienced as most helpful in mastery of a disorienting life event. Also, during the period after diagnosis, the family maintains the notion that family life can be returned to preillness normalcy through careful attention to treatment and rehabilitation requirements. In multifamily groups, families are exposed to the information about illness chronicity, news that they still hope will not apply to them. Even when families are intellectually clear and certain about the permanence of an illness (such as diabetes or cystic fibrosis), it typically takes them 2 years to accept that the illness will in fact not be going away.

It is at this point, 2 or more years after initial diagnosis, that families are ready to sit down with other families and discuss the specifics of family adaptation to chronic illness. This is a process marked by mourning losses, reallocating family resources, and reclaiming some cherished pieces of family identity within the limitations imposed by the chronic medical condition. With the crisis behind them, families can more easily arrange to attend group meetings and are more motivated to shift their focus from the illness to the family as a unit. After many months of chronic stress, the neglected needs of other family members, particularly the primary caregiver, are now apparent, motivating families to reassess and reorganize family life. In the transition to acceptance of illness chronicity, families need reassurance that no vital pieces of medical intervention have been missed. Families also need clarification of the permanent aspects of the disability, including education about why compensatory strategies rather than continued remediation efforts are preferable. Multifamily groups are uniquely suited to provide this input.

Yet even at this "transition to chronicity" point in the illness journey, it has been our experience that families are more easily enlisted in time-limited, structured multifamily groups by familiar, trusted members of the treatment team. Families are more likely to respond positively to recommendations by team members who know the story of their illness journey and can convey positive expectations regarding group participation. Recommendations of previously participating family members are also taken more seriously.

In later years, as families gain experience in dealing with the long-term effects of illness or disability, they are often interested in group participation to revisit and rework illness-related issues in light of new family developments or life-cycle transitions. These more experienced families benefit from being the experts in the multifamily group, sharing their perspective and wisdom with less experienced families. Treatment teams that maintain contact and involvement with patient families over the long term will provide the best opportunities for enlisting families in multifamily group treatment protocols and in measuring longer term outcomes of all family members.

The multifamily group for chronic medical conditions remains a promising and powerful intervention for families experiencing some of the most challenging stresses occurring in our culture at present. As we better understand the impact of these severe chronic conditions on families, multifamily group interventions can be tailored to meet specific family needs at different points in the illness journey. As we increasingly return to treatment models that put the family at the center of chronic patient care, multifamily group interventions provide a powerful tool in enabling families to meet these challenges.

Chapter 17

Implementing Multifamily Groups in the Real World

The New York State and Ohio Training and Dissemination Programs

LISA DIXON AND EDWARD DUNNE

In spite of their demonstrated effectiveness, multifamily groups are rarely used in typical clinical settings.[574, 575] Research on technology transfer has identified four fundamental conditions that must be met in order for individual or systems change to occur: dissemination of knowledge; evaluation of programmatic impact; availability of resources; and efforts to address the human dynamics of resisting change.[576] The ideal multifamily group technology transfer program would thus include these four elements. However, though limitations of resources, knowledge, or personnel lead to technology transfer efforts that fall short of the ideal, there is still much to learn from these imperfect efforts.

This chapter outlines two multifamily group technology transfer programs. The first was the New York State Family Support Demonstration Project. The second program took place in Ohio as part of the Schizophrenia Patient Outcomes Research Team (PORT). The New York and Ohio experiences are described in turn.

NEW YORK

The New York State Family Support Demonstration Project was initiated through a research grant funded by the State of New York, in cooperation with the New York State Alliance for the Mentally Ill, and continued through contracts following the research phase. The aim of the project was to demonstrate that previously reported positive research outcomes using family-based interventions with persons suffering from schizophrenia could be duplicated in actual clinical settings using line staff as the providers, independent of research studies and budgets.

The project was conceptualized as having three distinct phases, as described by McFarlane and colleagues.[259] First, a research phase was designed to contrast two different methods of delivering family-based interventions, either in multifamily psychoeducational groups or as single-family psychoeducation. The research project also assessed retrospectively the institution's standard care. The design included measurement of multiple outcomes of the intervention. The second, implementation, phase built upon the initial research. The treatment identified as superior in the research phase, psychoeducational multifamily group treatment, was taught to clinicians at the institutions that had participated in the research project. Project clinicians from Phase 1 became teachers and supervisors. The final, dissemination, phase sought to use these same teachers and supervisors of the preferred technology in other clinical settings throughout the State of New York.

Phase 1: Research

The research phase was conducted at five state-operated psychiatric centers and one city hospital, located in urban, suburban, and rural sections of New York State. Each site sponsored four clinicians who were taught one of the two methodologies (single- or multifamily psychoeducation). A total of 172 families and patients were enrolled in the study between September 1985 and June 1987. Each clinician carried a project caseload of no more than three families at any time, while continuing with regularly assigned responsibilities. The clinicians were at least master's-level social workers, nurses, or psychologists, most of whom had some prior training in family-based treatment, although none had prior experience with the models being researched. The clinicians who participated in the research phase received compensation in addition to their regular salaries.

Research constraints required strict adherence to the protocols of each of the treatment modalities in order for meaningful comparisons to be made. To ensure compliance, each contact with participating families was videotaped by the clinicians using equipment provided by the project. The tapes were sent to the senior supervisory staff of the project, who viewed them on a weekly basis. The clinicians received weekly telephone supervision of 45 minutes per family or multifamily group session, based upon the content of the videotapes. The supervisors were senior clinicians with strong backgrounds in family-based interventions and a thorough familiarity with the models being tested. Supervision on ways to recruit and maintain families, and to work within the system to ensure maximum outcomes were part of the model.

Participating clinicians received intensive training at the outset of the program through a 3-day workshop delivered in a training facility away from their usual workplace. This workshop was repeated annually throughout the life of the research phase (4 years), with content varied to reflect the maturing level of care provided to the families in the study. The clinicians received an additional day of booster training annually. Each site was visited quarterly for a full day of progress reports and additional training. Thus, clinicians in Phase 1 received approximately 88 hours of workshop training and a minimum 40 hours of direct supervision per annum.

Direct training of clinicians was augmented by orientation and training of facility administrators and other key personnel deemed to have potential impact on the likelihood of the program being carried out successfully. Designed as orientation programs to help the facility accommodate the research phase, this training was also helpful in overcoming resistance to a new technology, in that it encouraged facility administrators to "buy-in" to the new methodology at an early phase and then become advocates for its implementation. A final array of training was directed at the line staff of the facilities where the study was being conducted, as a way of helping to create an atmosphere conducive to the application of the new treatments. Thus, for each facility, there were approximately 4 hours per year of administrator training, coupled with a 3-hour presentation to the line staff.

Finally, each facility had a research unit consisting of a director and at least three interviewers who carried out the evaluations called for in the research protocol. These individuals also received extensive supervision and training and were compensated by the project. An overall project director at each site was also employed to ensure as smooth an implementation as possible.

The model developed to enhance the transfer of the new technology was based on the psychoeducational model itself. Several basic tenets of the model were identified and applied in working with both clinical and ad-ministrative staff. The first of these was the acknowledgment of the power of collegial relationships. The model takes the position that adults' attitudes and behaviors change to the extent that they feel empowered by the learn-ing situation, and that this is best accomplished by promoting a coopera-tive, collegial, and nonjudgmental relationship among all parties. The model postulates that this type of relationship between the clinician and the family supports familial change in the desired direction, that is, toward prevention of relapse.

The belief that families somehow cause schizophrenia was widely held by clinicians at the start of the project, and changing this belief system was viewed as the first task in disseminating the modern psychoeducational view. A collegial approach to both clinicians and administrators was adopted, inviting input on the model itself and on its implementation at the particular site. The supervisory sessions were always bracketed by periods of "chatting," mirroring the actual family sessions and following the tech-niques developed by Anderson and associates.[108] It was assumed that mod-eling the technique would be the most effective means of transferring this skill to the clinicians in the program. Administrators, included in the deci-sion making from the beginning, were invited to training sessions and con-sulted about problems that arose in the implementation of the model.

A second assumption of the model as it relates to families was also ap-plied to work with clinicians and supervisors: the assumption of least pa-thology. Clinicians were taught to view families as motivated by good inten-tions to help their ill relative but blocked from doing so by inadequate knowledge and limited resources. This assumption was replicated in deal-ing with clinicians and administrators: Their prior lack of engagement of families in collaborative treatment of their relatives was assumed to be due to factors such as inexperience with the methodology, lack of personnel or funds, and lack of knowledge. To promote this attitude, past failures were interpreted as signs of good intentions, which could now be built upon us-ing the new technology offered by the project. Project trainers and staff made themselves available to assist institutions and individuals in solving the inevitable problems that might be engendered by the adoption of a new attitude about the role of families in the treatment of schizophrenia.

A third tenet of the model is the value of taking small, incremental steps toward achieving change. Approaching problems in a stepwise fash-ion using formal problem-solving techniques was taught to families and cli-nicians. Clinicians were encouraged to use this methodology when dealing with problems within the institution that threatened to impede their implementation of the model. Both administrators and clinicians were encouraged to lower their expectations temporarily and to proceed at a moderate pace, avoiding unrealistic goals.

A final tenet of the model is the establishment of a network of like-thinking people. The psychoeducational model promotes connections between families as a means of reducing stigma and burden. The multiple-family group, which puts families with similar difficulties together in a collaborative enterprise, is specifically designed to promote this kind of network. In similar manner, the training programs, site visits, and conference calls offered by the project staff were conceptualized as nurturing a network across institutions, among all the individuals faced with the task of implementing the model.

Phase 2: Implementation

The research phase yielded evidence of clear superiority of family-based interventions over standard care and of multifamily groups over the single-family treatment modality in terms of relapse avoidance and rehospitalization.[313] Phase 2, the initial part of the dissemination effort, was initiated with the intention of emphasizing multifamily group treatment as the treatment of choice, although local circumstances were allowed to dictate whether multifamily groups would be the exclusive modality employed. Project clinicians initially trained and supervised in the single-family modality were taught the multifamily technology and received additional supervision from the senior staff in forming multifamily groups, using families from the research phase. Clinicians who had conducted multifamily groups during the research phase were assisted in forming additional ones. Both sets of clinicians also focused on training other staff at their own facilities.

Training models varied by site based on a number of factors, such as administrative interest, staff availability, and funding. Although the project supervisors remained available to them, the clinicians received considerably less support in this phase than they had in the research phase of the project. Additionally, the administrators were significantly less involved. In this phase, clinicians no longer received extra compensation for their work but were allowed to conduct their multifamily groups as part of their regular clinical responsibilities. Because research was no longer being conducted, the need for a site coordinator was obviated, as was that for the interviewers. Equipment and supplies, no longer obtainable from the research project, had to be requisitioned from the individual institutions, although clinicians were able to retain the equipment supplied to them during the research phase. Of the 26 original clinicians, 16 agreed to participate in Phase 2 of the project. Those who did not participate generally cited conflicts with their regular duties within the institution. The remaining clinicians represented each of the original sites.

As was done in the research phase, administrators were oriented to the methodology and goals of the project in a half-day training session. New clinicians were given 3 days of intense training in the techniques. In addition, new supervisors were given a 1-day training program in how to supervise within the constraints of the psychoeducational model. The clinicians were supervised in a group that met a half-day per month for at least 1 year. Administrative support varied by institution and ranged from enthusiasm to benign neglect. Two of the original sites had complete administrative turnovers during the course of Phase 2; in both instances, the new administrations were less committed to the project goals. Nevertheless, each of the original sites was successful in launching at least two new multifamily groups that ran for over 12 months, and some sites launched considerably more groups than that.

Phase 3: Dissemination

The dissemination phase sought to use these same teachers and supervisors in other clinical settings throughout the State of New York. Regional training was offered, using original project supervisors as well as the second generation of supervisors. The basic training model consisted of a "road show" type of orientation, geared toward upper levels of management in which the model and its benefits (particularly cost-effectiveness) were presented. Administrators then selected clinicians to participate in more intensive training conducted by the supervisors. This lasted 1½ days and was then followed by monthly supervision sessions in which all psychoeducational clinicians in the region were invited to participate. At least one annual, all-day booster training session was planned.

During the implementation phase, the nature of provision of care to the mentally ill changed radically in New York State. Private clinics began competing for Medicare reimbursement that had been going to public clinics handling the majority of the chronic cases. This compromised the dissemination phase, since these agencies were far less responsive to mandates from the State Office of Mental Health. Additionally, they were dependent for their survival on real income generated by clients, not state-controlled (and -distributed) budgets. Each participating agency was required to subsidize the entire effort, with the exception of the fee for the trainers. As another point of contrast, these agencies often had their own treatment philosophies that sometimes ran counter to the psychoeducational model. The clinicians tended to be pre-master's level, and many carried a caseload of more than 50 clients at any given time as part of their regularly assigned responsibilities. Most had no prior training in family-based treatment, and none had prior experience with the model being disseminated. No additional pay was given to the clinicians, who were expected not only to convert some of the individual cases they were carrying to family psychoeducational cases, but also to run multifamily groups during their regular work day. Most of the agencies dealt with patients who had long been discharged from the inpatient facility and were involved in either supportive employment or intensive case management. A substantial number of these individuals were completely out of contact with their families of origin. Thus, recruitment became a sizable barrier for this third generation of clinicians.

The second generation of supervisors was expected to deal with these difficulties, but generally came from systems that provided little preparation to do so. Eight regional sites were established with varying degrees of difficulty and generally limited success. When funding for the dissemination phase abruptly ended under an edict from the State Mental Health Commissioner, and support from the central supervisors was no longer available, most of the activity in the regional sites also ended.

Discussion

The New York approach clearly illustrates the importance of involving all levels of an institution in order to disseminate change. The most intense efforts apparently met with the most success. As the effort, money, and personnel resources became less available, change became less likely. Family psychoeducation as a treatment model is disadvantaged in its likelihood of rapid diffusion in that it meets only one of the criteria established by Rogers[577, 578]; it offers a clear, relative advantage in terms of relapse, rehospitalization, and rehabilitation outcomes compared to other treatment models. It is, however, more complex than competing models, at least at the onset. It is not usually compatible with the treatment philosophies of most of the clinicians expected to implement it. Its advantage is observable only after a long period of time. Also inhibiting its transfer is the problem of "front-loading" of effort. Simply put, all members of the endeavor must put in more time, money, and effort at the beginning in order to accomplish its considerable savings of these elements after the first year. Hence the pay-off frequently takes over a year to realize, a year which many agencies and clinicians do not feel they have.

OHIO

The Schizophrenia Patient Outcomes Research Team (PORT), a contract funded by the Agency for Health Care and Policy and Research and the National Institute of Mental Health, had several goals. The first was to develop recommendations for the treatment of persons with schizophrenia based upon a synthesis of the best scientific evidence. Psychopharmacological and psychosocial treatment recommendations were developed.[579] The second goal was to determine variations in the patterns of treatment for persons with schizophrenia receiving usual care, and the impact of these variations on outcome.[574] A final element of the PORT contract was that the recommendations and knowledge generated by the PORT be disseminated into the community.

The scope and scale of the PORT project required that the technology transfer component focus on a subset of the recommendations. The PORT chose to disseminate the recommendations focusing on services to families of persons with schizophrenia for two reasons. First, the research upon which the family psychosocial treatment recommendations were based was especially strong and rigorous. Second, PORT data suggested that there was virtually no implementation of family interventions in the community.[575] The PORT thus studied the relative effectiveness of two approaches to disseminating a recommendation for a family psychosocial intervention as follows:

> Patients who have ongoing contact with their families should be offered a family psychosocial intervention that spans at least 9 months and provides a combination of education about the illness, family support, crisis intervention, and problem-solving skills training. Such interventions should also be offered to nonfamily caregivers.

Selected as a model of services to families, the multifamily group, if offered, would comply with the treatment recommendation. Using a quasi-experimental design, the PORT aim was to determine whether two dissemination approaches led to changes in service delivery at the *agency level* and to enhanced family participation in treatment observable at the *patient level*.

The PORT also sought to determine agency factors or attitudes that impede or facilitate successful implementation of the model.

The PORT technology transfer study, having participated in other components of the PORT project, was conducted in the State of Ohio. A standard educational, didactic presentation ("road show") was compared to the standard presentation supplemented by intensive, site-level training in the multifamily group approach. The PORT study had defined two geographic regions that included several participating agencies. Site assignment was made according to geographic region to maximize comparability of conditions. Accordingly, five agencies were offered both the standard and intensive training. Four agencies were offered the standard training only and served as the control condition. All site agencies had participated in other components of the PORT study. By design, the PORT team made no other interventions at either the administrative or grassroots consumer level that might enhance the possibility of change taking place at the agencies.

The impact of the training was assessed by a comparison of services provided to families at each agency before and after the intensive training, using a key informant telephone interview. The agency interview solicited specific information from a key informant on the types of services provided to families, the number of families receiving each service, the funding of these services, and the type of personnel providing each service. When possible, the same interviewer–key informant pair participated in the interviews at both time points. After the interviews were conducted, written results were sent to the agency key informant to ensure accuracy. These interviews were conducted before the intensive training and then again, 9 months later. At the time of the intensive training, participants were asked a series of questions regarding perceived obstacles to implementation, in order to identify factors associated with adoption of the model.

The Interventions

The "Road Show"

The road show provided an approximately hour-long formal presentation highlighting the treatment recommendations related to families. Evidence was presented from the literature review, documenting the effectiveness of family interventions. The lecture focused on the multifamily group model. Short clips from training videotapes developed by the McFarlane team underscored how the multifamily group approach differs from what is generally perceived as standard care. Potential obstacles to implementation of family educational programs were paired with potential solutions to those problems. The "road show" included lectures and discussions about other PORT recommendations, including psychopharmacological treatments, and did not focus exclusively on family interventions.

This presentation concluded with two breakout group discussions at each site. The first group was organized around the type of intervention to be discussed, so any participant interested in family interventions was free to attend. The second group was organized around discipline or identified role. Family members and professionals thus had their own separate discussion groups. Discussions in the breakout sessions were generally enthusiastic about the implementation of the recommendations. Professionals expressed doubts that families were really willing to participate in these models. On several occasions, discussions between family members and professionals led to productive solutions. In one site, a few family members expressed anger that the presentation focused on treatment models that appeared to be oriented toward professional help rather than family self-help.

Intensive Training

The intensive training had two phases, the first a 2-day program conducted by the originators of the intervention on June 13–14, 1996. The training took place at a site central to the participating agencies. Didactic materials as well as role plays were used. Materials, including books, a treatment manual, and a video, were provided to all trainees. All five agencies from the target area were invited, all agencies were represented at the training (3–10 trainees from each site). Continuing Education Units were provided. Agency personnel were asked to have front-line clinicians and at least one administrator attend.

Participants in this phase were asked to fill out three sets of questionnaires: (1) a satisfaction survey at the end of the training; (2) a rigorous pre- and posttest designed to assess the knowledge of participants about the intervention; and (3) a survey of attitudes, expectations, and obstacles to implementation, filled out at the end of the 2-day program.

At the close of the 2-day program, participants at each site paired with one of four trainers to set up Phase 2. Participants in this second, "follow-up" phase, initially planned 3 months of technical assistance and support to each site by phone. An on-site training "booster" 3 months after the initial training was also planned. Personnel at each site were informed that the designated contact persons would have access to up to 5 hours of phone contact with the trainer, which could be used for whatever they felt they needed. Trainers were to provide a brief summary of all phone contacts. This initial design was modified, as described in the results section.

Results of the Technology Transfer Experiment

Phase 1: 2-Day Training

The satisfaction surveys revealed a high level of satisfaction with the 2-day program. Overall, 77% of the 35 participants rated the training as very good to outstanding. Of note, two of the study participants from one site expressed vocal dissatisfaction throughout the training, accounting for some of the lower ratings. These participants seemed to object to the model and felt that it was degrading to patients and families.

A 20-item pretest was given on the morning of the training and again at the end of the second day. All trainees were given a packet of reading materials and videotapes to view prior to the training. A total of 36 persons took the pretest, and 35 persons took the posttest. The mean number of items answered correctly by each trainee increased significantly from the pretest to the posttest, 15.56 (SD = 3.44) versus 17.80 (SD = 2.15), t = 10.81, df = 70, p = <.01. Trainees' considerable knowledge of the model prior to the formal training could have been a result of preparation required for the training. Trainees also acquired knowledge of the model from the training itself.

The participant survey revealed that the vast majority of staff participated in the training voluntarily (91%). A large majority of participants also reported that a designated individual in their agency was responsible for implementing multifamily groups (78%). Table 17.1 reports training participants' perspectives on the compatibility of multifamily group training with agency philosophy and priorities. Table 17.2 shows the obstacles to implementation of the multifamily group trainees anticipated at the end of the intensive 2-day program. The most important obstacles were lack of resources (e.g., money and time). Less important but significant obstacles emerged from participants' doubts about the effectiveness and feasibility of the model.

Phase 2: Follow-Up

During the summer months following the 2-day training, little contact occurred between the site participants and the trainers. Three sites had one

TABLE 17.1. Multifamily Group (MFG) Intensive Training: Participants' Responses

Question	Mean	SD
To what extent is MFG consistent with the *philosophy and mission* of your agency?[a]	1.61	0.66
To what extent are the methods and techniques of MFG consistent with the general mode of providing services at your agency?[a]	1.78	0.90
How much of a priority is the implementation of MFG in relation to the *short-term* goals of your agency?[b]	3.32	0.84
How much of a priority is the implementation of MFG in relation to the *long-term* goals of your agency?[b]	3.77	0.92
To what extent do you think MFG will be implemented by December 1996? Complete implementation means at least one fully operational MFG.[c]	3.33	1.19
To what extent do you think MFG will be implemented by June 1997? Complete implementation means at least one fully operational MFG.[c]	4.06	1.00

[a]1 = very consistent; 2 = somewhat consistent; 3 = mildly consistent; 4 = not consistent.
[b]1 = no priority; 2 = low priority; 3 = medium priority; 4 = high priority; 5 = very high priority.
[c]1 = not at all; 2 = almost not at all; 3 = moderate; 4 = almost completely; 5 = completely.

contact, and two had no contact. Participants in two of the sites expressed no interest in pursuing implementation of the model. One site, an academic center, was not committed to integrated psychosocial treatment. Another, a community mental health center, had relatively few patients with schizophrenia. Two of the sites were attempting to sort out problems related to implementation.

Given the limited amount of contact between sites and trainers, the on-site booster was essential; it was planned and conducted in September 1996. Trainers were enthusiastic about this, as were participants from three of the five sites. Staff from three sites participated. The agenda was informal, with participants at each site presenting their current status and problems. One agency had ongoing family groups and received feedback from the trainers on how to integrate multifamily group strategies (e.g., problem solving) into their ongoing groups. This agency rated the booster as "very helpful." Staff from a second agency focused on how to conduct joining sessions. They rated the session as "very helpful" with regard to the technical aspects of the intervention and "somewhat helpful" with regard to coping with administrative barriers. The third agency seemed to absorb many of the suggestions made by the other sites in getting started. This agency reported that participants were in the middle of a "(tax) levy" battle to pre-serve their basic program funding, and that they would move forward if the levy passed in November.

On the whole, the in-person booster training seemed to engage the participants and generate enthusiasm. The trainers addressed the specific concerns of the participants. In addition, during the interim, the trainers acquired more experience with a program replicating the multifamily group model in a different outpatient setting, and they could refer to this experi-ence. The trainers seemed well prepared to address the issues of imple-menting this model in an outpatient setting. The participants developed some *esprit de corps* and helped each other solve problems. Each site planned to continue working with the trainer on an as-needed basis.

After the September booster, contact between trainers and sites was er-ratic, but progress continued in sites that had participated in the booster. Between the fall of 1996 and spring of 1997, one of the agencies had started

TABLE 17.2. Multifamily Group (MFG) Intensive Training: Participants' Perceptions of Importance of Obstacles to Implementing Groups

Obstacle	Mean	SD	% with 3 or more
Intense work pressure on staff carrying out intervention	3.94	0.80	95
Uncertainty about financing of agency	3.67	1.46	80
Uncertainty about financing of MFG	3.39	1.42	71
Agency bureaucracy inhibiting ability to add a new service	2.83	1.04	68
Skepticism of staff about added value of MFG	2.67	1.09	60
Skepticism of staff about assumptions of MFG	2.56	0.86	55
Confidentiality	2.71	1.44	45
Inability to provide services on evenings and weekends to families	2.47	1.23	40
Lack of guidance and leadership to implement MFG	2.33	1.28	40
Lack of support for MFG among family members	2.41	1.00	40
Confusing nature of MFG	2.06	1.06	33
Lack of competent personnel to carry out MFG	2.11	0.83	28
Too few eligible patients and families	2.11	0.83	15
Low priority given to persons with serious mental illness in agency	1.39	0.85	10

Note. 1 = not at all; 2 = almost not at all; 3 = moderately important; 4 = very important; 5 = critically impor-tant.

a multifamily group, and in another, participants felt that they had successfully integrated multifamily group techniques into ongoing family groups. The levy at the final site passed, and participants anticipated starting a group soon.

Again, given the limited amount of contact, the consequent lack of consultation time used, and the success of the first on-site "booster," PORT staff decided to explore the possibility of conducting a second event. This idea was greeted enthusiastically by the three participating sites, and the second event was conducted on March 12, 1997. This booster was to be the last of the PORT-supported contacts between the sites and the trainers.

As in the first booster, the program was conducted at a site that was relatively convenient for all participants. Each of the sites sent two to three agency staff. Participants included both the front-line staff conducting the program and administrative supervisors. All sites reported receiving a great deal of administrative support from senior management at their agencies. One site had a single operating group and raised concerns about how to stick to the group format and engage consumers to participate. Another site, in the process of joining families, reported problems with changing the roles of case managers and reluctant families, and interfacing with community resources. Participants indicated that this model was having a major impact on how they assessed families in their agency. A final site reported success in starting a second group at its second hospital and was enthusiastically trying to integrate elements of the model into its ongoing program.

Trainers provided technical assistance for problems raised. The program concluded with trainers' offers to provide more assistance on an ad hoc basis. The group members also sought each other's phone numbers to continue contact.

Outcomes

The final postintervention agency assessment was conducted 1 year after the original "road show." The four agencies receiving the road show–only standard condition did not make any changes in the services provided to families. Of the five sites that received the intensive training, two sites implemented the multifamily group model, one modified existing programs in a manner that incorporated multifamily group principles, and two made no changes in services to families. The intensive training was thus partially successful in bringing about change in the services provided by participating agencies. It was quite successful in implementing family services in agencies that had historically worked with the appropriate patient population.

What factors explain the success of three sites and the failure of two sites? A closer examination of some of the variability in answers to questions asked at the time of the 2-day intensive training reveals some site differences that may shed light on differential adaptation of the model.

- Intensive training sites that did not implement the multifamily group model rated the *methods and techniques of the multifamily group* as significantly less consistent with the general mode of providing services at their agency than did sites that implemented multifamily groups.
- Intensive training sites that did not implement the multifamily group model rated the *implementation of multifamily group* as a lower short- and long-term priority when compared with implementing sites.
- Intensive training sites that did not implement the multifamily group model rated lack of competent staff, lack of leadership, confidentiality, skepticism regarding the assumptions of psychoeducational multifamily groups, and difficulties with agency bureaucracy as greater obstacles to implementation than implementing sites.

Discussion

Both arms of the PORT study disseminated some knowledge of an intervention with well-established programmatic impact via previous research. *The lack of change in the road show–only arm starkly illustrates the inadequacy of dissemination of knowledge alone in effecting technology transfer.* The intensive training arm partially addressed the human dynamics of resistance to change by the one-to-one approach, networking, and problem solving. However, the PORT approach did not address directly the availability of resources. What does the partial success of the intensive training arm tell us? In a hospitable environment, creative and committed staff can redeploy existing resources with some help and guidance. However, failure is more likely to occur in the absence of adequate attention to resource issues and where evidence of efficacy does not lead to attitudinal change.

CONCLUSIONS

Both the New York and Ohio efforts were partial successes and partial failures, with both achieving some uptake of the family psychoeducation models, at least for a period of time. New York had a particularly ambitious and comprehensive effort. To what extent did each state project provide the ideal fundamental conditions for systems change?[576] In both states, the protocol provided significant *dissemination of knowledge*. An *evaluation of programmatic (therapeutic) impact* was a specific component of the research phase of the New York study, to which the Ohio study was then able to refer. In the early phases, the New York effort provided additional *resources*. As those resources dwindled, moving from the research to the implementation to the dissemination phase, so did the uptake of the multifamily group treatment program. The PORT effort provided relatively few additional resources. Interestingly, in the absence of a comprehensive approach to addressing the *human dynamics of resisting change*, resources available in the PORT study were not initially used. In New York, the multifamily group model itself provided the framework for addressing the human dynamics of resisting change. However, attention to these dynamics required resources that were less available in the implementation and dissemination phases of the New York effort.

The partial successes and partial failures of these attempts to implement multifamily groups in the real world thus suggest several improvements in strategy for wide dissemination. When technology transfer efforts include dissemination of knowledge and evaluation of programmatic impact, but not sustained resources and attention to the human dynamics of resisting change, system change can begin but may not be sustained. Under such circumstances, system change can also occur in pockets of unusually committed staff, or where there is an especially good fit between the new program and the host, but system change will not occur in a predictable, widespread fashion.

Omitted from this model of system change is consideration of the explicit role of the stakeholders at both ends of the spectrum (i.e., the consumers, and the system leadership and payers). The New York experience clearly illustrates the vulnerability of implementation efforts to arbitrary changes in system leadership priorities, including decisions to support treatments that lack empirical support. The importance of the inclusion of a broad range of stakeholders in the process of implementation has been demonstrated by the results from two recent family psychoeducation dissemination programs in the states of Illinois and Maine.[580] In Maine, an initiative directed by key community mental health services and the Maine Medical Center introduced family advocates, consumers, mental health professionals, administrators, and policy leaders to the advantages of psychoeducational multifamily groups and trained clinical staff in the use of that approach. The project team pursued a three-step process: (1) Build consensus within the local and regional mental health community to adopt the model; (2) ensure that the human financial and technical resources are in place to implement the model; and (3) carry out concrete implementation plans, both statewide and site-specific, taking local complexities into account and making adaptations where necessary or desirable. Within 9 months of training, 14 of 15 participating agencies had implemented a psychoeducational multifamily group.

At the same time as the Maine initiative, the Maine Medical Center team received a mandate and funding from the Illinois Department of Mental Health to disseminate the model to clinicians in mental health centers and agencies throughout the state. Clinical staff at 51 of approximately 200 mental health agencies participated in training workshops. The Illinois effort was initiated by the central mental health authority through its regional offices. Incentives and encouragement were provided by central and regional state managers to adopt the approach and implement it within their routine clinical services. Orientation, training, and technical assistance were offered, using the same approaches as in Maine and New York. In contrast to Maine, 10% (5 of 51) of the sites in Illinois implemented multifamily groups.

What were the differences between the efforts in Maine and Illinois? Although the Illinois effort attempted to engage staff through the training, there was markedly less emphasis on local consensus building and leadership by mental health center administrators and clinical directors. The Illinois effort also put less effort into gaining clinician, family, and consumer acceptance than the effort in Maine. Surveys taken just after training demonstrated that Illinois trainees had much more skepticism about the approach than did their Maine counterparts, suggesting some between-state differences in acceptance of new models and empirical data about efficacy. Efforts at consensus building accounted for the increased expense in Maine relative to Illinois ($0.25 vs. $0.01 per capita). This ongoing project illustrates the importance of engaging participants at all levels in disseminating and implementing family psychoeducation. It also shows that there are approaches to implementation with greater and lesser effectiveness.

Future work on technology transfer must be a clear priority for family psychoeducation and other, more effective but less traditional treatments, and must consider each of these dimensions to optimize the chances of success and to learn from our failures.

Afterword

C. CHRISTIAN BEELS

It is difficult to imagine anything that could be added to this comprehensive volume, nor is it my task to sum up. That has been done admirably by the authors themselves. I have a few historical and social reflections to place here as a footnote to the extraordinary collection of evidence and experience in these chapters.

It is now a generation since the first international conference at Columbia University, in 1981, brought together what was then a contentious group of family therapists and researchers in schizophrenia and the family. McFarlane's first book[581] was in part a report of those proceedings. By the time the book came out, the clash of the "brain disease" and the "social deviance" factions at the conference was already beginning to yield to discussion and experiment. In 1986, McGlashan[582] was ready to declare in the *Annual Review of Psychiatry,* "In one decade, family therapy of schizophrenia has leaped forward as *the* . . . modality of greatest interest. . . . Mostly, interest exists because these methods have repeatedly proved to be effective in well-designed clinical trials" (p. 107). The family therapy he mentioned was represented by the psychoeducational designs of Anderson, Hogarty, Falloon, Leff, and McFarlane's group in New York, so well described in these pages. McFarlane designed his comparison of single- and multifamily psychoeducation without a comparison group receiving "family dynamic" or "systems" treatment, because, in 1985, to withhold a treatment of known effectiveness from research subjects would have been unethical. As far as the writers of books and granters of grants were concerned, the verdict was in.

But what was happening in what Dixon and Dunne call "the real world"? In New York and Ohio, and in other states where McFarlane's team has carried its message at the request of mental health authorities, the implementation of multifamily groups in clinical settings has died out after receiving an enthusiastic welcome. The analysis by Dixon and Dunne in Chapter 17 deserves a close reading. The main reasons given by staff for believing the approach will not be implemented have to do with perceptions of lack of support from their administration. There is something in the bones of mental health institutions in this country that does not really love this therapy—at least not enough to commit time, money, space, and teaching.

There must be many reasons for this. Harriet Lefley[583] has written a searching essay on the elements of our American culture that conflict with our willingness to give the families of those who suffer from mental illness the support they need and deserve. Against our cultural ideals of individual autonomy, agency, accountability, and mastery, the therapists and families described in this book have had to organize a counterculture that promotes belief in "comprehensive treatment, protection for the subject and social acceptance of an innate, biologically determined differentness without stigmatization"[583] (p. 338). Here, I think, we can see another reason why multifamily therapy is more effective than single-family therapy. One therapist and one family are not enough to make a culture—at least not one that effectively extends beyond the session.

And as Lefley and many of the authors in this book have noted, the new medical culture of managed care threatens even the pitifully little socially organized, long-term work with chronic illnesses that is still left from the reforms of 20 years ago. Van Noppen and Steketee, in Chapter 15 on obsessive–compulsive disorder, express the hope that the cost-effectiveness of multifamily treatment will make it attractive to the money managers, and we all say "Amen." But in general, the managers have not been interested in anything so "low tech" as this, just as they have not been interested in chronic illness and its management, or other outcomes that appear after they have sold the company.

McFarlane once told me that one of the origins of multifamily therapy was Peter Laqueur's observation that during visiting hours at Creedmoor State Hospital, patients and their families lingered to talk with each other and seemed to be getting something important out of it. Turning this communal consumer impulse into a therapy was an ingenious idea, because it

enabled the clinician to join in an activity that families had already initiated. This is still one of the simplest explanations, both for why it works
and why some psychiatric institutions have a hard time with it.

Here, in the later chapters, we have impressive evidence that those
who suffer from other chronic conditions—borderline personality disorder,
bipolar illness, obsessive–compulsive disorder, and chronic medical illness—also need to form their own subcultures and invent their own dis-
tinctive healing rituals. The adaptability of multifamily therapy to each of
these conditions is remarkable. By bringing out the unique courage and
skill of each family against a common enemy, multifamily groups bring realistic hope against despair.

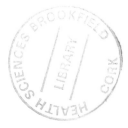

References

1. Solomon P. Moving from psychoeducation to family education for families of adults with serious mental illness. *Psychiatric Services* 1996;47:1364–1370.
2. Hatfield AB, Spaniol L, Zipple AM. Expressed emotion: A family perspective. *Schizophrenia Bulletin* 1987;13:221–226.
3. Weisman A. Understanding cross-cultural prognostic variability for schizophrenia. *Cultural Diversity and Mental Health* 1997;3:23–35.
4. Burland J. Family-to-family: A trauma-and-recovery model of family education. *New Directions for Mental Health Services* 1998;77: 33–41.
5. American Psychiatric Association. *Diagnostic and statistical manual of mental disorders*, 4th ed. Washington, DC: American Psychiatric Press, 1994.
6. Wolkowitz OW, Doran AR, Roy A, et al. Neuroleptic responsivity of negative and positive symptoms in schizophrenia. *American Journal of Psychiatry* 1987;144: 1549–1555.
7. Breier A, Wolkowitz O, Doran A, et al. Neuroleptic responsivity of negative and positive symptoms in schizophrenia. *American Journal of Psychiatry* 1987;144: 1549–1555.
8. Bleuler M. The long-term course of schizophrenia psychosis. *Psychological Medicine* 1974;4:244–254.
9. Ciompi L, Muller C. *Lebensweg und Alter der Schizophrennen: Eine Katamnestische Langseitstudies bisins Senium*. Berlin: Springer-Verlag, 1976.
10. Harding C, Brooks G, Ashikaga T, et al. The Vermont longitudinal study of persons with severe mental illness: I. Methodology, study sample, and overall status 32 years later. *American Journal of Psychiatry* 1987;144:718–726.
11. Lieberman J, Jody D, Geisler S, et al. Time course and biologic correlates of treatment response in first-epdisode schizophrenia. *Archives of General Psychiatry* 1993;50:369–376.
12. Szymanski SR, Cannon TD, Gallacher F, et al. Course of treatment response in first-episode and chronic schizophrenia. *American Journal of Psychiatry* 1996; 153:519–525.
13. Carpenter WJ, Heinrichs D, Wagman A. Deficit and nondeficit forms of schizophrenia: The concept. *American Journal of Psychiatry* 1988;145:578–583.

14. Bleuler E. *Dementia praecox or the group of schizophrenias*. New York: International Universities Press, 1950.

15. Leff J, Vaughn C. *Expressed emotion in families: Its significance for mental illness*. New York: Guilford Press, 1985.

16. McFarlane WR, Lukens EP. Insight, families and education: An exploration of the role of attribution in clinical outcome. In: Amador XF, David AS, eds. *Insight and psychosis*. New York: Oxford University Press, 1998:317–331.

17. Hwu HG, Tan H, Chen CC, et al. Negative symptoms at discharge and outcome in schizophrenia. *British Journal of Psychiatry* 1995;166:61–67.

18. Hogarty G, Ulrich R. Temporal effects of drug and placebo in delaying relapse in schizophrenic outpatients. *Archives of General Psychiatry* 1977;34:297–301.

19. Sullivan G, Marder SR, Liberman RP, et al. Social skills and relapse history in outpatient schizophrenics. *Psychiatry* 1990;53:340–345.

20. Stanley JA, Williamson PC, Drost DJ, et al. An *in vivo* study of the prefrontal cortex of schizophrenic patients at different stages of illness via phosphorus magnetic resonance spectroscopy. *Archives of General Psychiatry* 1995;52:399–406.

21. Bleuler M. A 23 year longitudinal study of 208 schizophrenics and impressions in regard to the nature of schizophrenia. *Journal of Psychosomatic Research* 1968; 6(Suppl.):3–14.

22. Lieberman JA, Koreen AR, Chakos M, et al. Factors influencing treatment response and outcome of first-episode schizophrenia: Implications for understanding the pathophysiology of schizophrenia. *Journal of Clinical Psychiatry* 1996; 57:5–9.

23. McGorry PD. EPPIC: An evolving system of early detection and optimal management. *Schizophrenia Bulletin* 1996;22:305–326.

24. Van Kammen DP, Van Kammen WB, Naum LS, et al. Dopamine metabolism in the cerebrospinal fluid of drug-free schizophrenic patients with and without cortical atrophy. *Archives of General Psychiatry* 1986;43:978–983.

25. Losonczy MF, Davidson M, Davis K. The dopamine hypothesis of schizophrenia. In: Meltzer HE, ed. *Psychopharmacology: The third generation of progress*. New York: Raven Press, 1987:715–726.

26. Kapur S, Remington G. Serotonin–dopamine interaction and its relevance to schizophrenia. *American Journal of Psychiatry* 1996;153:466–476.

27. Burnet PW, Eastwood SL, Harrison PJ. 5–HT1A and 5–HT2A receptor mRNAs and binding site densities are differentially altered in schizophrenia. *Neuropsychopharmacology* 1996;15:442–455.

28. Aparicio-Legarza MI, Cutts AJ, Davis B, et al. Deficits of [^{3}H] D-aspartate binding to glutamate uptake sites in striatal and accumbens tissue in patients with schizophrenia. *Neuroscience* 1997;232:13–16.

29. Tamminga C. Glutamatergic aspects of schizophrenia. *British Journal of Psychiatry* 1999;37(Suppl.):12–15.

30. Olney JW, Farber NB. Glutamate receptor dysfunction and schizophrenia. *Archives of General Psychiatry* 1995;52:998–1007.

31. Adler C, Malhotra A, Elman I, et al. Comparison of ketamine-induced thought disorder in healthy volunteers and thought disorder in schizophrenia. *American Journal of Psychiatry* 1999;156:1646–1649.

32. Bunney W, Bunney B. Evidence for a compromised dorsolateral prefrontal cortical parallel circuit in schizophrenia. *Brain Research Reviews* 2000;**31**:138–146.

33. Le CS, Harper C, Lopez P, et al. Increased levels of expression of an NMDARI splice variant in the superior temporal gyrus in schizophrenia. *NeuroReport* 2000; **11**:983–986.

34. Weinberger D. Cell biology of the hippocampal formation in schizophrenia. *Biological Psychiatry* 1999;**45**:395–402.

35. Heresco LU, Javitt D, Ermilov M, et al. Efficacy of high-dose glycine in the treatment of enduring negative symptoms of schizophrenia. *Archives of General Psychiatry* 1999;**56**:29–36.

36. Tsai G, Yang P, Chung L, et al. D-serine added to antipsychotics for the treatment of schizophrenia [see comments]. *Biological Psychiatry* 1998;**44**:1081–1089.

37. Volk DW, Austin MC, Pierri JN. Decreased glutamic acid decarboxylase-67 messenger RNA expression in a subset of prefrontal cortical GABA neurons in subjects with schizophrenia. *Archives of General Psychiatry* 2000;**57**:237–245.

38. Farber N, Newcomer J, Olney J. The glutamate synapse in neuropsychiatric disorders: Focus on schizophrenia and Alzheimer's disease. *Progress in Brain Research* 1998;**116**:421–437.

39. Aghajanian G, Marek G. Serotonin model of schizophrenia: Emerging role of glutamate mechanisms. *Brain Research Review* 2000;**31**:302–312.

40. Duncan G, Sheitman B, Lieberman J. An integrated view of pathophysiological models of schizophrenia. *Brain Research Reviews* 1999;**29**:250–264.

41. Freedman R, Hall M, Adler LE, et al. Evidence in postmortem brain tissue for decreased numbers of hippocampal nicotinic receptors in schizophrenia. *Biological Psychiatry* 1995;**38**:22–33.

42. Maier M, Ron MA, Barker GJ, et al. Proton magnetic resonance spectroscopy: An *in vivo* method of estimating hippocampal neuronal depletion in schizophrenia. *Psychological Medicine* 1995;**25**:1201–1209.

43. Nuechterlein KH, Dawson ME. A heuristic vulnerability/stress model for schizophrenic episodes. *Schizophrenia Bulletin* 1984;**10**:300–312.

44. Karper LP, Freeman GK, Grillon C, et al. Preliminary evidence of an association between sensorimotor gating and distractibility in psychosis. *Journal of Neuropsychiatry and Clinical Neuroscience* 1996;**8**:60–66.

45. Buchsbaum MS, Someya T, Teng CY, et al. PET and MRI of the thalamus in never-medicated patients with schizophrenia. *American Journal of Psychiatry* 1996; **153**:191–199.

46. Sabri O, Erkwoh R, Schreckenberger M, et al. Correlation of positive symptoms exclusively to hyperperfusion or hypoperfusion of cerebral cortex in never-treated schizophrenics. *Lancet* 1997;**349**:1735–1739.

47. Sabri O, Erkwoh R, Schreckenberger M, et al. Regional cerebral blood flow and negative/positive symptoms in 24 drug-naive schizophrenics. *Journal of Nuclear Medicine* 1997;**38**:181–188.

48. Schroder J, Buchsbaum MS, Siegel BV, et al. Cerebral metabolic activity correlates of subsyndromes in chronic schizophrenia. *Schizophrenia Research* 1996;**19**:41–53.

49. Tecce J, Cole J. The distraction–arousal hypothesis, CNV and schizophrenia. In:

Mostofsky D, ed. *Behavior control and modification of psychological activity.* Englewood Cliffs, NJ: Prentice-Hall, 1976.

50. Johnstone E, Crow T, Frith C, et al. Cerebral ventricular size and cognitive impairment in chronic schizophrenia. *Lancet* 1976;11:924–926.

51. Schlaepfer TE, Harris GJ, Tien AY, et al. Decreased regional cortical gray matter volume in schizophrenia. *American Journal of Psychiatry* 1994;151:842–848.

52. Breier A, Buchanan RW, Elkashef A, et al. Brain morphology and schizophrenia: A magnetic resonance imaging study of limbic, prefrontal cortex, and caudate structures. *Archives of General Psychiatry* 1992;49:921–926.

53. Barta PE, Pearlson GD, Powers RE, et al. Auditory hallucinations and smaller superior temporal gyral volume in schizophrenia. *American Journal of Psychiatry* 1990;147:1457–1462.

54. Aylward EH, Brettschneider PD, McArthur JC, et al. Magnetic resonance imaging measurement of gray matter volume reductions in HIV dementia. *American Journal of Psychiatry* 1995;152:987–994.

55. Pearlson GD, Barta PE, Powers RE, et al. Ziskind–Somerfeld Research Award 1996: Medial and superior temporal gyral volumes and cerebral asymmetry in schizophrenia versus bipolar disorder. *Biological Psychiatry* 1997;41:1–14.

56. DeQuardo JR, Bookstein FL, Green WD, et al. Spatial relationships of neuroanatomic landmarks in schizophrenia. *Psychiatry Research* 1996;67:81–95.

57. Lieberman J, Bogerts B, Degreef G, et al. Qualitative assessment of brain morphology in acute and chronic schizophrenia. *American Journal of Psychiatry* 1992; 149:784–794.

58. Rapoport JL, Giedd J, Kumra S, et al. Childhood-onset schizophrenia: Progressive ventricular change during adolescence. *Archives of General Psychiatry* 1997; 54:897–903.

59. Andreasen NC, Smith MR, Jacoby CG, et al. Ventricular enlargement in schizophrenia: Relationship to positive and negative symptoms. *American Journal of Psychiatry* 1982;139:297–302.

60. Weinberger D. Implications of normal brain development for the pathogenesis of schizophrenia. *Archives of General Psychiatry* 1987;44:660–669.

61. Andreasen NC, O'Leary DS, Flaum M, et al. Hypofrontality in schizophrenia: Distributed dysfunctional circuits in neuroleptic-naive patients. *Lancet* 1997; 349: 1730–1734.

62. Berman K, Zec R, Weinberger D. Physiological dysfunction of dorsolateral prefrontal cortex in schizophrenia: II Role of medication, attention, and mental effort. *Archives of General Psychiatry* 1986;43:126–143.

63. Yurgelun-Todd DA, Waternaux CM, Cohen BM, et al. Functional magnetic resonance imaging of schizophrenic patients and comparison subjects during word production. *American Journal of Psychiatry* 1996;153:200–205.

64. Goldsmith SK, Shapiro RM, Joyce JN. Disrupted pattern of D2 dopamine receptors in the temporal lobe in schizophrenia: A postmortem study. *Archives of General Psychiatry* 1997;54:649–658.

65. Carter CS, Robertson LC, Nordahl TE, et al. Perceptual and attentional asymmetries in schizophrenia: Further evidence for a left hemisphere deficit. *Psychiatry Research* 1996;62:111–119.

66. Katz M, Buchsbaum MS, Siegel BV, Jr., et al. Correlational patterns of cerebral glu-
cose metabolism in never-medicated schizophrenics. *Neuropsychobiology* 1996;
33:1–11.

67. Nordahl TE, Kusubov N, Carter C, et al. Temporal lobe metabolic differences in
medication-free outpatients with schizophrenia via the PET-600. *Neuropsychopharmacology* 1996;15:541–554.

68. Tune L, Barta P, Wong D, et al. Striatal dopamine D2 receptor quantification and
superior temporal gyrus: Volume determination in 14 chronic schizophrenic subjects. *Psychiatry Research* 1996;67:155–158.

69. Stefansson SB, Jonsdottir TJ. Auditory event-related potentials, auditory digit
span, and clinical symptoms in chronic schizophrenic men on neuroleptic medication. *Biological Psychiatry* 1996;40:19–27.

70. Trestman RL, Horvath T, Kalus O, et al. Event-related potentials in schizotypal
personality disorder. *Journal of Neuropsychiatry and Clinical Neuroscience* 1996;
8:33–40.

71. Gupta S, Andreasen NC, Arndt S, et al. Neurological soft signs in neuroleptic-
naive and neuroleptic-treated schizophrenic patients and in normal comparison
subjects. *American Journal of Psychiatry* 1995;152:191–196.

72. Rossi A, De Cataldo S, Di Michele V, et al. Neurological soft signs in schizophrenia. *British Journal of Psychiatry* 1990;157:735–739.

73. Harrow M, Quinlan D. Is disordered thinking unique to schizophrenia? *Archives
of General Psychiatry* 1977;34:15–21.

74. Mueser KT, Penn DL, Blanchard JT, et al. Affect recognition in schizophrenia: A
synthesis of findings across three studies. *Psychiatry* 1997;60:310–308.

75. Sullivan EV, Shear PK, Zipursky RB, et al. A deficit profile of executive, memory,
and motor functions in schizophrenia. *Biological Psychiatry* 1994;36:641–653.

76. Scully PJ, Coakley G, Kinsella A, et al. Psychopathology, executive (frontal) and
general cognitive impairment in relation to duration of initially untreated versus
subsequently treated psychosis in chronic schizophrenia. *Psychological Medicine*
1997;27:1303–1310.

77. Wiersma D, Nienhuis FJ, Giel R, et al. Stability and change in needs of patients
with schizophrenic disorders: A 15– and 17–year follow-up from first onset of
psychosis, and a comparison between "objective" and "subjective" assessments of
needs for care. *Social Psychiatry and Psychiatric Epidemiology* 1998;33:49–56.

78. Harrison G, Croudace T, Mason P, et al. Predicting the long-term outcome of
schizophrenia. *Psychological Medicine* 1996;26:697–705.

79. Torgalsboen AK, Rund BR. "Full recovery" from schizophrenia in the long term: A
ten-year follow-up of eight former schizophrenic patients. *Psychiatry* 1998; 61:
20–34.

80. Kendler K. The genetics of schizophrenia. *APA Annual Review* 1986;5:25–41.

81. Gottesman II, Shields J. *Schizophrenia, the Epigenetic Puzzle.* Cambridge, UK:
Cambridge University Press, 1982.

82. Kendler K, Gruenberg A. An independent analysis of the Danish Adoption Study
of Schizophrenia: VI. The relationship between psychiatric disorder as defined by
DSM-III in the relatives and adoptees. *Archives of General Psychiatry* 1984;41:555–
564.

83. Kety S. Mental illness in the biological and adoptive relatives of schizophrenic adoptees: Findings relevant to genetic environmental factors in etiology. *American Journal of Psychiatry* 1983;**140**:720–727.

84. Cannon TD, Kaprio J, Lonnquist J, et al. The genetic epidemiology of schizophrenia in a Finnish twin cohort: A population-based modeling study. *Archives of General Psychiatry* 1998;**55**:67–74.

85. Akbarian S, Bunney WEJ, Potkin SG, et al. Altered distribution of nicotinamide–adenine dinucleotide–diaphorase cells in frontal lobes of schizophrenics implies disturbance of cortical development. *Archives of General Psychiatry* 1993;**50**:227–230.

86. Keshavan MS, Anderson S, Pettegrew JW. Is schizophrenia due to excessive synaptic pruning in the prefrontal cortex?: The Feinberg hypothesis revisited. *Journal of Psychiatric Research* 1994;**28**:239–265.

87. Hoffman RE, Dobscha SK. Cortical pruning and the development of schizophrenia: A computer model. *Schizophrenia Bulletin* 1989;**15**:477–490.

88. Mednick S, Cannon T. Fetal development, birth and the syndromes of adult schizophrenia. In: Mednick S, Cannon T, Barr C, Lyon M, eds. *Fetal neural development and adult schizophrenia.* New York: Cambridge University Press, 1991.

89. Wright P, Takei N, Rifkin L, et al. Maternal influenza, obstetric complications, and schizophrenia. *American Journal of Psychiatry* 1995;**152**:1714–1720.

90. Verdoux H, Geddes JR, Takei N, et al. Obstetric complications and age at onset in schizophrenia: An international collaborative meta-analysis of individual patient data. *American Journal of Psychiatry* 1997;**154**:1220–1227.

91. Chengappa KN, Nimgaonkar VL, Bachert C, et al. Obstetric complications and autoantibodies in schizophrenia. *Acta Psychiatrica Scandinavica* 1995;**92**:270–273.

92. Kendell RE, Juszczak E, Cole SK. Obstetric complications and schizophrenia: A case control study based on standardised obstetric records. *British Journal of Psychiatry* 1996;**168**:556–561.

93. Kunugi H, Nanko S, Takei N, et al. Perinatal complications and schizophrenia: Data from the Maternal and Child Health Handbook in Japan. *Journal of Nervous and Mental Disease* 1995;**184**:542–546.

94. Smith GN, Honer WG, Kopala L, et al. Obstetric complications and severity of illness in schizophrenia. *Schizophrenia Research* 1995;**14**:113–120.

95. Geddes JR, Lawrie SM. Obstetric complications and schizophrenia: A meta-analysis. *British Journal of Psychiatry* 1995;**167**:786–793.

96. Kunugi H, Nanko S, Takei N, et al. Schizophrenia following in utero exposure to the 1957 influenza epidemics in Japan. *American Journal of Psychiatry* 1995;**152**:450–452.

97. Bersani G, Taddei I, Venturi P, et al. Familial occurrence and obstetric complications in siblings discordant for schizophrenia. *Minerva Psichiatria* 1995;**36**:127–132.

98. Bradbury T, Miller G. Season of birth in schizophrenia: A review of evidence, methodology and etiology. *Psychological Bulletin* 1985;**98**:569–594.

99. Franzek E, Beckmann H. Gene–environment interaction in schizophrenia: Season-of-birth effect reveals etiologically different subgroups. *Psychopathology* 1996;**29**:14–26.

100. McGrath JJ, Pemberton MR, Welham JL, et al. Schizophrenia and the influenza epidemics of 1954, 1957 and 1959: A southern hemisphere study. *Schizophrenia Research* 1994;**14**:1–8.
101. Takei N, Van Os J, Murray RM. Maternal exposure to influenza and risk of schizophrenia: A 22 year study from the Netherlands. *Journal of Psychiatric Research* 1995;**29**:435–445.
102. Barr CE, Mednick SA, Munk-Jorgensen P. Exposure to influenza epidemics during gestation and adult schziophrenia. *Archives of General Psychiatry* 1990;**47**: 869–874.
103. Ganguli R, Brar JS, Chengappa KN, et al. Autoimmunity in schizophrenia: A review of recent findings. *Annals of Medicine* 1993;**25**:489–496.
104. Noy S, Achiron A, Laor N. Schizophrenia and autoimmunity—a possible etiological mechanism? *Neuropsychobiology* 1994;**30**:157–159.
105. Yang ZW, Chengappa KN, Shurin G, et al. An association between anti-hippocampal antibody concentration and lymphocyte production of IL-2 in patients with schizophrenia. *Psychological Medicine* 1994;**24**:449–455.
106. Hollister JM, Laing P, Mednick SA. Rhesus incompatibility as a risk factor for schizophrenia in male adults. *Archives of General Psychiatry* 1996;**53**:19–24.
107. Susser E, Neugebauer R, Hoek HW, et al. Schizophrenia after prenatal famine: Further evidence. *Archives of General Psychiatry* 1996;**53**:25–31.
108. Anderson CM, Reiss DJ, Hogarty GE. *Schizophrenia and the family: A practitioner's guide to psychoeducation and management.* New York: Guilford Press, 1986.
109. Lehman AF, Thompson JW, Dixon LB, et al. Schizophrenia: Treatment outcomes research [Editors' introduction]. *Schizophrenia Bulletin* 1995;**21**:561–566.
110. Zubin J, Steinhauer SR, Condray R. Vulnerability to relapse in schizophrenia. *British Journal of Psychiatry* 1992;**161**(Suppl. 18):13–18.
111. McFarlane WR, Lukens EP. Systems theory revisited: Research on family expressed emotion and communication deviance. In: Lefley HP, Wasow M, eds. *Helping families cope with mental illness.* Chur, Switzerland: Harwood Academic, 1994:79–104.
112. McFarlane WR, Lukens EP. Insight, families, and education: An exploration of the role of attribution in clinical outcome. In: Amador XF, David AS, eds. *Insight and pychosis.* New York: Oxford University Press, 1998.
113. Hatfield AB, Lefley HP. *Families of the mentally ill: Coping and adaptation.* New York: Guilford Press, 1987.
114. Nicholson I, Neufeld R. A dynamic vulnerability perspective on stress and schizophrenia. *American Journal of Orthopsychiatry* 1992;**62**:117–130.
115. Zubin J, Spring B. Vulnerability: A new view of schizophrenia. *Journal of Abnormal Psychology* 1977;**86**:103–126.
116. Cohen S, Wills TA. Stress, social support, and the buffering hypothesis. *Psychological Bulletin* 1985; **98**:310–357.
117. Heinrichs D, Carpenter W. The coordination of family therapy with other treatment modalities. In: McFarlane WR, ed. *Family therapy in schizophrenia.* New York: Guilford Press, 1983:267–288.
118. Duckworth K, Nair V, Patel JK, Goldfinger SM. Lost time, found hope and sorrow: The search for self, connection and purpose during "awakenings" on the new antipsychotics. *Harvard Review of Psychiatry* 1997;**5**:227–233.

119. Mueser KT, Bellack AS, Wade JH, et al. An assessment of the educational needs of chronic psychiatric patients and their relatives. *British Journal of Psychiatry* 1992;**160**:674–680.

120. Mueser KT, Valentiner DP, Agresta J. Coping with negative symptoms of schizophrenia: Patient and family perspectives. *Schizophrenia Bulletin* 1997;**23**:329–339.

121. Brekke JS, Levin S, Wolkon G, et al. Psychosocial functioning and subjective experience in schizophrenia. *Schizophrenia Bulletin* 1993;**19**:599–608.

122. Davidson L, Strauss JS. Sense of self in recovery from severe mental illness. *British Journal of Medical Psychology* 1992;**65**:131–145.

123. Penn DL, Mueser KT, Spaulding W, et al. Information processing and social competence in chronic schizophrenia. *Schizophrenia Bulletin* 1995;**21**:269–281.

124. Sarti P, Cournos F. Medication and psychotherapy in the treatment of chronic schizophrenia. *Psychiatric Clinics of North America* 1990;**13**:215–228.

125. Amador XF, David AS, eds. *Insight and psychosis*. New York: Oxford University Press, 1998.

126. House JS, Landis KR, Umberson D. Social relationships and health. *Science* 1988;**241**:540–545.

127. Breier A, Strauss J. The role of social relationships in the recovery from psychotic disorders. *American Journal of Psychiatry* 1984;**141**:949–955.

128. Sullivan WP, Poertner J. Social support and life stress: A mental health consumers perspective. *Community Mental Health Journal* 1989;**25**:21–32.

129. Cresswell CM, Kuipers L, Power MJ. Social networks and support in long-term psychiatric patients. *Psychological Medicine* 1992;**22**:1019–1026.

130. Meeks S, Murrell SA. Service providers in the social networks of clients with severe mental illness. *Schizophrenia Bulletin* 1994;**20**:399–406.

131. Tausig M, Fisher GA, Tessler RC. Informal systems of care for the chronically mentally ill. *Community Mental Health Journal* 1992;**28**:413–425.

132. Hammer M. Social supports, social networks, and schizophrenia. *Schizophrenia Bulletin* 1981;**7**:45–57.

133. Wasylenki D, James S, Clark C, et al. Clinical care update: Clinical issues in social network therapy for clients with schizophrenia. *Community Mental Health Journal* 1992;**28**:427–440.

134. Beels CC. Social support and schizophrenia. *Schizophrenia Bulletin* 1981;**7**:58–72.

135. Amador XF, Strauss DH, Yale SA, et al. Awareness of illness in schizophrenia. *Schizophrenia Bulletin* 1991;**17**:113–132.

136. Cassel J. The contribution of the social environment to host resistance. *American Journal of Epidemiology* 1976;**104**:107–123.

137. Mueller DP. Social networks: A promising direction for research on the relationship of the social environment to psychiatric disorder. *American Journal of Psychiatry* 1980;**14**:147–161.

138. Penninx BWJH, Kriegsman DMW, van Eijk JTM, et al. Differential effect of social support on the course of chronic disease: A criterion-based literature review. *Families, Systems and Health* 1996;**14**:223–244.

139. Jed J. Social support for caretakers and psychiatric rehospitalization. *Hospital and Community Psychiatry* 1989;**49**:1297–1299.

140. Solomon P, Draine J. Subjective burden among family members of mentally ill adults: Relation to stress, coping, and adaptation. *American Journal of Orthopsychiatry* 1995;**65**:419–427.

141. Pattison E, Llama R, Hurd G. Social network mediation of anxiety. *Psychiatric Annals* 1979;**9**:56–67.

142. Garrison V. Support systems of schizophrenic and nonschizophrenic Puerto Rican women in New York City. *Schizophrenia Bulletin* 1978;**4**:561–596.

143. Brown GW, Birley JLT, Wing JK. Influence of family life on the course of schizophrenic disorders: A replication. *British Journal of Psychiatry* 1972;**121**:241–258.

144. Anderson C, Hogarty G, Bayer T, et al. Expressed emotion and social networks of parents of schizophrenic patients. *British Journal of Psychiatry* 1984;**144**:247–255.

145. Lipton F, Cohen C, Fischer E, et al. Schizophrenia: A network crisis. *Schizophrenia Bulletin* 1981;**7**:144–151.

146. Tolsdorf C. Social networks, support and coping: An explanatory study. *Family Process* 1976;**15**:407–417.

147. Biegel DE, Yamatani H. Self-help groups for families of the mentally ill: Research perspectives. In: Goldstein MZ, ed. *Family involvement in the treatment of schizophrenia*. Washington, DC: American Psychiatric Press, 1986.

148. Cohen CI, Sokolovsky J. Schizophrenia and social networks: Ex-patients in the inner city. *Schizophrenia Bulletin* 1978;**4**:546–555.

149. Sokolovsky J, Cohen CI. Toward a resolution of methodological dilemmas in network mapping. *Schizophrenia Bulletin* 1981;**7**:109–118.

150. Dozier M, Harris M, Bergman H. Social network density and rehospitalization among young adult patients. *Hospital and Community Psychiatry* 1987;**38**:61–64.

151. Kawachi I, Colditz GA, Ascherio A, et al. A prospective study of social networks in relation to total mortality and cardiovascular disease in men in the USA. *Journal of Epidemiology and Community Health* 1996;**50**:245–251.

152. Brown GW, Harris T. *Social origins of depression: A study of psychiatric disorder in women.* New York: Free Press, 1978.

153. Lin N, Ensel W. Depression-mobility and its social etiology: The role of life events and social support. *Journal of Health and Social Behavior* 1984;**25**:176–188.

154. Fenton WS, Blyler CR, Heinssen RK. Determinants of medication compliance in schizophrenia: Empirical and clinical findings. *Schizophrenia Bulletin* 1997;**23**:637–651.

155. Haynes RB. Physician interventions to improve compliance. *Geriatric Consultant* 1986:20–29.

156. Heller T, Roccoforte JA, Hsieh K, et al. Benefits of support groups for families of adults with severe mental illness. *American Journal of Orthopsychiatry* 1997;**67**:187–198.

157. Hultman CM, Ohlund LS, Wieselgren IM, et al. Electrodermal activity and social network as predictors of outcome of episodes in schizophrenia. *Journal of Abnormal Psychology* 1996;**105**:626–636.

158. Becker T, Leese M, Clarkson P, et al. Links between social network and quality of life: An epidemiologically representative study of psychotic patients in south London. *Social Psychiatry and Psychiatric Epidemiology* 1998;**33**:229–304.

159. Koivumaa Honkanen HT, Viinamaki H, Honkanen R, et al. Correlates of life satisfaction among psychiatric patients. *Acta Psychiatrica Scandinavica* 1996;**94**: 372–378.
160. Viinamaki H, Niskanen L, Jaaskelainen J, et al. Factors predicting psychosocial recovery in psychiatric patients. *Acta Psychiatrica Scandinavica* 1996;**94**:365–371.
161. Solomon P, Draine J. Subjective burden among family members of mentally ill adults: Relation to stress, coping, and adaptation. *American Journal of Orthopsychiatry* 1995;**65**:419–427.
162. Solomon P, Draine J. Adaptive coping among family members of persons with serious mental illness. *Psychiatric Services* 1995;**46**:1156–1160.
163. Perlick D, Stastny P, Mattis S, et al. Contribution of family, cognitive and clinical dimensions to long-term outcome in schizophrenia. *Schizophrenia Research* 1992;**6**:257–265.
164. Hamilton NG, Ponzoha CA, Cutler DL, et al. Social networks and negative versus positive symptoms of schizophrenia. *Schizophrenia Bulletin* 1989;**15**:625–633.
165. Macdonald EM, Jackson HJ, Hayes RL, et al. Social skill as determinant of social networks and perceived social support in schizophrenia. *Schizophrenia Research* 1998;**29**:275–286.
166. Brugha TS, Wing JK, Brewin CR, et al. The relationship of social network deficits with deficits in social functioning in long-term psychiatric disorders. *Social Psychiatry and Psychiatric Epidemiology* 1993;**28**:218–24.
167. Leff J, Sartorius N, Jablensky A, et al. The International Pilot Study of Schizophrenia: Five-year follow-up findings. *Psychological Medicine* 1992;**22**:131–145.
168. Pasamanick B, Scarpetti F, Dinit S. *Schizophrenics in the community: An experimental study in the prevention of hospitalization.* New York: Appleton–Century–Crofts, 1967:301–306.
169. Stein LI, Test MA. Alternative to mental hospital treatment I: Conceptual model, treatment program and clinical evaluation. *Archives of General Psychiatry* 1980; **37**:392–397.
170. Kopeikin H, Marshall V, Goldstein M. Stages and impact of crisis-oriented family therapy in the aftercare of acute schizophrenia. In: McFarlane WR, ed. *Family therapy in schizophrenia.* New York: Guilford Press, 1983:69–98.
171. McFarlane WR, Link B, Dushay R, et al. Psychoeducational multiple family groups: Four-year relapse outcome in schizophrenia. *Family Process* 1995; **34**: 127–144.
172. Steinberg H, Durell J. A stressful social situation as a precipitant of schizophrenia. *British Journal of Psychiatry* 1968;**114**:1097–1105.
173. Scheflen AE. *Body language and social order.* Englewood Cliffs, NJ: Prentice-Hall, 1972.
174. Bowen L, Wallace CJ, Glynn SM, et al. Schizophrenic individuals' cognitive functioning and performance in interpersonal interactions and skills training procedures. *Journal of Psychiatric Research* 1994;**28**:289–301.
175. Nuechterlein KH, Snyder KS, Mintz J. Paths to relapse: Possible transactional processes connecting patient illness onset, expressed emotion, and psychotic relapse. *British Journal of Psychiatry* 1992;**18**(Suppl.):88–96.

176. Silverstein SM. Information processing, social cognition, and psychiatric rehabilitation in schizophrenia. *Psychiatry* 1997;**60**:327–340.

177. Bellack AS, Morrison RL, Wixted JT, et al. An analysis of social competence in schizophrenia. *British Journal of Psychiatry* 1990;**156**:809–818.

178. Falloon IRH, Boyd JL, McGill CW. *Family care of schizophrenia: A problem-solving approach to the treatment of mental illness.* New York: Guilford Press, 1984.

179. McFarlane WR. Multiple family therapy in schizophrenia. In: McFarlane WR, ed. *Family therapy in schizophrenia.* New York: Guilford Press, 1983:141–172.

180. Liberman R. Coping and competence as protective factors in the vulnerability–stress model of schizophrenia. In: Goldstein MJ, Hand I, Hahlweg K, eds. *Treatment of schizophrenia: Family assessment and intervention.* Berlin: Springer, 1986:201–216.

181. Liberman RP, Corrigan PW. Designing new psychosocial treatments for schizophrenia. *Psychiatry* 1993;**56**:238–249.

182. Hogarty GE, Kornblith SJ, Greenwald D, et al. Personal therapy: A disorder-relevant psychotherapy for schizophrenia. *Schizophrenia Bulletin* 1995;**21**:379–393.

183. Hogarty G, Kornblith S, Greenwald D, et al. Three-year trials of personal therapy among schizophrenic patients living with or independent of family: I. Description of study and effects on relapse rates. *American Journal of Psychiatry* 1997;**154**:1504–1513.

184. Hogarty GE, Greenwald D, Ulrich RF, et al. Three-year trials of personal therapy among schizophrenic patients living with or independent of family: II. Effects on adjustment of patients. *American Journal of Psychiatry* 1997;**154**:1514–1524.

185. Anderson C. A psychoeducational program for families of patients with schizophrenia. In: McFarlane WR, ed. *Family therapy in schizophrenia.* New York: Guilford Press, 1983:99–116.

186. Marsh DT. The psychodynamic model and services for families: Issues and strategies. In: Lefley H, Wasow M, eds. *Helping families cope with mental illness.* Chur, Switzerland: Harwood Academic Publishers, 1994:105–128.

187. McCubbin HI, McCubbin MA. Typologies of resilient families: Emerging roles of social class and ethnicity. *Family Relations* 1988;**37**:247–254.

188. Lefley HP. *Family caregiving in mental illness.* Thousand Oaks, CA: Sage, 1996.

189. Marsh DT, Lefley HP, Evans-Rhodes D, et al. The family experience of mental illness: Evidence for resilience. *Psychiatric Rehabilitation Journal* 1996;**20**:3–12.

190. Willick MS. Schizophrenia: A parent's experience: Mourning without end. In: Andreasen N, ed. *Schizophrenia: From mind to molecule.* Washington DC: American Psychiatric Press, 1994.

191. Marsh DT, Dickens RM, Koeske RK, et al. Troubled journey: Siblings and children of people with mental illness. *Innovations and Research* 1993;**2**:17–28.

192. Lightburn A, Kemp SP. Family-support programs: Opportunities for community-based practice. *Families in Society: The Journal of Contemporary Human Services* 1994:16–26.

193. Moos R, Tsu V. The crisis of physical illness. In: Moos R, ed. *Coping with physical illness.* London: Plenum Press, 1977.

194. Pearlin LI, Lieberman MA, Menaghan EG, et al. The stress process. *Journal of Health and Social Behavior* 1981;**22**:337–356.

195. Rosenfield S. Labeling mental illness: The effects of received services and perceived stigma on life satisfaction. *American Sociological Review* 1997;**62**:660–672.
196. Link BG, Mirotznik J, Cullen FT. The effectiveness of stigma coping orientations: Can negative consequences of mental illness labeling be avoided? *Journal of Health and Social Behavior* 1991;**32**:302–320.
197. Freeman H, Simmons O. Feeling of stigma among relatives of former mental patients. *Social Problems* 1961;**8**:312–321.
198. Lefley HP. Family burden and family stigma in major mental illness. *American Psychologist* 1989;**44**:556–560.
199. Sommer R. Family advocacy and the mental health system: The recent rise of the alliance for the mentally ill. *Psychiatric Quarterly* 1990;**61**:205–221.
200. Yarrow M, Clausen J, Robbins P. The social meaning of mental illness. *Journal of Social Issues* 1955;**11**:33–48.
201. Phelan JC, Bromet EJ, Link BG. Psychiatric illness and family stigma. *Schizophrenia Bulletin* 1998;**24**:115–126.
202. Friedmann MS, McDermut WH, Solomon DA, et al. Family functioning and mental illness: A comparison of psychiatric and non-clinical families. *Family Process* 1997;**36**:357–367.
203. Lefley H. Aging parents as caregivers of mentally ill adult children: An emerging social problem. *Hospital and Community Psychiatry* 1987;**38**:1063–1070.
204. Maurin JT, Boyd CB. Burden of mental illness on the family: A critical review. *Archives of Psychiatric Nursing* 1990;**4**:99–107.
205. Jackson HJ, Smith N, McGorry P. Relationship between expressed emotion and family burden in psychotic disorders: An exploratory study. *Acta Psychiatrica Scandinavica* 1990;**82**:243–249.
206. Smith J, Birchwood M, Cochrane R, et al. The needs of high and low expressed emotion families: A normative approach. *Social Psychiatry and Psychiatric Epidemiology* 1993;**28**:11–16.
207. Potasznik H, Nelson G. Stress and social support: The burden experienced by the family of a mentally ill person. *American Journal of Community Psychology* 1984;**12**:589–595.
208. Winefield HR, Harvey EJ. Needs of family caregivers in chronic schizophrenia. *Schizophrenia Bulletin* 1994;**20**:557–566.
209. Birchwood M, Cochrane R. Families coping with schizophrenia: Coping styles, their origins and correlates. *Psychological Medicine* 1990;**20**:857–865.
210. Stueve A, Vine P, Struening EL. Perceived burden among caregivers of adults with serious mental illness: Comparison of black, Hispanic and white families. *American Journal of Orthopsychiatry* 1997;**67**:199–209.
211. Beels C, McFarlane W. Thoughts on family therapy and schizophrenia. In: McFarlane WR, ed. *Family therapy in schizophenia*. New York: Guilford Press, 1983:17–40.
212. Mintz L, Nuechterlein K, Goldstein M, et al. The initial onset of schizophrenia and family expressed emotion: Some methodological considerations. *British Journal of Psychiatry* 1989;**154**:212–217.
213. MacGregor P. Grief: The recognized parental response to mental illness in a child. *Social Work* 1994;**39**:160–166.

214. Struening EL, Stueve A, Vine P, et al. Factors associated with grief and depressive symptoms in caregivers of people with serious mental illness. *Research in Community Mental Health* 1995;8:91–94.

215. Willick MS. Schizophrenia: The family's experience. In: Kaufmann C, Gorman J, eds. *Schizophrenia: New directions for clinical research and treatment.* Larchmont, NY: Mary Ann Liebert, 1996:177–187.

216. Johnson D. The family's experience of living with mental illness. In: Lefley HP, Johnson DJ, eds. *Families as allies in treatment of the mentally ill.* Washington, DC: American Psychiatric Association Press, 1990:31–64.

217. Clark RE. Family costs associated with severe mental illness and substance use. *Hospital and Community Psychiatry* 1994;45:808–813.

218. Amador X, Andreasen N, Flaum M, et al. Awareness of illness in schizophrenia, schizoaffective and mood disorders. *Archives of General Psychiatry* 1994;51:826–836.

219. Mishne J. *The evolution and application of clinical theory.* New York: Free Press, 1993.

220. Fromm-Reichmann F. Notes on the development of treatment of schizophrenics by psychoanalytic psychotherapy. *Psychiatry* 1948;2:263–273.

221. Kasinin J, Knight E, Sage P. The parent–child relationship in schizophrenia. *Journal of Nervous and Mental Disorders* 1934;79:249–263.

222. Levy DM. Maternal overprotection and rejection. *Archives of Neurology and Psychiatry* 1931;25:886–889.

223. Levy D. *Maternal overprotection.* New York: Columbia University Press, 1943.

224. Tietz T. A study of mothers of schizophrenic patients. *Psychiatry* 1949;12:55–65.

225. Bateson G, Jackson D, Haley J, et al. Towards a theory of schizophrenia. *Behavioral Science* 1956;1:251–264.

226. Lidz T, Cornelison AR, Fleck S, et al. The intrafamilial environment of the schizophrenic patient: II. Marital schism and marital skew. *American Journal of Psychiatry* 1957;114:241–248.

227. Fellin P. *Mental health and mental illness: Policies, programs, and services.* Itasca, IL: Peacock, 1996.

228. Starr P. *The social transformation of American medicine.* New York: Basic Books, 1982.

229. Brown GW, Monck EM, Carstairs GM, et al. Influence of family life on the course of schizophrenic illness. *British Journal of Society and Medicine* 1958;16:55–68.

230. Brown GW, Rutter M. The measurement of family activities and relationships. *Human Relations* 1966;19:241–263.

231. Leff J, Vaughn C. The role of maintenance therapy and relatives' expressed emotion in the relapse of schizophrenia: A two-year follow-up. *British Journal of Psychiatry* 1981;139:102–104.

232. Vaughn CE, Leff JP. The influence of family and social factors on the course of psychiatric illness: A comparison of schizophrenic and depressed neurotic patients. *British Journal of Psychiatry* 1976;129:125–137.

233. Bebbington P, Kuipers L. The predictive utility of expressed emotion in schizophrenia: An aggregate analysis. *Psychological Medicine* 1994;24:707–718.

234. Miklowitz D, Goldstein M, Doane J, et al. Is expressed emotion an index of a

transactional process?: I. Parent's affective style. *Family Process* 1989;28:153–156.

235. Miklowitz D, Goldstein M, Falloon I, et al. Interactional correlates of expressed emotion in the families of schizophrenics. *British Journal of Psychiatry* 1984; 144:482–487.

236. Hatfield A. Taking issue: The expressed emotion theory: Why families object. *Hospital and Community Psychiatry* 1987;38:341.

237. Hatfield A. Issues in psychoeducation for families of the mentally ill. *International Journal of Mental Health* 1988;17:48–64.

238. Kanter J, Lamb H, Loeper C. Expressed emotion in families: A critical review. *Hospital and Community Psychiatry* 1987;38:374–380.

239. Leff J, Tress K, Edwards B. The clinical course of depressive symptoms in schizophrenia. *Schizophrenia Research* 1988;8:25–30.

240. Lefley HP. Expressed emotion: Conceptual, clinical, and social policy issues. *Hospital and Community Psychiatry* 1992;43:591–598.

241. Birchwood MJ, Smith J. Schizophrenia and the family. In: Orford J, ed. *Coping with disorder in the family.* Kent, UK: Croom Helm, 1987:7–38.

242. Gottschalk L, Falloon I, Marder S, Lebell M, et al. The prediction of relapse of schizophrenic patients using emotional data obtained from their relatives. *Psychiatry Research* 1988;25:261–276.

243. MacMillan J, Gold A, Crow T, et al. Expressed emotion and relapse. *British Journal Psychiatry* 1986;148:133–143.

244. Hogarty G, Anderson C, Reiss Dea. Family psychoeducation, social skills training and maintenance chemotherapy in the aftercare treatment of schizophrenia. *Archives of General Psychiatry* 1986;43:633–642.

245. Kuipers L, Bebbington P. Expressed emotion research in schizophrenia. *Psychological Medicine* 1988;18:893–909.

246. Hyde A, Goldman C. Use of a multi-modal multiple family group and the comprehensive treatment and rehabilitation of people with schizophrenia. *Psychosocial Rehabilitation Journal* 1992;15:77–86.

247. Leff J. Review Article: Controversial issues and growing points in research on relatives' expressed emotion. *International Journal of Social Psychiatry* 1989;35: 133–145.

248. Strachan A, Feingold D, Goldstein M, et al. Is expressed emotion an index of a transactional process?: II. Patient's coping style. *Family Process* 1989;28:169–181.

249. Goldstein M, Rosenfarb I, Woo S, et al. Intrafamilial relationships and the course of schizophrenia. *Acta Psychiatrica Scandanavica* 1994;384(Suppl.):60–66.

250. Wuerker AM. Communication patterns and expressed emotion in families of persons with mental disorders. *Schizophrenia Bulletin* 1996;22:671–690.

251. Wuerker AM. Relational control patterns and expressed emotion in families of persons with schizophrenia and bipolar disorder. *Family Process* 1994;33:389–407.

252. Brewin C, MacCarthy B, Duda R, et al. Attribution and expressed emotion in the relatives of patients with schizophrenia. *Journal of Abnormal Psychology* 1991; 100:546–555.

253. Hooley JM, Licht DM. Expressed emotion and causal attributions in the spouses of depressed patients. *Journal of Abnormal Psychology* 1997;106:298–306.

254. Carter B, McGoldrick M. *The changing family life cycle: A framework for family therapy.* Boston: Allyn & Bacon, 1989.
255. Terkelsen K. Schizophrenia and the family: II. Adverse effects of family therapy. *Family Process* 1983;**22**:191–200.
256. King S, Dixon M. The influence of expressed emotion, family dynamics, and symptom type on the social adjustment of schizophrenic young adults. *Archives of General Psychiatry* 1996;**53**:1098–1104.
257. Pescosolido B, Wright E, Sullivan W. Communities of care: A theoretical perspective on case management models in mental health. *Advances in Medical Sociology* 1995;**6**:37–79.
258. Kinsella KB, Anderson RA, Anderson WT. Coping skills, strengths, and needs as perceived by adult offspring and siblings of people with mentla illness: A retrospective study. *Psychiatric Rehabilitation Journal* 1996;**20**:24–32.
259. McFarlane WR, Dunne E, Lukens E, et al. From research to clinical practice: Dissemination of New York State's family psychoeducation project. *Hospital and Community Psychiatry* 1993;**44**:265–270.
260. Borkman T. Experiential knowledge: A new concept for the analysis of self-help groups. *Social Service Review* 1976;**50**:445–456.
261. Laqueur HP, LaBurt HA, Morong E. Multiple family therapy. In: Masserman J, ed. *Current psychiatric therapies*, Vol. 4. New York: Grune & Stratton, 1964.
262. Detre T, Sayer J, Norton A, et al. An experimental approach to the treatment of the acutely ill psychiatric patient in the general hospital. *Connecticut Medicine* 1961;**25**:613–619.
263. O'Shea MD. Multiple family therapy: Current status and critical appraisal. *Family Process* 1985;**24**:555–582.
264. Lehman AF, Carpenter WT, Jr., Goldman HH, Steinwachs DM. Treatment outcomes in schizophrenia: Implications for practice, policy, and research. *Schizophrenia Bulletin* 1995;**21**:669–675.
265. Mosher L, Keith S. Research on the psychosocial treatment of schizophrenia: A summary report. *American Journal of Psychiatry* 1979;**136**:623–631.
266. Granovetter M. The strength of weak ties. *American Journal of Sociology* 1973;**78**:1360–1380.
267. Reiss D, Costell R. The multiple family group as a small society: Family regulation of interaction with nonmembers. *American Journal of Psychiatry* 1977;**134**:21–24.
268. Falloon I, Boyd J, McGill C, et al. Family management in the prevention of morbidity of schizophrenia. *Archives of General Psychiatry* 1985;**42**:887–896.
269. Spiegel D, Wissler T. Family environment as a predictor of psychiatric rehospitalization. *American Journal of Psychiatry* 1986;**143**:56–60.
270. McFarlane WR. Social networks, expressed emotion and stigma in the families of persons with schizophrenia. Unpublished data, 1985.
271. Harrow M, Astrachan B, Becker R, et al. An investigation into the nature of the patient–family therapy group. *American Journal of Orthopsychiatry* 1967;**37**:888–899.
272. Singer M, Wynne L. Thought disorder and family relations of schizophrenics: III. Methodology using projective techniques. *Archives of General Psychiatry* 1965;**12**:187–200.

273. Wagener DK, Hogarty GE, Goldstein MJ, et al. Information processing and communication deviance in schizophrenic patients and their mothers. *Psychiatry Research* 1986;**18**:365–377.

274. Asch S. *Social psychology.* Englewood Cliffs, NJ: Prentice-Hall, 1952.

275. Festinger L. A theory of social comparison processes. *Human Relations* 1957;**7**: 117–140.

276. Hackman JR. Group influences in individuals. In: Dunnette M, ed. *Handbook of industrial and organization psychology.* Chicago: Rand McNally, 1976.

277. Schachter S. Deviation, rejection and communication. *Journal of Abnormal and Social Psychology* 1951;**46**:190–207.

278. Nugter MA, Dingemans PM, Linszen DH, et al. Parental communication deviance: Its stability and the effect of family treatment in recent-onset schizophrenia. *Acta Psychiatrica Scandinavica* 1997;**95**:199–204.

279. Laqueur HP, LaBurt H, Morong E. Multiple family therapy: Further developments. *International Journal of Social Psychiatry* 1964;**10**:69–80.

280. Beels CC. Family and social management of schizophrenia. *Schizophrenia Bulletin* 1975;**13**:97–118.

281. Berman K. Multiple family therapy: Its possibilities in preventing readmission. *Mental Hygiene* 1966;**50**:367–370.

282. Levin E. Therapeutic multiple family groups. *International Journal of Group Psychotherapy* 1966;**19**:203–208.

283. Lurie A, Ron H. Socialization program as part of aftercare planning. *General Psychiatric Association Journal* 1972;**17**:157–162.

284. Lansky M, Bley C, McVey G, et al. Multiple family group as aftercare. *International Journal Group Psychotherapy* 1978;**29**:211–224.

285. Falloon IRH, Lieberman R, Lillie F. Family therapy for relapsing schizophrenics and their families: A pilot study. *Family Process* 1981;**20**:211–221.

286. Benningfield AB. Multiple family therapy systems. *Advances in Family Psychiatry* 1980;**2**:411–424.

287. Strelnick AH. Multiple family group therapy: A review of the literature. *Family Process* 1977;**16**:307–325.

288. Goldstein MJ, Rodnick EH, Evans JR, et al. Drug and family therapy in the aftercare of acute schizophrenics. *Archives of General Psychiatry* 1978;**35**:1169–1177.

289. Brown GW, Monck EM, Carstairs GM, et al. Influence of family life on the course of schizophrenic illness. *British Journal of Psychiatry* 1962;**16**:55–68.

290. Schaeffer DS. Effects of frequent hospitalizations on behavior of psychotic patients in multiple family therapy. *Journal of Clinical Psychology* 1969;**25**:104–105.

291. Spitzer RL, Endicott J, Robins E. *Research Diagnostic Criteria (RDC) for a selected group of functional disorders.* New York State Psychiatric Institute, New York, 1978.

292. American Psychiatric Association. *Diagnostic and statistical manual of mental disorders,* 3rd ed., rev. Washington, DC: American Psychiatric Press, 1987.

293. Vaughn CE, Snyder KS, Jones S, et al. Family factors in schizophrenic relapse. *Archives of General Psychiatry* 1984;**41**:1169–1177.

294. Young JL, Zonana HV, Shepler L. Medication noncompliance in schizophrenia: Codification and update. *American Academy of Psychiatry and the Law* 1986;**14**: 105–122.

295. McFarlane WR, Stastny P, Deakins S. Family-aided assertive community treatment: A comprehensive rehabilitation and intensive case management approach for persons with schizophrenic disorders. *New Directions in Mental Health Services* 1992;**53**:43–54.

296. McFarlane WR, Stastny P, Deakins SM, et al. *Employment outcomes in Family-aided Assertive Community Treatment.* American Psychiatric Association Institute on Psychiatric Services, Boston, October 1995.

297. McFarlane WR, Dushay RA, Deakins SM, et al. Employment outcomes in Family-aided Assertive Community Treatment. *American Journal of Orthopsychiatry* 2000;**70**:203–214.

298. Kay S, Fiszbein A, Opler L. The positive and negative syndrome scale (PANSS) for schizophrenia. *Schizophrenia Bulletin* 1987;**13**:261–276.

299. Anthony WA, Cohen MR, Vitalo R. The measurement of rehabilitation outcome. *Schizophrenia Bulletin* 1978;**4**:365–383.

300. Bond GR, Boyer SL. Rehabilitation programs and outcomes. In: Ciardello JA, Bell MD, eds. *Vocational rehabilitation of persons with prolonged mental illness.* Baltimore: Johns Hopkins University Press, 1988:231–263.

301. Test MA, Stein LI. Alternatives to mental hospital treatment: III. Social cost. *Archives of General Psychiatry* 1980;**37**:409–412.

302. Hoult J, Reynolds I, Charbonneau Powis M, et al. A controlled study of psychiatric hospital versus community treatment-the effect on relatives. *Australian and New Zealand Journal of Psychiatry* 1981;**15**:323–328.

303. Cardin VA, McGill CW, Falloon IRH. An economic analysis: Costs, benefits, and effectiveness. In: Falloon IRH, ed. *Family management of schizophrenia: A study of clinical, social, family, and economic benefits.* Baltimore: Johns Hopkins University Press, 1985:115–123.

304. Dyck D, Short RA, Hendryx MS, et al. Management of negative symptoms among patients with schizophrenia attending multiple-family groups. *Psychiatric Services* 2000;**51**:512–519.

305. Leff J, Berkowitz N, Shavit N, et al. A trial of family therapy v. a relatives group for schizophrenia. *British Journal of Psychiatry* 1989;**145**:58–66.

306. Schooler NR, Keith SJ, Severe JB, et al. Relapse and rehospitalization during maintenance treatment of schizophrenia: The effects of dose reduction and family treatment. *Archives of General Psychiatry* 1997;**54**:453–463.

307. Smith J, Birchwood M. Specific and non-specific educational intervention with families living with a schizophrenic relative. *British Journal of Psychiatry* 1987; **150**:645–652.

308. Reilly J, Rohrbaugh M, Lachner J. A controlled evaluation of psychoeducation workshops for relatives of state hospital patients. *Journal of Marital and Family Therapy* 1988;**14**:429–432.

309. Abramowitz IA, Coursey RD. Impact of an educational support group on family participants who take care of their schizophrenic relatives. *Journal of Consulting and Clinical Psychology* 1989;**57**:232–236.

310. Posner C, Wilson K, Kral M, et al. Family psychoeducational support groups in schizophrenia. *American Journal of Orthopsychiatry* 1992;**62**:206–218.

311. Solomon P, Draine J, Mannion E, et al. Impact of brief family psychoeducation on self-efficacy. *Schizophrenia Bulletin* 1996;**22**:41–50.

312. Solomon P, Draine J, Mannion E, et al. Effectiveness of two models of brief family education: Retention of gains by family members with serious mental illness. *American Journal of Orthopsychiatry* 1997;67:177–186.

313. McFarlane, WR, Lukens, E, Link, B, et al. Multiple-family groups and psychoeducation in the treatment of schizophrenia. *Archives of General Psychiatry* 1995;52:679–687.

314. Leff J, Vaughn C. The interaction of life events and relatives' expressed emotion in schizophrenia and depressive neurosis. *British Journal of Psychiatry* 1980; 136:146–153.

315. Chung R, Langeluddecke P, Tennant C. Threatening life events in the onset of schizophrenia, schizophreniform psychosis and hypomania. *British Journal of Psychiatry* 1986;148:680–685.

316. Day R. Stressful life events preceding the acute onset of schizophrenia: A cross-national study from the World Health Organization. *Culture, Medicine and Psychiatry* 1987;11:123–205.

317. Hirsch S, Bowen J, Emami J, et al. A one year prospective study of the effect of life events and medication in the aetiology of schizophrenic relapse. *British Journal of Psychiatry* 1996;168:49–56.

318. Miller WR, Rollnick S. *Motivational interviewing: Preparing people to change addictive behavior.* New York: Guilford Press, 1991.

319. Vaughn C, Leff J. Patterns of emotional response in relatives of schizophrenic patients. *Schizophrenia Bulletin* 1981;7:43–44.

320. North CS, Pollio DE, Sachar B, et al. The family as caregiver: A group psychoeducation model for schizophrenia. *American Journal of Orthopsychiatry* 1998; 68:39–46.

321. Mueser KT, Gingerich S. *Coping with schizophrenia: A guide for families.* Oakland, CA: New Harbinger, 1994.

322. Hatfield AB. *Family education in mental illness.* New York: Guilford Press, 1990.

323. Torrey EF. *Surviving schizophrenia.* New York: Harper & Row, 1983.

324. Knoedler WH. How the Training in Community Living program helps patients to work. *New Directions for Mental Health Services* 1979;2:57–66.

325. Field G, Allness D, Knoedler W. Application of the Training in Community Living program to rural areas. *Journal of Community Psychology* 1980;8:9–15.

326. Witheridge TF, Dincin J. An assertive outreach program in an urban setting. *New Directions for Mental Health Services* 1985;26:65–76.

327. Bond GR, Miller LD, Krumwied RD, et al. Assertive case management in three CMHCs: A controlled study. *Hospital and Community Psychiatry* 1988;39:411–418.

328. Stein LI, Ganser LJ. Wisconsin's system for funding mental health services. *New Directions for Mental Health Services* 1983;18:25–32.

329. Test MA, Knoedler WH, Allness DJ. The long-term treatment of young schizophrenics in a community support program. *New Directions for Mental Health Services* 1985;26:17–27.

330. Olfson M. Assertive community treatment: An evaluation of the experimental evidence. *Hospital and Community Psychiatry* 1990;41:634–641.

331. Thompson KS, Griffith EEH, Leaf PS. A historical review of the Madison model of community care. *Hospital and Community Psychiatry* 1990;41:625–634.

332. Test MA. *Long-term employment outcome in the Program for Assertive Community Treatment*. American Psychiatric Association Institute on Psychiatric Services, Boston, October 1995.
333. Marx AJ, Ludwig AM. Resurrection of the family of the chronic schizophrenic. *American Journal of Psychotherapy* 1969;23:37–57.
334. Marx AJ, Test MA, Stein LI. Extrohospital management of severe mental illness. *Archives of General Psychiatry* 1973;29:505–511.
335. Allness D, Knoedler W. Personal communication, 1988.
336. Taube CA, Marlock L, Burus BJ. New directions in research on assertive community treatment. *Hospital and Community Psychiatry* 1990;41:642–647.
337. Reynolds I, Hoult JE. The relatives of the mentally ill: A comparative trial of community-oriented and hospital-oriented psychiatric care. *Journal of Nervous and Mental Disease* 1984;172:480–489.
338. Cook WL, Strachan AM, Goldstein MJ, et al. Expressed emotion and reciprocal affective relationships in families of disturbed adolescents. *Family Process* 1989;28:337–348.
339. Stein LI, Santos AB. *Assertive community treatment of persons with severe mental illness*. New York: Norton, 1998.
340. Strauss JS, Carpenter WT. Prediction of outcome in schizophrenia. *Archives of General Psychiatry* 1977;34:159–163.
341. Falloon IRH, McGill CW, Boyd JL. Family management in the prevention of morbidity in schizophrenia: Social outcome of a two-year longitudinal study. *Psychological Medicine* 1992;17:59–66.
342. Hogarty GE, Anderson CM, Reiss DJ, et al. Family psychoeducation, social skills training, and maintenance chemotherapy in the aftercare treatment of schizophrenia: II. Two-year effects of a controlled study on relapse and adjustment. *Archives of General Psychiatry* 1991;48:340–347.
343. McFarlane WR, Dushay RA, Stastny P, et al. A comparison of two levels of Family-aided Assertive Community Treatment. *Psychiatric Services* 1996;47:744–750.
344. Bond GR. Vocational rehabilitation. In: Liberman RP, ed. *Handbook of psychiatric rehabilitation*. New York: MacMillan, 1992:244–263.
345. Bachrach LL. Service planning for chronic mental patients: Some principles. *International Journal of Group Psychotherapy* 1991;41:23–31.
346. Becker DR, Drake RE. Individual placement and support: A community mental health center approach to vocational rehabilitation. *Community Mental Health Journal* 1994;30:519–532.
347. Drake RE, Becker DR, Biesanz JC, et al. Rehabilitative day treatment vs supported employment: I. Vocational outcomes. *Community Mental Health Journal* 1994;30:519–532.
348. Drake RE, McHugo GJ, Becker DR, et al. The New Hampshire study of supported employment for people with severe mental illness. *Journal of Consulting and Clinical Psychology* 1996;64:391–399.
349. Chandler D, Meisel J, Hu TW, et al. Client outcomes in a three-year controlled study of an integrated service agency model. *Psychiatric Services* 1996;47:1337–1343.
350. Bachrach LL. Perspectives on work and rehabilitation. *Hospital and Community Psychiatry* 1991;42:890–891.

351. Arns PG, Linney JA. Work, self and life satisfaction for persons with severe and persistent mental disorders. *Psychosocial Rehabilitation Journal* 1993;17:63–79.
352. Balser R, Harvey B. *Vocational Pathways: A manual*. Portland, ME: Maine Medical Center, 1996.
353. Granovetter MS. *Getting a job: A study of contacts and careers*. Cambridge, MA: Harvard University Press, 1974.
354. Granovetter MS. Placement as brokerage—information problems in the labor market for rehabilitated workers. In: Vandergoot D, Worrall J, eds. *Placement in rehabilitation*. Baltimore, MD: University Park Press, 1979.
355. Lamb HR, Goertzel V. Are they really in the community? *Archives of General Psychiatry* 1971;24:29–34.
356. Carpenter M. Residential placement for the chronic psychiatric patient: A review and evaluation of the literature. *Schizophrenia Bulletin* 1978;4:384–398.
357. Linn N, Klett C, Caffey E. Foster home characteristics and psychiatric patient outcome. *Archives of General Psychiatry* 1980;37:129–132.
358. Kruzich J, Kruzich S. Milieu factors influencing patients' integration into community residential facilities. *Hospital and Community Psychiatry* 1985;36:378–382.
359. Segal S, Aviram U. *The mentally ill in community-based sheltered care: A study of community care and social integration*. New York: Wiley, 1978.
360. Cournos F. The impact of environmental factors on outcome in residential programs. *Hospital and Community Psychiatry* 1987;38:848–852.
361. Segal S, Holschuh J. Effects of sheltered care environments and resident characteristics on the development of social networks. *Hospital and Community Psychiatry* 1991;42:1125–1131.
362. McFarlane WR, Dunne E. Family psychoeducation and multi-family groups in the treatment of schizophrenia. *Directions in Psychiatry* 1991;11:2–7.
363. Drake R, Osher F. Family psychoeducation when there is no family. *Hospital and Community Psychiatry* 1987;38:274–277.
364. Lehman A, Newman S. Housing. In: Breakey WR, ed. *Integrated mental health services*. New York: Oxford University Press, 1996.
365. Ranz JM, Horen BT, McFarlane WR, et al. Creating a supportive environment using staff psychoeducation in a supervised residence. *Hospital and Community Psychiatry* 1991;42:1154–1159.
366. Miklowitz DJ, Goldstein MJ, Nuechterlein KH, et al. Family factors and the course of bipolar disorder. *Archives of General Psychiatry* 1988;45:225–231.
367. Sturgeon D, Kuipers L, Berkowitz R, et al. Psychophysiological responses of schizophrenic patients to high and low expressed emotion relatives. *British Journal of Psychiatry* 1981;138:40–45.
368. Tarrier N, Vaughn C, Lader MH, et al. Bodily responses to people and events in schizophrenics. *Archives of General Psychiatry* 1979;36:311–315.
369. Patterson G, Reid J, Jones R, et al. *A social learning approach to family intervention*. Eugene, OR: Castalia, 1975.
370. Venables PH. Schizophrenia: Towards a new synthesis. In: Wing JK, ed. *Cognitive disorder*. New York: Academic Press, 1978.
371. Linn N, Caffey E, Klett C, et al. Day treatment and psychotropic drugs in the aftercare of schizophrenic patients. *Archives of General Psychiatry* 1979;36:1055–1066.

372. Carling PJ. Housing and supports for persons with mental illness: Emerging approaches to research and practice. *Hospital and Community Psychiatry* 1993; 44:439–444.

373. Nagy M, Fisher G, Tessler R. Effects of facility characteristics on the social adjustment of mentally ill residents of board-and-care homes. *Hospital and Community Psychiatry* 1988;39:1281–1286.

374. McCarthy J, Nelson G. An evaluation of supportive housing for current and former psychiatric patients. *Hospital and Community Psychiatry* 1991;42:1254–1256.

375. Moos R. *Community-Oriented Programs Environment Scale manual*, 2nd ed. Palo Alto: Consulting Psychologists Press, 1988.

376. Falloon I, Lieberman R. Behavioral family interventions in the management of chronic schizophrenia. In: McFarlane WR, ed. *Family therapy in schizophrenia*. New York: Guilford Press, 1983:141–172.

377. Steinglass P. Psychoeducational family therapy for schizophrenia: A review essay. *Psychiatry* 1987;50:14–23.

378. Goodwin FK, Jamison KR. *Manic–depressive illness*. New York: Oxford University Press, 1990.

379. Miklowitz D, Goldstein M. Family factors and the course of bipolar affective disorder. *Archives of General Psychiatry* 1988;45:225–231.

380. O'Connell R, Mayo J. Social support and long-term lithium outcome. *British Journal of Psychiatry* 1985;147:272–275.

381. Rosenfarb IS, Miklowitz DJ, Goldstein MJ, et al. Family transactions and relapse in bipolar disorder. *Family Process* 2001;40:5–14.

382. Strakowski SM, Keck JPE, McElroy SL, et al. Twelve-month outcome after a first hospitalization for affective psychosis. *Archives of General Psychiatry* 1998; 55:49–55.

383. Coryell W, Scheftner W, Keller M, et al. The enduring psychosocial consequences of mania and depression. *American Journal of Psychiatry* 1993;150: 720–727.

384. Bauwens F, Tracy A, Pardoen D, et al. Social adjustment of remitted bipolar and unipolar out-patients: A comparison with age- and sex-matched controls. *British Journal of Psychiatry* 1991;159:239–244.

385. Janowski D, Leff M. Playing the manic game. *Archives of General Psychiatry* 1970;22:252–261.

386. Moltz D. Bipolar disorder and the family: An integrative model. *Family Process* 1993;32:409–423.

387. Holder D, Anderson C. Psychoeducational family intervention for depressed patients and their families. In: Keitner GI, ed. *Depression and families: Impact and treatment*. Washington, DC: American Psychiatric Press, 1989.

388. van Gorp WG, Altshuler L, Theberge DC, et al. Cognitive impairment in euthymic bipolar patients with and without prior alcohol dependence: A preliminary study. *Archives of General Psychiatry* 1998;55:41–46.

389. Coyne JC. Depression and the response of others. *Journal of Abnormal Psychology* 1976;85:186–193.

390. Coyne JC. Interpersonal processes in depression. In: Keitner GI, ed. *Depression and families: Impact and treatment*. Washington, DC: American Psychiatric Press, 1989.

391. Coyne JC, Kessler RC, Tal M, et al. Living with a depressed person. *Journal of Consulting and Clinical Psychology* 1987;**55**:347–352.

392. Beardslee WR, Hoke L, Wheelock I, et al. Initial findings on preventive intervention for families with parental affective disorders. *American Journal of Psychiatry* 1992;**149**:1335–1340.

393. Clarkin JF, Haas GL, Glick ID. Inpatient family intervention. In: Clarkin JF, Haas GL, Glick ID, eds. *Affective disorders and the family: Assessment and treatment.* New York: Guilford Press, 1988:134–152.

394. Clarkin JF, Carpenter D, Hull D, et al. Effects of psychoeducational intervention for married patients with bipolar disorder and their spouses. *Psychiatric Services* 1998;**49**:531–533.

395. Goldstein MJ, Miklowitz DJ. Family intervention for persons with bipolar disorder. *New Directions in Mental Health Services* 1994;**62**:23–35.

396. Miklowitz DJ, Frank E, George EL. New psychosocial treatments for the outpatient management of bipolar disorder. *Psychopharmacology Bulletin* 1996;**32**:613–621.

397. Miklowitz DJ, Goldstein MJ. *Bipolar disorder: A family-focused treatment approach.* New York: Guilford Press, 1997.

398. Miklowitz DJ, Simoneau TL, George EL, et al. Family-focused treatment of bipolar disorder: 1–year effects of a psychoeducational program in conjunction with pharmacotherapy. *Biological Psychiatry* 2000;**48**:582–592.

399. Anderson CM, Griffin S, Rossi A, et al. A comparative study of the impact of education vs. process groups for families of patients with affective disorders. *Family Process* 1986;**25**:185–205.

400. McFarlane WR, Deakins SM, Gingerich SL, et al. *Multiple-family psychoeducational group treatment manual.* New York: New York State Psychiatric Institute, 1991.

401. White M. *Selected papers.* Adelaide: Dulwich Centre, 1989.

402. Wehr TA, Sack DA, Rosenthal NE. Sleep reduction as a final common pathway in the genesis of mania. *American Journal of Psychiatry* 1987;**144**:201–204.

403. Blacker D, Tsuang MT. Contested boundaries of bipolar disorder and the limits of categorical diagnosis in psychiatry. *American Journal of Psychiatry* 1992;**149**:1473–1483.

404. Merikangas KR. Assortive mating for psychiatric disorders and psychological traits. *Archives of General Psychiatry* 1982;**39**:1173–1180.

405. Keitner GI, Miller IW. Family functioning and major depression: An overview. *American Journal of Psychiatry* 1990;**147**:1128–1137.

406. Crowther JH. The relationship between depression and marital maladjustment: A descriptive study. *Journal of Nervous and Mental Disease* 1985;**173**:227–231.

407. Miller IW, Kabacoff RI, Keitner GI, et al. Family functioning in the families of psychiatric patients. *Comprehensive Psychiatry* 1986;**27**:302–312.

408. Jacob M, Frank E, Kupfer D, et al. Recurrent depression: An assessment of family burden and family attitudes. *Journal of Clinical Psychiatry* 1987;**48**:395–400.

409. Fadden G, Bebbington P, Kuipers L. Caring and its burdens: A study of the spouses of depressed patients. *British Journal of Psychiatry* 1987;**151**:660–667.

410. Keitner GI, Ryan CE, Miller IW, et al. 12–month outcome of patients with major

depression and comorbid psychiatric or medical illness (compound depression). *American Journal of Psychiatry* 1991;**148**:345–50.

411. Bouras N, Vanger P, Bridges PK. Marital problems in chronically depressed and physically ill patients and their spouses. *Comprehensive Psychiatry* 1986;**27**:127–130.

412. Merikangas RK, Prusoff BA, Kupfer DJ, et al. Marital adjustment in major depression. *Journal of Affective Disorders* 1985;**9**:5–11.

413. Hinchcliffe MK, Vaughan PW, Hooper D, et al. The melancholy marriage: An inquiry into the interaction of depression: II. Expressiveness. *British Journal of Medical Psychology* 1977;**50**:125–142.

414. Billings AG, Moos RH. Life stresors and social resources affect posttreatment outcomes among depressed patients. *Journal of Abnormal Psychology* 1985;**94**:140–153.

415. Krantz SE, Moos RH. Functioning and life context among spouses of remitted and nonremitted depressed patients. *Journal of Consulting and Clinical Psychology* 1987;**55**:353–360.

416. Keitner GI, Miller IW, Epstein NB, et al. Family functioning and the course of major depression. *Comprehensive Psychiatry* 1987;**28**:54–64.

417. Swindle RWJ, Cronkite RC, Moos RH. Life stressors, social resources, coping and the 4–year course of unipolar depression. *Journal of Abnormal Psychology* 1989;**98**:468–477.

418. George LK, Blazer DG, Hughes DC, et al. Social support and the outcome of major depression. *British Journal of Psychiatry* 1989;**154**:478–485.

419. Moos RF. Depressed outpatients' life contexts, amount of treatment, and treatment outcome. *Journal of Nervous and Mental Disease* 1990;**178**:105–112.

420. Goering PN, Lancee WJ, Freeman SJ. Marital support and recovery from depression. *British Journal of Psychiatry* 1992;**160**:76–82.

421. McLeod JD, Kessler RC, Landis KR. Speed of recovery from major depressive episodes in a community sample of married men and women. *Journal of Abnormal Psychology* 1992;**101**:277–286.

422. Keitner GI, Ryan CE, Miller IW, et al. Recovery and major depression: Factors associated with twelve-month outcome. *American Journal of Psychiatry* 1992;**149**:93–99.

423. Keitner GI, Ryan CE, Miller IW, et al. Psychosocial factors and the long-term course of major depression. *Journal of Affective Disorders* 1997;**44**:57–67.

424. Vaughn C, Leff J. The measurement of expressed emotion in the families of psychiatric patients. *British Journal of Social and Clinical Psychology* 1976;**15**:157–165.

425. Hooley J, Orley J. Levels of expressed emotion and relapse in depressed patients. *British Journal of Psychiatry* 1986;**148**:642–647.

426. Hooley JM, Teasdale JD. Preditors of relapse in unipolar depressives: Expressed emotion, marital distress and percieved criticism. *Journal of Abnormal Psychology* 1989;**98**:229–235.

427. Miller IW, Keitner GI, Schatzberg A, et al. Psychosocial functioning of chronically depressed patients before and after treatment with sertraline or imipramine. *Journal of Clinical Psychiatry* 1998;**59**:608–619.

428. McCullough JP, McCune KJ, Kay AL, et al. One-year prospective replication study of an untreated sample of community dysthymia subjects. *Journal of Nervous and Mental Disease* 1994;**182**:396–401.

429. Merikangas KR, Bromet EJ, Spiker DG. Assortative mating, social adjustment, and course of illness in primary affective disorder. *Archives of General Psychiatry* 1983;**40**:795–800.

430. Stewart JW, Quitkin FM, McGrath PJ, et al. Social functioning in chronic depression: Effect of 6 weeks of antidepressant treatment. *Psychiatry Research* 1988; **25**:213–222.

431. Kocsis JH, Frances AJ, Voss C, et al. Imipramine and social–vocational adjustment in chronic depression. *American Journal of Psychiatry* 1988;**145**:997–999.

432. Kocsis JH, Zisook S, Davidson J, et al. Double-blind comparison of sertraline, imipramine, and placebo in the treatment of dysthymia: Psychosocial outcomes. *American Journal of Psychiatry* 1997;**154**:390–395.

433. Friedman RA, Markowitz JC, Parides M, et al. Acute response of social functioning in dysthymic patients with desipramine. *Journal of Affective Disorders* 1995;**34**:85–88.

434. Agosti V, Stewart JW, Quitkin FM. Life satisfaction and psychosocial functioning in chronic depression: Effect of acute treatment with antidepressants. *Journal of Affective Disorders* 1991;**23**:35–41.

435. Markowitz JC, Friedman RA, Miller N, et al. Interpersonal improvement in chronically depressed patients treated with desipramine. *Journal of Affective Disorders* 1996;**41**:59–62.

436. Brown GW, Moran P. Clinical and psychosocial origins of chronic depressive episodes: I. A community survey. *British Journal of Psychiatry* 1994;**165**:447–456.

437. Henck JW, Frahm DT, Anderson JA. Validation of automated behavioral test systems. *Neurotoxicology and Teratology* 1996;**18**:189–197.

438. Miller IW, Norman WH, Keitner GI, et al. Compounded depression and family functioning. *Behavior Therapy* 1989;**20**:25–47.

439. Glick ID, Clarkin JF, Haas GL, et al. A randomized clinical trial of inpatient family intervent: VI. Mediating variables and outcome. *Family Process* 1991;**30**:85–99.

440. Antonuccio DO, Akins WT, Chatham PM, et al. An exploratory study: The psychoeducational group treatment of drug-refractory unipolar depression. *Journal of Behavioral Therapy and Experimental Psychiatry* 1984;**15**:309–313.

441. Barrara M. An evaluation of a brief group therapy for depression. *Journal of Consulting and Clinical Psychology* 1979;**47**:413–415.

442. Brown RA, Lewinsohn PM. A psychoeducational approach to the treatment of depression: Comparison of group, individual, and minimal contact procedures. *Journal of Clinical and Consulting Psychology* 1984;**52**:774–783.

443. Comaz-Diaz L. Effects of cognitive and behavioral group treatment on the depressive symptomology of Puerto Rican women. *Journal of Consulting and Clinical Psychology* 1981;**49**:627–632.

444. Covi L, Lipman RS. Cognitive behavioral group psychotherapy combined with imipramine in major depression. *Psychopharmacology Bulletin* 1987;**23**:173–176.

445. Fleming B, Thorton D. Coping skills training as a component in the short-term

treatment of depression. *Journal of Consulting and Clinical Psychology* 1980; 48:652–654.

446. Fuchs CZ, Rehm LP. A self-control behavior therapy program for depression. *Journal of Consulting and Clinical Psychology* 1977;45:206–215.

447. Hogg J, Deffenbacher J. A comparison of cognitive and interpersonal-process group therapies in the treatment of depression among college students. *Journal of Counseling Psychology* 1988;35:304–310.

448. LaPointe K, Rimm D. Cognitive, assertive, and insight-oriented group therapies in the treatment of reactive depression in women. *Psychotherapy: Theory, Research and Practice* 1980;17:312–321.

449. Lewinsohn P, Antonuccio D, Steinmetz J, et al. *The coping with depression course: A psychoeducational intervention for unipolar depression.* Eugene, OR: Castalia, 1984.

450. Neimeyer R, Feixas G. The role of homework and skill acquisition in the outcome of group cognitive therapy for depression. *Behavior Therapy* 1990;21: 281–292.

451. Nezu AM. Efficacy of a social problem-solving therapy approach for unipolar depression. *Journal of Consulting and Clinical Psychology* 1986;54:196–202.

452. Nezu AM, Perri MG. Social problem-solving therapy for unipolar depression: An initial dismantling investigation. *Journal of Consulting and Clinical Psychology* 1989;57:408–413.

453. Rehm L, Fuchs C, Roth D, et al. A comparison of self-control and assertion skills treatment of depression. *Behavior Therapy* 1979;10:429–442.

454. Rehm LP, Kaslow NJ, Rabin AS. Cognitive and behavioral targets in a self-control therapy program for depression. *Journal of Consulting and Clinical Psychology* 1987;55:60–67.

455. Rude SS. Relative benefits of assertion or cognitive self-control treatment for depression as a function of proficiency in each domain. *Journal of Consulting and Clinical Psychology* 1986;54:390–394.

456. Sanchez VC, Lewinsohn PM, Larson DW. Assertion training: Effectiveness in the treatment of depression. *Journal of Clinical Psychology* 1980;36:526–529.

457. Shaw BF. Comparison of cognitive therapy and behavior therapy in the treatment of depression. *Journal of Consulting and Clinical Psychology* 1977;45:543–551.

458. Steuer JL, Mintz J, Hammen CL, et al. Cognitive-behavioral and psychodynamic group psychotherapy in treatment of geriatric depression. *Journal of Consulting and Clinical Psychology* 1984;52:180–189.

459. Teri L, Lewinsohn P. Individual and group treatment of unipolar depression: Comparison of treatment outcome and identification of predictors of successful treatment outcome. *Behavior Therapy* 1986;17:215–228.

460. Thompson LW, Gallagher D, Nies G, et al. Evaluation of the effectiveness of professionals and nonprofessionals as instructors of "coping with depression" classes for elders. *Gerontologist* 1983;23:390–396.

461. Wierzbicki M, Bartlett T. The efficacy of group and individual cognitve therapy for mild depression. *Cognitive Therapy and Research* 1987;11:337–342.

462. Zettle RD, Rains JC. Group cognitive and contextual therapies in treatment of depression. *Journal of Clinical Psychology* 1989;45:436–445.

463. Frank E, Kupfer DJ, Wagner EF, et al. Efficacy of interpersonal psychotherapy as a maintenance treatment of recurrent depression. *Archives of General Psychiatry* 1991;48:1053–1059.

464. Basco MR, Rush AJ. *Cognitive-behavioral therapy for bipolar disorder.* New York: Guilford Press, 1996.

465. Yalom ID. *The theory and practice of group psychotherapy.* New York: Basic Books, 1995.

466. Anderson, C. *Guidelines for patients and families living with an affective disorder.* Lecture at the Cape Cod Institute, August 24, 1985.

467. Schou M. *Lithium treatment of manic depressive illness: A practical guide,* 5th rev. ed. New York: Karger, 1993.

468. National Depressive and Manic–Depressive Association. *A guide to depressive and manic–depressive illness: Diagnosis, treatment and support.* NDMDA, 1998.

469. Gonzalez S, Steinglass P, Reiss D. Putting the illness in its place: Discussion groups for families with chronic medical illnesses. *Family Process* 1989;28:69–87.

470. Keitner GI, Solomon DA, Ryan CE, et al. Prodromal and residual symptoms in bipolar I disorder. *Comprehensive Psychiatry* 1996;37:362–367.

471. Linehan MM, Heard HL, Armstrong HE. Naturalistic follow-up of a behavioral treatment for chronically parasuicidal borderline patients. *Archives of General Psychiatry* 1993;50:971–974.

472. Gunderson JG, Englund DW. Characterizing the families of borderlines. *Psychiatric Clinics of North America* 1981;4:159–168.

473. Gunderson J, Sabo A. The phenomenological and conceptual interface of borderline personality disorder and post-traumatic stress disorder. *American Journal of Psychiatry* 1993;150:19–27.

474. Young DW, Gunderson JG. Family images of borderline adolescents. *Psychiatry* 1995;58:164–172.

475. Schwartz CE, Dorer DJ, Beardslee WR, et al. Maternal expressed emotion and parental affective disorder: Risk for childhood depressive disorder, substance abuse, or conduct disorder. *Journal of Psychiatric Research* 1990;24:231–250.

476. Hooley J, Richters J, Weintraub S, et al. Psychopathology and marital distress: The positive side of positive symptoms. *Journal of Abnormal Psychology* 1987; 96:27–33.

477. Kernberg OF. Borderline personality organization. *Journal of the American Psychoanalytic Association* 1967;15:641–685.

478. Siever LJ, Frucht W. *The new view of self.* New York: Simon & Schuster/Macmillan, 1997.

479. Kimble CR, Oepen G, Weinberg E, et al. Neurological vulnerability and trauma in borderline personality disorder. In: Zanarini MC, ed. *Role of sexual abuse in the etiology of borderline personality disorder.* Washington, DC: American Psychiatric Press, 1997:165–180.

480. Modell AH. Primitive object relationships and the predisposition to schizophrenia. *International Journal of Psychoanalysis* 1963;44:282–292.

481. Masterson J, Rinsley D. The borderline syndrome: The role of the mother in the genesis and psychic structure of the borderline personality. *International Journal of Psychoanalysis* 1975;56:163–177.

482. Adler G, Buie DH, Jr. Aloneness and borderline psychopathology: The possible relevance of child development issues. *International Journal of Psychoanalysis* 1979;60:83–96.

483. Gunderson JG. *Borderline personality disorder.* Washington, DC: American Psychiatric Press, 1984.

484. Gunderson J. The borderline patient's intolerance of aloneness: insecure attachments and therapist availability. *American Journal of Psychiatry* 1996;153:752–758.

485. Bowlby J. *A secure base: Parent–child attachment and healthy human development.* New York: Basic Books, 1988.

486. Ruiz-Sancho A, Fogler J, Gunderson JG. *Factors that influence the family involvement in a study of a psychoeducational treatment of borderline personality disorder.* Paper presented at the 5th International Congress on the Disorders of Personality, Vancouver, BC, Canada, June 1997.

487. Hafner RJ. Anxiety disorders and family therapy. *Australian and New Zealand Journal of Family Therapy* 1992;13:99–104.

488. Hibbs ED, Hamburger SD, Lenane M, et al. Determinants of expressed emotion in families of disturbed and normal children. *Journal of Psychology and Psychiatry* 1991;32:757–770.

489. Marks IM. The reduction of fear: Towards a unifying theory. *Journal of the Canadian Psychiatric Association* 1973;18:9–12.

490. Leonard HL, Swedo SE, Lenane MC, et al. A 2- to 7–year follow-up study of 54 obsessive–compulsive children and adolescents. *Archives of General Psychiatry* 1993;50:429–439.

491. Steketee G. Social support and treatment outcome of obsessive compulsive disorder at 9–month follow-up. *Behavioural Psychotherapy* 1993;21:81–95.

492. Van Noppen B, Steketee G, McCorkle BH, et al. Group and multi-family behavioral treatment for obsessive compulsive disorder: A pilot study. *Journal of Anxiety Disorders* 1997;11:431–446.

493. Nymberg JH, Van Noppen B. Obsessive–compulsive disorder: A concealed diagnosis. *American Family Physician* 1994;49:1129–1137.

494. Karno M, Golding JM, Sorenson SB, et al. The epidemiology of obsessive compulsive disorder in five U.S. communities. *Archives of General Psychiatry* 1988; 45:1094–1099.

495. Hollander E, Kwon JH, Stein DJ, et al. Obsessive–compulsive and spectrum disorders: Overview and quality of life issues. *Journal of Clinical Psychiatry* 1996;57:3–6.

496. Weissman MM, Bland RC, Canino GJ, et al. The cross national epidemiology of obsessive–compulsive disorder: The Cross-National Collaborative Group. *Clinical Psychiatry* 1994;55:5–10.

497. Black DW, Noyes R, Goldstein RB, et al. A family study of obsessive–compulsive disorder. *Archives of General Psychiatry* 1992;49:362–368.

498. Coryell W. Obsessive–compulsive disorder and primary unipolar depression: Comparisons of background, family history, course, and mortality. *Journal of Nervous and Mental Disease* 1981;169:220–224.

499. Hafner RJ. Anxiety disorders. In: Falloon IRH, ed. *Handbook of behavioral family therapy.* New York: Guilford Press, 1988:203–230.

500. U.S. Bureau of the Census. *Statistical abstract of the United States: 1996.* Washington, DC: U.S. Government Printing Office, 1996.
501. Steketee G, Grayson JB, Foa EB. A comparison of characteristics of obsessive–compulsive disorder and other anxiety disorders. *Journal of Anxiety Disorders* 1987;1:325– 335.
502. Khanna S, Rajendra PN, Channabasavanna SM. Sociodemographic variables in obsessive compulsive disorder in India. *International Journal of Social Psychiatry* 1986;32:47–54.
503. Lo WH. A follow-up study of obsessional neurotics in Hong Kong Chinese. *British Journal of Psychiatry* 1967;113:823–832.
504. Ingram IM. Obsessional illness in mental hospital patients. *Journal of Mental Science* 1961;107:382–402.
505. Eisen J, Steketee G. Course of illness of OCD. In: Pato M, Steketee G, Dickstein LJ, et al., eds. *Obsessive–compulsive disorder across the life cycle*, Vol. 16. Washington, DC: American Psychiatric Press, 1997:73–95.
506. Miller I, Epstein NB, Bishop DS, et al. McMaster Family Assessment Device: Reliability and validity. *Journal of Marital and Family Therapy* 1985;11:345–356.
507. Livingston-Van Noppen B, Rasmussen SA, Eisen J, et al. Family function and treatment in obsessive–compulsive disorder. In: Jenike M, Baer L, Minichiello WE, eds. *Obsessive–compulsive disorder: Theory and treatment.* Chicago: Year Book Medical Publishers, 1990:325–340.
508. Calvocoressi L, Lewis B, Harris M, et al. Family accommodation in obsessive–compulsive disorder. *American Journal of Psychiatry* 1995;152:441–443.
509. Shafran R, Ralph J, Tallis F. Obsessive–compulsive symptoms and the family. *Bulletin of the Menninger Clinic* 1995;59:472–479.
510. Tynes LL, Salins C, Winstead DK. Obsessive–compulsive patients: Familial frustration and criticism. *Journal of Louisiana State Medical Society* 1990;142:24–29.
511. Kobak KA, Rock AL, Greist JH. Group behavior therapy for obsessive–compulsive disorder. *Journal for Specialists in Group Work* 1995;20:26–32.
512. Van Balkom A, van Oppen P, Vermeulen A, et al. A meta-analysis on the treatment of obsessive compulsive disorder: A comparison of antidepressants, behavior, and cognitive therapy. *Clinical Psychology Review* 1994;14:359–381.
513. Turner SM, Beidel DC, Spaulding SA, et al. The practice of behavior therapy: A national survey of cost and methods. *Behavior Therapist* 1995;18:1–4.
514. Hafner RJ. Marital interaction in persisting obsessive–compulsive disorders. *Australian and New Zealand Journal of Psychiatry* 1982;16:171–178.
515. Hafner RJ, Gilchrist P, Bowling J, et al. The treatment of obsessional neurosis in a family setting. *Australian and New Zealand Journal of Psychiatry* 1981;15:145–151.
516. Hoover CF, Insel T. Families of origin in obsessive–compulsive disorder. *Journal of Nervous and Mental Disease* 1984;172:223–228.
517. Riggs DS, Hiss H, Foa EB. Marital distress and the treatment of obsessive compulsive disorder. *Behavior Therapy* 1992;23:585–597.
518. Emmelkamp PMG, de Haan E, Hoogduin CAL. Marital adjustment and obsessive–compulsive disorder. *British Journal of Psychiatry* 1990;156:55–60.
519. Cobb J, McDonald R, Marks I, et al. Marital versus exposure therapy: Psychological treatment of co-existing marital and phobic–obsessive problems. *Behavioural Analysis and Modification* 1980;4:3–16.

520. Emmelkamp PMG, Kloek J, Blaauw E. Obsessive–compulsive disorders in principles and practice of relapse prevention. In: Wilson PH, ed. *Principles and practice of relapse prevention*. New York: Guilford Press, 1992:213–234.

521. Hooley JM, Rosen LR, Richters JE. Expressed emotion: Toward clarification of a critical construct. In: Miller GA, ed. *The behavioral high-risk paradigm in psychopathology*. New York: Springer Verlag, 1995:88–120.

522. Chambless D, Steketee G. *Expressed emotion and the outcome of treatment for agoraphobia and obsessive compulsive disorder*. Paper presented at the Association for Advancement of Behavior Therapy, Miami, 1997.

523. Liberman RP. Behavioral approaches to family and couple therapy. *American Journal of Orthopsychiatry* 1970;40:106–118.

524. Patterson GR. *Families: Applications of social learning to family life*. Champaign, IL: Research Press, 1971.

525. Stuart RB. Operant–interpersonal treatment for marital discord. *Journal of Consulting and Clinical Psychology* 1969;33:675–682.

526. Jackson DD. Family rules. *Archives of General Psychiatry* 1965;12:589–594.

527. Jacobson NS. The modification of cognitive processes in behavioral marital therapy: Integrating cognitive and behavioral intervention strategies. In: Hahlweg K, Jacobson NS, eds. *Marital interaction: Analysis and modification*. New York: Guilford Press, 1984.

528. Anderson C, Hogarty G, Reiss D. Family treatment of adult schizophrenic patients: A psychoeducational approach. *Schizophrenia Bulletin* 1980;6:490–505.

529. Tynes LL, Salins C, Skiba W, et al. A psycho-educational and support group for obsessive–compulsive disorder patients and their significant others. *Comprehensive Psychiatry* 1992;33:197–201.

530. Marks IM, Hodgson R, Rachman S. Treatment of chronic obsessive–compulsive neurosis by in-vivo exposure: A two-year follow-up and issues in treatment. *British Journal of Psychiatry* 1975;127:349–364.

531. Black DW, Blum NS. Obsessive–compulsive disorder support groups: The Iowa model. *Comprehensive Psychiatry* 1992;33 :65–71.

532. Cooper M. A group for families of obsessive–compulsive persons. *Families in Society: The Journal of Contemporary Human Services* 1993:301–307.

533. Dalton P. Family treatment of an obsessive–compulsive child: A case report. *Family Process* 1983;22:99–108.

534. Fine S. Family therapy: A behavioral approach to childhood obsessive compulsive neurosis. *Archives of General Psychiatry* 1973;28:695–697.

535. March JS, Mulle K, Herbel B. Behavioral psychotherapy for children and adolescents with obsessive–compulsive disorder: An open trial of a new protocol-driven treatment package. *Journal of the American Academy of Child and Adolescent Psychiatry* 1994;33:333–341.

536. Thornicroft G, Colson L, Marks IM. An inpatient behavioural psychotherapy unit description and audit. *British Journal of Psychiatry* 1991;158:362–367.

537. Emmelkamp PMG, DeLange I. Spouse involvement in the treatment of obsessive–compulsive patients. *Behaviour Research and Therapy* 1983;21:341–346.

538. Mehta M. A comparative study of family-based and patient-based behavioural management in obsessive–compulsive disorder. *British Journal of Psychiatry* 1990;157:133–135.

539. Falloon IRH, ed. *Handbook of behavioral family therapy.* New York: Guilford Press, 1988.

540. Steketee G, White K. *When once is not enough.* Oakland, CA: New Harbinger, 1990.

541. Biegel DE, Sales E, Schulz R. *Family caregiving in chronic illness: Alzheimer's disease, cancer, heart disease, mental illness and stroke.* Newbury Park, CA: Sage, 1991.

542. Cole RE, Reiss D. *How do families cope with chronic illness?* Hillsdale, NJ: Erlbaum, 1993.

543. Czaczkes JW, Kaplan-DeNour A. *Chronic hemodialysis as a way of life.* New York: Brunner/Mazel, 1980.

544. Ostroff J, Steinglass P. Psychosocial adaptation following treatment: A family systems perspective on cancer survivorship. In: Baider L, Cooper CL, De-Nour AK, eds. *Cancer and the family.* New York: Wiley, 1996:129–147.

545. Patterson JM, Garwick AW. The impact of chronic illness on families: A family systems perspective. *Annals of Behavioral Medicine* 1994;16:131–142.

546. Campbell TL. Family's impact on health: A critical review. *Family Systems Medicine* 1986;4:135–328.

547. Fisher L, Ransom DC, Terry HE, et al. The California Family Health Project: I. Introduction and a description of adult health. *Family Process* 1992;31:231–250.

548. Litman TJ. The family as a basic unit in health and medical care: A social–behavioral overview. *Social Science and Medicine* 1974;8:495–519.

549. Stuber ML, Gonzalez S, Meeske K, et al. Post-traumatic stress after childhood cancer: II. A family model. *Psycho-Oncology* 1994;3:313–319.

550. Wamboldt MZ, Levin L. Utility of multifamily psychoeducational groups for medically ill children and adolescents. *Family Systems Medicine* 1995;13:151–161.

551. Pomeroy EC, Rubin A, Walker RJ. A psychoeducational task-centered group intervention for family members of persons with HIV/AIDS: Strategies for intervention. *Family Process* 1996;35:299–312.

552. Steinglass P. Multiple family discussion groups for patients with chronic medical illness. *Families, Systems and Health* 1998;16:55–70.

553. Satin W, LaGreca AM, Zigo MA, et al. Diabetes in adolescence: Effects of multifamily group intervention and parent simulation of diabetes. *Journal of Pediatric Psychology* 1989;14:259–275.

554. Fisher L, Weihs KL. Can addressing family relationships improve outcomes in chronic disease?: Report on the National Working Group on Family-Based Interventions in Chronic Disease. *Journal of Family Practice* 2000;49:561–566.

555. Campbell TL, Patterson JM. The effectiveness of family interventions in the treatment of physical illness. *Journal of Marital and Family Therapy* 1995; 21:545–583.

556. Schooler NR, Keith CM. The clinical research base for the treatment of schizophrenia. *Psychopharmacology Bulletin* 1993;29:431–436.

557. Burman B, Margolin G. Analysis of the association between marital relationships and health problems: An interactional perspective. *Psychological Bulletin* 1992;112:39–63.

558. Franks P, Campbell T. Social relationships and health: The relative roles of family functioning and social support. *Social Science and Medicine* 1992;34:779–788.
559. Spiegel D, Yalom I. A support group for dying patients. *International Journal of Group Psychotherapy* 1978;28:233–245.
560. Rolland JS. *Families, illness and disability: An integrative treatment model.* New York: Basic Books, 1994.
561. Stuber ML. Psychiatric sequelae in seriously ill children and their families. *Journal of Consulting and Clinical Psychology* 1996;65:120–129.
562. Kazak AE, Stuber ML, Barakat LP, et al. Predicting posttraumatic stress symptoms in mothers and fathers of survivors of childhood cancers. *Journal of the American Academy of Child and Adolescent Psychiatry* 1998;37:823–831.
563. Steinglass P, Bennett LA, Wolin SJ, et al. *The alcoholic family.* New York: Basic Books, 1987.
564. Steinglass P, Gonzalez S, Dosovitz I, et al. Discussion groups for chronic hemodialysis patients and their families. *General Hospital Psychiatry* 1982;4:7–14.
565. Gonzalez S, Steinglass P, Reiss D. *Family-centered interventions for the chronically disabled: The 8-session multiple-family discussion group program: Treatment manual.* Washington, DC: George Washington University Rehabilitation Research and Training Center, 1986.
566. Stuber ML, Gonzalez S, Benjamin H, et al. Fighting for recovery: Group interventions for adolescents with cancer and their parents. *Journal of Psychotherapy Practice and Research* 1995;4:286–296.
567. Wellisch D, Mosher M, Scoy C. Management of family emotional stress: Family group therapy in a private oncology practice. *International Journal of Group Psychotherapy* 1978;28:225–231.
568. Kazak AE, Simms S, Barakat L, et al. Surviving Cancer Competently Intervention Program (SCCIP): A cognitive-behavioral and family therapy intervention for adolescent survivors of childhood cancer and their families. *Family Process* 1999;38:175–191.
569. Kazak AE. in press.
570. Holder B, Turner-Musa J, Kimmel PL, et al. Engagement of African American families in research on chronic illness: A multisystem recruitment approach. *Family Process* 1998;37:127–151.
571. Boise L, Heagery B, Eskenazi L. Facing chronic illness: The family support model and its benefits. *Patient Education and Counseling* 1996;27:75–84.
572. Brown DG, Krieg K, Belluck F. A model for group intervention with the chronically ill: Cystic fibrosis and the family. *Social Work Health Care* 1995;21:81–94.
573. Takacs LF, Kollman CE. An inflammatory bowel support group for teens and their parents. *Gastroenterology Nursing* 1994;17:11–13.
574. Lehman AF, Steinwachs DM, Dixon LB, et al. Patterns of usual care for schizophrenia: Initial results from the Schizophrenia PORT client survey. *Schizophrenia Bulletin* 1998;24:11–19.
575. Dixon L, Lyles A, Scott J, et al. Services to families of adults with schizophrenia: From treatment recommendations to dissemination. *Psychiatric Services* 2001;52:935–942.

576. Backer TE, Liberman RP, Kuehnel T. Dissemination and adoption of innovative psychosocial interventions. *Journal of Clinical and Consulting Psychology* 1986; 1:111–118.

577. Rogers EM. New product adoption and diffusion. *Journal of Consumer Research* 1976;2:290–301.

578. Rogers EM. The diffusions of innovations perspective. In: Weinstein D, ed. *Taking care: Understanding and encouraging self protective behavior.* New York: Cambridge University Press, 1987.

579. Lehman AF, Steinwachs DM, Buchanan R, et al. Translating research into practice: The Schizophrenia Patient Outcomes Research Team (PORT) treatment recommendations. *Schizophrenia Bulletin* 1998;24:1–10.

580. McFarlane WR, McNary S, Dixon L, et al. Predictors of dissemination of family psychoeducation in community mental health centers in Maine and Illinois. *Psychiatric Services* 2001;52:935–942.

581. McFarlane W. Multiple family therapy in schizophrenia. In: McFarlane WR, ed. *Family therapy in schizophrenia.* New York: Guilford Press, 1983:141–172.

582. McGlashan TH. Schizophrenia: Psychosocial treatments and the role of psychosocial factors in its etiology and pathogenesis. In: Frances AJ, Hales RE, eds. *Psychiatry update: American Psychiatric Association Annual Review,* Vol. 5. Washington, DC: American Psychiatric Press, 1986.

583. Lefley HP. Families, culture, and mental illness: Constructing new realities. *Psychiatry* 1998;61:335–356.

584. Van Noppen B, Steketee G. Individual, group and multifamily cognitive-behavioral treatment of obsessive–compulsive disorder. In Pato MT, Zohar, J, eds. *Current treatments of obsessive–compulsive disorder,* 2nd ed. Washington, DC: American Psychiatric Press, 2001.

Index

Page numbers followed by "f" indicate figure, "t" indicate table.

ACT (Assertive Community Treat-
    ment), 58, 175, 180
  elements, 175–176
  limitations, 176–178
  pace, 186–187
  and psychoeducational multifamily
    groups, 178, 182–187
  synopsis, 181–182
American culture of individuality, vs.
    family support, 360
AMI (Alliance for the Mentally Ill), 33
Amygdala, 10
Anderson, Carol, 15
Anderson, Reiss, and Hogarty
  joining process, 104
  psychoeducational approach, 50
    and hope/motivation, 116
  workshop themes, 117

B

Bergen County outcome trial, 51
  design/method, 51–52
  results, 52–53
Biosocial theory, 7
  biosocial hypothesis, 75
  as foundation of psychoeducational
    multifamily groups, 75

cognitive dysfunction, 78–79
life events, 79
psychophysiological dysfunction,
    76–78
Bipolar illness
  challenges to group formation/
    IndMaintenance, 240
  diagnostic ambiguity, 240
  group structure IndMaintenance,
    241
  psychiatric conditions in family
    members, 241
  and psychoeducational approaches
    to treatment, 220, 221t, 242
  educational workshop, 231, 235–
    237
  educational workshop/outline,
    232t–235t
  group guidelines, 236t
  group meetings (ongoing), 237–239
  joining, 228t–229t
  joining/content, 227, 229
  joining/structure, 226–227
  similarities with schizophrenia
    biopsychosocial, 221
  burden, 222
  course, 221–222
  stigma, 222–223

Bipolar illness (*continued*)
  specific issues, 223
    affect, 224
    episodic course, 223–224
    influence on personality, 225
    practical effects, 225–226
Borderline personality disorder (BPD),
      268, 289–290
  deficits
    affect and impulse dyscontrol,
        273–274
    dichotomous thinking, 274
    intolerance of aloneness, 274
  dialectical behavioral therapy (DBT),
      269
  and family treatments, 270
  multifamily group role, 277–279
    case example, 279–280
    "overinvolvement," 279
  psychoeducational multifamily
      treatment, 268–269, 270
    and alienation, 271–272
    and EE, 272–273
    family guidelines, 284t
    joining phase, 281–282
    multifamily groups, 285–286
    psychoeducational workshop,
        282–283, 285
    rationale, 275–277
    stages of change, 287–288
    structure, 280
  treatment outcome, 288–289
Brain function alterations, 6–7
  brain stem and midbrain, 7, 9
  higher cortical areas (prefrontal,
      superior temporal gyri,
      postcentral areas), 11–12
    and cognitive dysfunctions, 78
  limbic system and thalamus, 10–11.
      See also Amygdala; Cingulate
      cortex; Hippocampus
  neurotransmitters, 7–9, 8f, 12. *See
      also* Dopamine; GABA;
      Glutamate; NMDA;
      Noradrenaline; Serotonin
  and psychological functioning, 13–
      14

C

CFI (crisis family intervention), 59
Chronic medical disorders and PMFG,
      315, 339–340
  implementation obstacles, 316–317
    biomedical bias of medical
        settings, 317–318
    demonstrations of group's
        effectiveness, 318–319
    recruitment of participant
        families, 319–320
  issues at stages of medical illness,
      316
  MFDG (multifamily discussion
      group) model, 327–329, 337–
      338
    educational component, 329–332
    problem-solving component, 336–
        337
    social network component, 332–336
  supportive research, 338–339
  theoretical framework, 320–321
    emotional and social isolation,
        324–326
    "familiness" of chronic illness,
        321–323
    family "identity," 326–327
    overallocation of resources, 323–
        324
Cingulate cortex, 10
Clinical approach to the PMFG model
  biosocial theory foundation, 75–76
    cognitive dysfunction, 78–79
    life events, 79
    psychophysiological dysfunction,
        76–78
  clinicians. *See* Therapists
  course of recovery and treatment,
      80–82
    relapse risk, 82f
    stages of treatment, 91
  "devil's pact" principle, 80
  family social structure and
      treatment, 82–83
  goals, 76
  group climate, 101–102

group membership, 99
  and other clinicians/programs,
    100–101
  logistics examples
    patients' participation, 98–99
    rural settings issues, 98
    significant substance abuse (as
      additional problem), 96–97
    as stable outpatient, 95–96
    typical application (point of
      relapse), 94–95
  realms, 76
  techniques. *See* Intervention tech-
    niques in multifamily group con-
    text; Phase-oriented techniques
Clozapine, 8
Cognitive processing and
    schizophrenia, 78–79
  deficits of internal/external cue
    modulation and symptomatic
    behavior/functional disability, 25–
    26
Coping capabilities
  development of as environmental
    interventions, 26–27
  as a function of affirming social
    support, 24, 40
  "indirect learning," 41–42
  as intermediate outcome of multi-
    family group treatment, 73
  and strategies for handling family
    stress, 27–28

D

DBT (dialectical behavioral therapy), 269
Distraction–arousal hypothesis, 11
Dopamine, 7–8
  levels during acute episodes, 8, 12
  and substantia nigra, 7
  and ventral tegmentum, 7
Double bind, 31

E

Expressed emotion, 31–33
  and borderline personality disorder,
    269, 272

controversy and research, 34
  and family responses, 33–34, 42,
    114
Employment. *See also* FACT/results
  as family motivation for PMFG, 95–
    96
EOI (emotional overinvolvement), 32
  and successful interventions, 43
ERP (exposure and response preven-
    tion) treatment. *See* Obsessive–
    compulsive disorder
Expressed emotion research
  and FACT, 179–180
  insights, 77

F

FACT (Family-aided Assertive Commu-
    nity Treatment), 58, 187, 197
  additive effects, 182
  case example, 188–189
  and coordination, 182–183
  and crisis intervention, 184
  and cross-family relationships, 185–
    186
  design/methods, 59
  and expressed emotion, 179–180
  and multiple interventions, 183–184
  pace/stepwise approach, 186–187
  primary justification, 178
  relapse risk, 184
  results, 59–60
    effectiveness, 67
    employment activity increase, 59–60
    and family burden reduction, 60–61
  studies, 58–59
  as vocational rehabilitation, 194
    case example, 196–197
    employment specialist role, 192
    goal, 190–191, 194–196
    phases, 193–194
    PMFG goal, 194
    PMFG meeting format, 193
    program modifications toward
      employment goal, 191–192
  as vocational rehabilitation/prior
    outcome studies, 190

FACT (*continued*)
as vocational rehabilitation/study, 61
design/methods, 61–62
qualitative outcomes, 64
results, 62–63, 63f
Falloon and Liberman, family
behavioral management, 50
Family. *See also* Multifamily groups;
Psychoeducational interven-
tions/educating families; Psychoeducational multifamily
group model
advocacy movement, 114–115
attitudes toward, 30–31
and chronic illness, 321–323
and family "identity," 327
"communication deviance"
characteristic, 45
experiences during episodes of
schizophrenia, 107–108
index family, 88–89
interactions and psychiatric illness,
30
"double bind," 31
responses to EE, 33–34
and isolation, 39
and obsessive–compulsive disorder,
293–294
family-assisted treatment, 300–
302
family functioning, 294–296
family support groups, 300
and treatment outcome, 297–298
and professional alliances, 34–35
quality of life/experienced burden,
29–30
sense of loss, 110
social structure in PMFG treatment,
82–83
and stigma, 28–29
stress of illness, 27–28
support vs. American culture of
individuality, 360
supportive approach to
schizophrenia, 4
and long-term outcome, 24
Family behavioral management, 50

Family Guidelines, 123–125, 124t
information for patients, 125–
126
Family therapy, 247, 263–264
and BPD, 270
family crisis therapy model, 50
Freud, influence of theory of
schizophrenia, 4
Functioning, two-tiered model, 21

G

GABA (gamma-aminobutyric acid), 9
Glutamate, 9
Goldstein, family crisis therapy model,
50

H

Hippocampus, 10

I

IBT (individual behavioral treatment).
See Obsessive–compulsive
disorder
Initial sessions of a PMFG, 127–128,
141
first meeting/introduction, 128
agenda setting, 129
explicit rules (case example),
132–133
goal, 128
group leader's approach/tech-
niques, 131–132
introductions (case examples),
129–131
second meeting/life impacts of
schizophrenia, 133–134
case examples, 135–136
meeting wrap-up, 137–138
mood of meeting, 136–137
socializing importance, 134
clinician guidelines, 138
communication/group interaction
rules, 140–141
crises/emergencies, 140
late-arriving guidelines, 139

new members, 138–139
reminders about attending, 139–
140
Intervention techniques in multifamily
group context, 83
cross-family linkage, 88–89
cross-parenting, 89–90
group interpretation, 86
interfamily assistance (positive
reinforcement of), 87
intragroup social conversation
support, 87–88
theme definitions, 86–87
interfamily management, 90–91
self-triangulation, 84
attendance monitoring, 85–86
controlling extreme affect, 86
family management guideline
linkage, 84
interactional information definition, 84
interruption blocking, 85
problem-solving sequences direction, 85

J

Joining, 104
as first stage of PMFG treatment,
104
guiding process, 109–112
role of clinicians, 105
sessions/steps, 105
session 1—information gathering
(early symptoms/precipitants),
106–107
session 2—relationship building
with family, 107–108
session 3—goal planning/
educational workshop introduction, 108–109

L

La belle indifférence, 13
Laqueur and Detre, pioneers of multi-
family group modality, 49, 360
Long-term effects of psychotic state, 6

M

Major depressive disorder, 244, 266–
267
common themes/concerns
collaboration with mental health/
other professionals, 264–265
difficult family interactions, 265–
266
empowerment and responsibility,
266
illness stages/coping strategies,
264
patient in crisis, 265
and family functioning, 244–246
family therapy, 247, 263–264
group therapy, 247
multifamily group treatment, 247
multifamily group treatment guidelines, 248
clinical procedures, 251
family composition, 249–250
goals/structure overview, 248–249
group composition, 250
screening session, 251–252
screening session/outline, 252–
253
therapists, 250–251
pharmacotherapy, 246–247
psychoeducation group sessions
one–six
goals, 253, 255, 257, 259, 260, 262
outline, 254–255, 256–257, 258–
260, 262–263
preparation, 253, 255, 258, 259,
261, 262
"Marital schism and skew," 31
Mental health professionals' role, 35
MFBT (multifamily behavioral treatment). See Obsessive–
compulsive disorder
Multifamily groups (MFGs)
empirical studies of outcomes. See
also Bergen County outcome
trial; FACT studies; New York
State Family Psychoeducation
Study

Multifamily groups, empirical studies
of outcomes (continued)
clinical and theoretical
implications, 65–67
early studies, 49
methodological limitations, 49–50
PMFG outcomes, 58
therapist skill level, 66
origins, 360–361
technology transfer program
elements, 341
case examples, 355–357. See also
New York State Family Support
Demonstration Project; Schizophrenia Patient Outcomes
Research Team (Ohio)

N

NAMI (National Alliance for the
Mentally Ill), 69, 290
and family advocacy movement,
114–115
NEPDA (New England Personality
Disorders Association), 290
New York State Family Psychoeducation in Schizophrenia Study, 53
design/method, 53–54
and FACT development, 187
results, 54–58, 54f, 55f
New York State Family Support
Demonstration Project, 342,
347–348
dissemination phase, 342
impact of regulatory changes,
346–347
regional training, 346
implementation phase, 342
multifamily emphasis, 345–346
as multifamily group technology
transfer program, 341
research phase, 342
assumptions in model, 344–345
clinician training, 343
constraints, 342–343
scope, 342
structure for transfer, 343–344

NMDA (N-methyl-D-aspartate), 9, 119
Noradrenaline, and the locus
coeruleus, 7
Nutritional treatment for
schizophrenia, 9

O

Obsessive–compulsive disorder (OCD),
291
behavioral treatments (individual/
IBT and multifamily/MFBT),
292, 313–314
exposure and response prevention
(ERP), 296–297
models, 299–300
diagnosis/prevalence, 292–293
and the family, 293–294
family variables treatment outcome predictors, 291, 295,
297–298
impact on family functioning,
294–296
support groups, 300
as symptom modifiers, 299
multiple-family group treatment,
301–302
case example/overview, 303–305
case example/first session, 305–
307
case example/second session,
307–308
case example/third session, 309
case example/fourth session, 310–
311
case example/fifth(eleventh
sessions, 311–312
case example/twelfth (last)
session, 312–313
features and procedures, 303
single-family interventions, 300–
301

P

PACT (Program of Assertive Community Treatment), 176–177, 180
Personal Therapy, 26–27

Phase-oriented techniques
   community reentry, 92–93
   social and vocational rehabilitation,
      93–94
Problem-solving approach, 144, 170
   as an essential part of PMFG treat-
      ment, 113, 142, 186
   group session format, 144–145
      initial socializing, 146–147
      go-round, 147–149, 150–152
      selecting problem to solve, 152–
         155
      solving a problem, 155. See also
         Six-step method of problem
         solving
      closing (socializing), 165
   guidelines for clinicians
      "generic problem solving," 168
      leadership changes, 169
      meetings with small attendance,
         167–168
      problem solving with intractable
         family disagreement, 165–167
      techniques for longer term
         groups, 168–169
   in multifamily groups, 143–144
   as a social prosthesis, 142–143
   in supportive housing programs
      training, 209–210
   worksheet, 171a
Psychoeducational interventions, 4, 27,
      35, 50. See also Distraction-
      arousal hypothesis; Staff train-
      ing (of supportive housing pro-
      grams)
   counterintuitive coping skills, 75
   educating families, 113
      absence of education, 113–114
      and hope/motivation, 116
      physiology and psychology of
         schizophrenia, 115
      rationale, 114–116
   educating patients, 125–126
   educational and directive processes,
      46–48
   for high EE families, 32–33
   optimal environment, 15–16

stigma implications, 29
studies, 69
workshop. See also Survival Skills
      Workshop
   clinician guidelines, 118–119
   goals, 116–117
   information sources, 118
   themes/polling method, 117–118
Psychoeducational multifamily group
      model, 4, 16–17. See also
      Biosocial theory; Bipolar illness;
      Borderline personality disorder;
      Chronic medical disorders;
      Clinical approach to the PMFG
      model; Major depressive disor-
      der; Multifamily groups
      (MFGs); Obsessive–compulsive
      disorder
   comparative studies
      vs. other family intervention stud-
         ies, 67–69
      vs. single-family psychoeducation-
         al treatment, 37
   congruence with social/clinical prob-
      lems in schizophrenia, 37
   cross-parenting, 44
   effectiveness; in empirical studies,
      58, 66
   establishment of, 42–23
   family communication promotion,
      45–46
   goals, 73
   history, 36
      early studies (MFG), 49
      MFG with psychoeducation, 50
      and theoretical underpinnings,
         41–42
      traditional social form, 47
   indirect learning, 41–42
   intra- and interfamily boundaries,
      43–44
   mastery-based group identity, 39–40
   medical vs. psychiatric groups, 317
   relapse study, 24
   vs. self-help or advocacy groups, 74
   as a therapeutic social network, 37–
      39, 47, 69–70

Psychoeducational multifamily group
model (*continued*)
treatment components, 113. *See also*
Initial sessions of a PMFG;
Joining; Problem-solving
approach; Psychoeducational
interventions/educating families
treatment groups, 75–76
treatment stages, 91
underlying assumptions, 74
"weak ties," 39
Psychosocial influences on schizophrenia. *See also* Biosocial theory;
Cognitive deficits and schizophrenia
continuity of social context, 25, 38
reciprocal model of cognitive processing, 26
and core strategy of rehabilitation,
18
environmental impacts, 19, 26
multifamily group as therapeutic
social network, 37–39, 69–70
social networks, 22
diminished size, 23
social support, 74
and coping capabilities, 24
dimensions, 21
in traditional cultures, 24

S

Schizophrenia
biological basis, 3, 4. *See also*
Biosocial theory; Brain function
alterations
and modern imaging methods, 11
causes, 14–15
diseases causing disorder, 3
clinical symptoms
negative, 5, 14, 40–41
positive, 4–5
courses, 6
recovery from acute episode, 5–6
relapse risk, 24
as a disorder of sensory stimulation
processing, 14

domains of outcome, 20
symptomology vs. social functioning, 21
history of concept, 4,359
information resources, 118,121
interaction of principal factors, 30f
rehabilitation. *See* Psychosocial
influences on schizophrenia
and relationships, 19. *See also*
Cognitive processing and
schizophrenia
prosthetic ego need, 25
social support as symptom status
predictor, 24
and stress, 19–20
family stress, 27–28
therapy. *See* Personal Therapy
and transitions, 41
Schizophrenia Patient Outcomes
Research Team (PORT), 341,
355
assessment mechanism, 349
and outcomes, 354–355
goals, 348
interventions
intensive training, 350–351
"road show," 349–350
regions, 349
technology transfer experiment
results
first phase, 351, 352t, 353t
follow-up, 351–354
Serotonin
and the raphe nuclei, 7
and schizophrenia, 8
Single-family treatment model
vs. multifamily group model, 37
vulnerabilities of, 38
Six-step method of problem solving,
155–156
advantages/disadvantages of each
solution discussion, 161–162
choice of best solution, 162
plan to implement solution, 162–
164
implementation review, 164–
165

list all solutions, 160–161
problem definition, 156–160
Staff training (of supportive housing
programs), 219
areas of focus, 200
client choice, 205
criticism avoidance, 202–203
flexible social milieu, 206–207
graduated performance expectations, 205–206
positive reinforcement, 203–204
staff psychoeducational guidelines, 201, 201t
stimulation intensity adjustment,
204–205
general issues, 217–218
historical background, 198–199
model overview, 201–202
and psychoeducational model, 199–
200
joining and education, 207–208
Stigma, 28–29
vs. mastery-based group identity,
39–40
reduction in multifamily group,
74
Stress
and schizophrenia, 19
stress–diathesis –stress(vulnerability)
model, 20
Substance abuse, 188. See also Clinical
approach to the PMFG model/
logistics examples
Supportive housing programs
psychoeducation approach
components, 207. See also
Staff training (of supportive
housing programs)
general interventions, 213–214
problem solving, 209–210
psychoeducational groups, 210
psychoeducational groups/
medication groups format, 211
psychoeducational groups/
positive socialization groups
format, 210–211

psychoeducational groups/
problemsolving groups format,
211–213
staff supervision, 208–209
psychoeducational model adaptations (case examples), 214–217
Survival Skills Workshop
curriculum, 121, 122t, 123
Family Guidelines, 123–125, 124t
meeting summary/conclusion, 125
practicalities/procedures, 119–121

T

TARA (Treatment and Research
Advances), 290
Therapists, 250–251. See also Joining;
Staff training (of supportive
housing programs)
requirements for PMFG for major
depression
roles in PMFG treatment, 100–101
approach/techniques in initial sessions, 131–132
family–professional alliance creation, 105
guidelines, 118–119
guiding process, 109–112
and style, 101–102
skill level and MFG outcomes, 66
social/personal stance as MFG leaders, 102–103
Treatment approaches. See also ACT;
FACT
behavioral treatments for OCD
(individual/IBT and multifam-
ily/MFBT), 292
confinement, 30
high-risk patients, 187
associated problems, 187–188
therapeutic social environment. See
Psychoeducational multifamily
group model
Treatment Strategies in Schizophrenia Study (National Institute of
Mental Health), 68

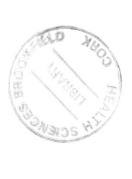